Register Now for Online Access to Your Book!

SPRINGER PUBLISHING
CONNECT™

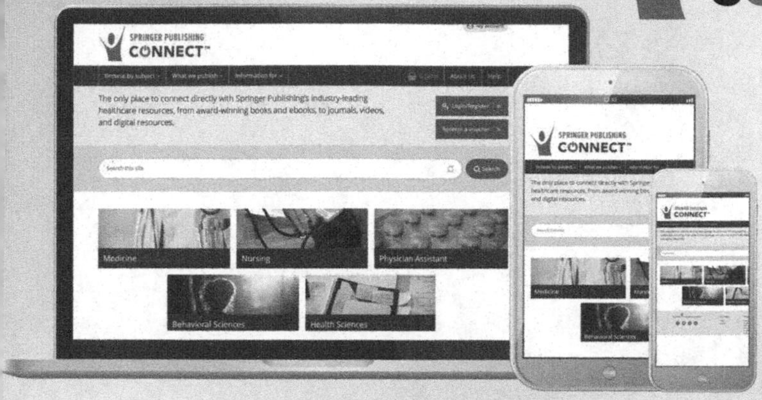

'our print purchase of *CMSA's Integrated Case Management: A Manual for Case Managers by Case Managers, Second Edition,* **includes online access to the :ontents of your book**—increasing accessibility, portability, and searchability!

\ccess today at:

ıttp://connect.springerpub.com/content/book/978-0-8261-8834-2

ır scan the QR code at the right with your smartphone. Log in or egister, then click "Redeem a voucher" and use the code below.

FS31T25Y

Scan here for quick access.

laving trouble redeeming a voucher code?
io to https://connect.springerpub.com/redeeming-voucher-code

f you are experiencing problems accessing the digital component of his product, please contact our customer service department at cs@ pringerpub.com

ne online access with your print purchase is available at the publisher's discretion nd may be removed at any time without notice.

'ublisher's Note: New and used products purchased from third-party sellers are not uaranteed for quality, authenticity, or access to any included digital components.

SPRINGER PUBLISHING
View all our products at springerpub.com

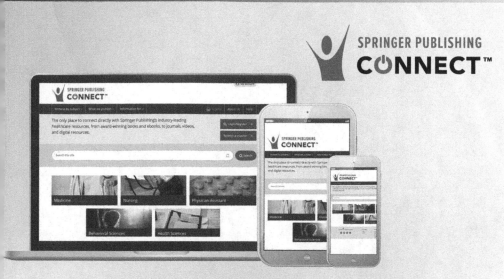

CMSA's Integrated Case Management

Rebecca Perez, MSN, RN, CCM, FCM, is an experienced registered nurse with a master's degree in nursing, a certified case manager, and a member of the Omega Gamma Chapter of Sigma Theta Tau International Nursing Honor Society, the Capella University National Society of Leadership and Success, and the National Quality Forum Leadership Consortium. Her most recent works include *Case Management Society of America Integrated Case Management: A Manual for Case Managers by Case Managers*, Second Edition; *CMSA's Case Management Adherence Guide 2020*; *CMSA's Case Management Adherence and Transition of Care Guide for* Clostridioides difficile; and *CMSA's Case Management Adherence and Transitions of Care Guide for Hepatic Encephalopathy*. She is the author of numerous professional articles and resources for CMSA and is a speaker on case management topics. She is the senior manager of education for CMSA and executive director for the Case Management Society Foundation. She was recently awarded a fellow in case management designation.

CMSA's Integrated Case Management

A Manual for Case Managers by Case Managers

Second Edition

Rebecca Perez, *MSN, RN, CCM, FCM*

SPRINGER PUBLISHING

CMSA Case Management Society of America

First Springer Publishing edition 978-0-8261-8833-5

Springer Publishing Company, LLC
11 West 42nd Street, New York, NY 10036
www.springerpub.com
connect.springerpub.com

Acquisitions Editor: John Zaphyr
Compositor: diacriTech

ISBN: 978-0-8261-8833-5
ebook ISBN: 978-0-8261-8834-2
DOI: 10.1891/9780826188342

Printed by BnT

Library of Congress Control Number: 2023937620

Printed in the United States of America.

Contents

SECTION V: Interdisciplinary Teams and Using Integrated Case Management to Improve Outcomes

Appendices

Foreword

There have been so many changes within our evolving healthcare system, but we did not expect the rapid shift to the uncharted territory of the COVID-19 pandemic. We were not prepared for the unexpected. The pandemic heightened human suffering, caused unprecedented economic instability and a break in physical and mental health services for people of all socioeconomic levels. The world was turned upside down causing an interruption in all domains of care and a break in socialization that continues to impact health outcomes today. Our professional case managers played an essential role coordinating patient care at the pandemic front lines. As we move forward, leaving the pandemic twilight zone behind, we need to continue to provide critical interventions for patients experiencing complex physical conditions, behavioral health difficulties, including the increase in the use of opioids, and newly added contemporary social problems.

Case managers need to grasp the opportunity of the unexpected and embrace the strategies of an Integrated Case Management (ICM) model required to meet the challenges of today's complex patients and their families. The Case Management Society of America (CMSA), a multidisciplinary organization, has provided continued support for the profession of case management through educational forums since it was founded in 1990. Understanding that case managers needed guidance to implement an integrated model, they launched the first and second editions of *CMSA's Integrated Case Management: A Manual for Case Managers by Case Managers*, guided by the CMSA's *Standards of Practice.*

I was fortunate to spend most of my professional case management career in a leadership role working for a not-for-profit New York State Medicaid managed-care organization that focused on health equity, quality improvement, client satisfaction, and innovative programs. Our membership primarily consisted of underserved vulnerable populations. Unfortunately, our case management model was a prime example of a disconnected patient outreach approach with limited positive outcomes. An obvious need to break down the silos between our behavioral health and clinical case management programs was apparent, but the organization did not have the infrastructure, tools, or in-depth training to implement a plan.

I was privileged to work under the guidance and mentorship of forward-thinking and insightful leaders and colleagues who were not afraid to explore new methods and concepts. When CMSA launched its ICM program, our organization was one of the first to implement the program. We were introduced to the new philosophy of "one" primary case manager coordinating patient care across all domains of health: biological, psychological, social, and navigating the health system. Our training included the use of motivational interviewing techniques to establish ongoing trusting patient relationships enabling case managers to identify all barriers to care and promote advocacy. We studied the innovative Integrated Case Management Complexity Assessment Grid (ICM-CAG) tool that classified and tracked the patient's level of complexity and prioritized their urgent needs requiring immediate intervention. We were enlightened! Our mission was to implement the ICM program within our organization.

We had a positive partnership with CMSA and our behavioral health department and moved forward with the development of a well-trained interdisciplinary team composed of registered nurses, licensed social workers, peer support specialists, case manager extenders, and physician advisors. Our award-winning integrated program made a significant impact on our most complex patients' holistic health outcomes and their quality of life. Our successful model still exists today.

I was honored to be asked to write the foreword for this second edition of *CMSA's Integrated Case Management: A Manual for Case Managers by Case Managers*. I am dedicated to the philosophy and delivery of the integrated model and am pleased that I had the opportunity to share my experiences and successes with you. I would like to acknowledge Rebecca Perez. The success of our integrated program and all future programs would not be possible without her dedication, knowledge, and expert ICM training. Enjoy your new learning experience and start making a difference!

Sheilah McGlone, RN, CCM
CMSA Member since 1998
Former Senior Director, Hudson Health Plan
Case Management Consultant and Educator

Preface

As the current Case Management Society of America (CMSA) national president, it is my distinct honor to introduce this update to the seminal *CMSA's Integrated Case Management: A Manual for Case Managers by Case Managers.* CMSA has been a pioneer in the pursuit of true patient-centered care using an integrated approach, beginning with the development of content and curriculum in 2008. Fifteen years later, Integrated Case Management (ICM) has become even more relevant to the practice of professional case management and the healthcare system overall.

The goal of ICM is to provide a seamless, holistic care experience for our patients/clients/members by integrating physical and mental health case management principles and assessment tools. Through this approach, the foundational principles of case management (right care, right setting, right time, reduction of duplication of services, resolution of care gaps, and patient advocacy) are optimized.

Too often, patients/clients/members are treated in silos when the best practice is to treat the whole person. ICM strives to bridge that practice gap, providing the professional case manager with the knowledge base and tools to promote optimal outcomes and be the advocate through the care continuum.

The Triple Aim and now the Quadruple Aim, moving to the Quintuple Aim, all put "improving the experience of healthcare and improving the health of populations" at their core. ICM is a key to doing just that, with the additional benefit of reducing cost of care.

ICM is an advanced practice model that focuses on relationship development, engagement, retention, communication, and risk identification and prioritization. Since its introduction in 2008, over 1,000 individual and organizational case managers have been trained. These represent Veteran's Affairs, Indian health services, health plans, hospital systems, and accountable care organizations. The importance of the ICM model cannot be downplayed as the demand for training continues to rise, year after year, as more and more states make integrated case management a requirement for their Medicaid plans.

The integration of concepts, built on the proven foundational tenets of case management, will be a phenomenal addition to your case manager's toolbox!

Colleen Morley, DNP, RN, CCM, CMAC, CMCN, ACM, RN, FCM
President, Case Management Society of America

Acknowledgments

The Case Management Society of America would like to acknowledge and express its sincere gratitude to the following professionals for their invaluable contributions to the development of this manual:

Melanie A. Prince, MSS, MSN, BSN, NE-BC, CCM, FAAN, FCM

Kathleen M. Moriarity, MSN, RN, CCDS, CCM

SECTION I

The Role of Integrated Case Management in Addressing Complexity

CHAPTER 1

Defining Healthcare Complexity

Rebecca Perez

OBJECTIVES

- Discover what defines complexity
- Explore the impact of health complexity
- Define the attributes of integrated case management

Introduction

Since 2006, the Case Management Society of America (CMSA) has been building and nurturing the Integrated Case Management Program. The integrated model has been in practice and has been studied for over 20 years in Europe. The decision to bring this advanced case management practice model to the United States resulted in CMSA becoming a leader in the care of individual challenged with complex health conditions. The literature published overwhelmingly demonstrates health improvements when this patient-centered, holistic approach reduces health risks. The recent focus on complex care models in the United States has resulted in the muddling of terms. Complexity, comorbidity, and multimorbidity are often confused or used interchangeably. To focus on complex care, the correct definitions must be grasped.

Comorbidity

Comorbidity indicates the presence of at least two conditions that can be acute or chronic. Comorbidity does not necessarily indicate complexity, however. For example, the individual with controlled type 2 diabetes and controlled hypertension, living independently with strong social support, does not experience complexity. These chronic conditions carry a risk for future worsening health, but at present, complexity is not present. Alternately, the individual with uncontrolled type 2 diabetes, elevated blood pressure, disability due to chronic foot ulcers alienated from friends and family due to persistent complaining and lack of motivation to self-manage does indeed demonstrate complexity.

Multimorbidity

Multimorbidity presents as the co-occurrence of multiple chronic or acute medical and/or behavioral conditions. Multimorbidity often results in complexity because the number and severity of the conditions makes it difficult to self-manage. But multimorbidity does not necessarily equate to complexity. An individual in recovery for a substance use disorder, professionally managed depression, and controlled hypertension fits the definition of multimorbidity but is not complex. The presence of risk for future health challenges must be monitored, and complexity could quickly develop if any of these conditions were not well controlled. An individual with substance use disorder, serious mental illness, and cachexia would fall under the label of complex. Serious mental illness is a challenge to manage and significantly increases the risk for worsening health. In this case, complexity is present.

Complexity

Complexity is characterized by multidimensional and multifaceted medical conditions complicated by age, fragility, socioeconomic challenges, unavailable or limited culture and language needs, environment, behavior, and health system factors (Tortajada et al., 2017).

CASE STUDY

Sergeant Major K.

Sergeant Major K. returned home after several tours of duty in the Middle East. He was in a vehicle that drove over an improvised explosive device (IED) and suffered a mild traumatic brain injury and loss of both lower limbs below the knee. His acute phase of care took place at Walter Reed Medical Center, and he was discharged to the Veterans Affairs health system near his hometown. His physical recovery was not progressing as expected due to negative behaviors. His behavior alternated between being argumentative and uncooperative to apologetic and tearful. Sergeant Major K. returned to his home shared with his wife and two children. His wife attended physical therapy sessions and medical appointments to better understand her husband's needs, willingly taking the role of caregiver. However, mood swings that included angry outbursts alternating with withdrawn, depressed behavior were becoming increasingly difficult for his wife to manage. He experienced several falls because he would not use the assistive devices prescribed as a support while learning to ambulate on his new prosthetics. His wife noticed he was drinking alcohol at all hours of the day, so she stopped buying alcohol. His aggressive behavior progressed and occurred more often, frightening the children. After an especially violent outburst, his wife took the children and left. Sergeant Major K. contacted an old high school friend known to sell opiates and arranged a buy. Sergeant Major K. is now taking street opiates, is without social support, and is not keeping physical therapy or follow-up medical appointments.

To reduce the risks associated with the level of complexity shown by the subject in this case study, a systematic and targeted approach will be needed and is facilitated by identifying where the greatest risk lies and prioritizing the interventions needed to reduce the risk. If an attempt to address all the patient's health challenges at one time is attempted, little to no success can be expected. An integrated case management approach focuses on all risk but prioritizes where to begin so that the greatest risk is mitigated. All risk will be addressed by priority.

Five percent of the United States population accounts for 50% of healthcare costs and are challenging to manage (Hardin et al., 2021). Individuals challenged with complexity may have multiple providers who are not collaborating, frequent the emergency department, do not take medications as prescribed, have financial issues that make affording care difficult, dwell in unsafe environments, and have little to no or unavailable social supports. While not an exhaustive list of potential challenges, these examples provide a sampling of contributors to complexity.

With complexity comes risk. Challenges to reducing complexity require determining the actual root cause and what concern to address first. Where does the greatest risk lie? What is most concerning for the patient? How are the risks and challenges prioritized? The health concerns of the complex individual can be overwhelming, not just for the individual, but also for the healthcare professional.

Interventions

Complexity results in not just poor health but inadequate quality of life, an increased risk of mortality, disability, and psychological stress (Tortajada et al., 2017). Internationally, case management and multidisciplinary team collaboration are recognized as the most common organizational interventions (Tortajada et al., 2017). Identification and engagement of complex individuals are required for positive health outcomes. How identification is conducted is dependent on the tools and data used. Many organizations have developed comprehensive analytic tools that include the social determinants of health, while others may only consider claims data. The more sophisticated analytic programs easily identify those experiencing risk and those that are anticipated to experience risk. The resources and services provided by case management are most effective when offered to those that will benefit the most.

Engagement

Identification of those that will benefit the most from case management intervention must also be engaged in the process. Engagement starts with relationships. Individuals challenged with complexity may be hesitant to engage with healthcare professionals due to distrust. That distrust may originate from a lack of respect, condescension and judgment, bias, little to no clinician-demonstrated empathy, demonstrated inequities, and poor health literacy with no attempts by professionals to improve. To expect engagement, the healthcare professional must make every effort to learn, understand, demonstrate empathy, recognize, and remove biases and judgments, and, above all, demonstrate respect.

Engagement is best accomplished when the patient can be met face-to-face. Inclusion of family or caregivers will strengthen engagement. When possible, patients and their support systems should be met in person to conduct a comprehensive assessment. The first few encounters may be lengthy—it is not unusual to last upward of 45 to 60 minutes. There will be much to learn from your patient and building trust takes time. The assessment should translate to the patient's story. Everyone has a story, and that story helps others understand who and where they are on the life and health journey. More time may be needed to learn if there are significant social or behavioral concerns (Hardin et al., 2021). Once trust is established, encounters may not require as much time.

Complex Care Delivery

Delivering "complex care" is an emerging healthcare discipline. *Blueprint for Complex Care*, published in 2018 by the National Center for Complex Strategies and the Institute for Healthcare Improvement, reinforced the need to develop programs and tools to uniformly measure utilization, cost, and clinical outcomes (Silverman, 2021). Two studies from 2020 demonstrated conflicting results on cost and utilization for complex patients and the need for better strategies (Silverman, 2021).

The National Center for Complex Health and Social Needs and the Camden Coalition of Healthcare Providers identified populations that would benefit from care integration of physical, behavioral, and social needs. They include children with complex needs; the nonelderly disabled; those with presence of multiple chronic conditions; those with major, complex conditions; and the frail elderly (Hardin et al., 2021). Programs to address complexity can be operated by health plans, primary care clinics, health systems, and community-based organizations to serve these diverse subpopulations. Hardin et al. (2021) outline the elements for development of a complex care program, including the following:

- Person-centered
- Team-based/cross-sector
- Equitable
- Data driven

Case Management Society of America's Integrated Case Management Model

CMSA's Integrated Case Management model includes these elements as will be demonstrated. One of the program's driving tenets is a primary case manager collaborating with an individual challenged with complexity, implementing the case management process starting with a comprehensive assessment that examines four domains of health: biological, psychological, social, and health system. Based on the comprehensive assessment, risk is identified and prioritized for targeted goals and interventions. Elements within the four domains of health are systematically reviewed to reveal connections in risk resulting in a greater understanding of the patient's challenges.

The model requires case managers and their affiliated organizations to think differently about how not only to engage the complex patient, but how to address their needs. The traditional medical model of "sick care" or crisis management is replaced by prioritizing risk, developing interventions to reduce risk, and collaboration with all team members, the patient, and their support system. The integrated case manager also prioritizes the patient's preferences: Instead of focusing on diseases and conditions and forcing education, the case manager asks the patient to share what is important to them, what concerns they have, what they know, what they want to know versus telling them what they should do, or giving condition education without asking permission.

Ever evolving payment models may cause some healthcare entities to shy away from implementing such a program, especially one that lacks incentives. However, emerging payment models make a case for challenging traditional fee-for-service care delivery. Fee-for-service care delivery allows reimbursement for every event or service; for example, hospital admissions or expensive diagnostics. The Centers for Medicare & Medicaid Services has introduced reimbursement for care quality, patient-reported outcomes, and demonstrated patient-centered care. Recent provider incentives include bundled payments and direct contracting. Value-based care reimburses for health improvements versus paying for every service rendered with no evidence of improvement (Hardin et al., 2021). Value-based care and payments incentivize the provider to promote prevention and improve health outcomes. By focusing on health-related factors, value-based care expands strategies to include addressing social risk factors (National Academies of Sciences Engineering Medicine [NASEM], 2019). Health systems are paying attention to upstream factors, that is, social determinants of health, but must also include strategies to mitigate social risks, improve primary prevention, and treatment of acute and chronic conditions (NASEM, 2019).

Throughout this revised edition of *CMSA's Integrated Case Management: A Manual for Case Managers by Case Managers, Second Ediiton,* the integrated case management process will share evidence-based strategies to address complexity and reduce risk to prevent worsening health and improve health outcomes and patient satisfaction (Hardin et al., 2021).

REFERENCES

Hardin, L., Humowiecki, M., & Sale, V. (2021). *Building the value case for complex care*. National Center for Complex Health and Social Needs and Camden Coalition of Healthcare Providers.

National Academies of Sciences Engineering Medicine. (2019). *Integrating social care into the delivery of health care: Moving upstream to improve the nation's health*. The National Academies Press. https://doi.org/10.17226/25467

Silverman, K. D. (2021). *Assessing the impact of complex care models: Opportunities to fill the gaps*. Center for Healthcare Strategies. www.chs.org

Tortajada, S., Giménez-Campos, M. S., Villar-López, J., Faubel-Cava, R., Donat-Castelló, L., Valdivieso-Martínez, B., Soriano-Melchor, E., Bahamontes-Mulió, A., & García-Gómez, J. M. (2017). Case management for patients with complex multimorbidity: Development and validation of a coordinated intervention between primary and hospital care. *International Journal of Integrated Care, 17*(2), 1–8. https://doi.org/10.5334/ijic.2493

CHAPTER 2

The Mechanics of an Integrated Case Management Approach

Rebecca Perez

OBJECTIVES

- Discover how to identify medically complex populations
- Define the integrated case management (ICM) process
- Explore the qualifications and training

Introduction

Working with complex patients may be one of the greatest challenges a case manager can face. Complex patients require multidimensional assistance in order to reduce complexity. The historical biomedical approach is ineffective in helping complex patients regain stability as the focus has been on diseases and conditions. The integrated case management (ICM) model teaches case managers to focus on the person challenged with medical, behavioral, and social issues to help them regain health and function.

Identifying the Individual Challenged With Complexity

People with complex health and social needs are a heterogeneous population and engagement must be targeted at those who will benefit the most from case management interventions. Identification of these individuals requires analysis of more than utilization, cost, diagnosis, and insurance status. Gaining an understanding of the populations and their needs are the only way to target and tailor interventions that will result in health improvements. How these populations are identified varies because there is no standard definition or description.

According to Davis et al. (2021), defining patients with complex needs remains an ongoing discussion. The needs of complex patients are often framed around the biopsychosocial model of disease which describes how biological and psychological factors interact and determine the potential for health and wellness (Davis et al., 2021). Davis et al. (2021) found common themes in how some organizations defined complexity:

- 83% of complex population definitions included a cost-based criterion, a utilization-based criterion, or both.
- 38.9% of complex definitions included a health conditions-based criterion.
- 19% to 20% of these population definitions also included a subjective component such as referral or screening of the candidate patient list.

The National Center for Complex Health and Social Needs and the Camden Coalition of Healthcare Providers produced a Complex Care Toolkit in 2021. The toolkit was created and designed to support healthcare organizations, funders, and payers make the business case for transforming the delivery of care to individuals with complex healthcare needs. In their toolkit, they define complexity as having the following attributes (Hardin et al., 2021):

- *For children*: Severe, sustained impairment such as ventilator dependence, enteral feedings and deficits in learning, mental functions, communication, motor skills, self-care, hearing, and vision.
- *For nonelderly disabled*: Those under the age of 65 with a condition such as end-stage renal disease or a disability based on the receipt of Supplemental Security Income (SSI).
- *Multiple chronic conditions*: Those with only one complex condition and/or between one and five noncomplex conditions.
- *Major complex chronic conditions*: Those with two or more complex conditions or at least six noncomplex conditions.
- *Frail elderly*: Those over the age of 65 with two or more frailty indicators such as gait abnormality, malnutrition, failure to thrive, cachexia, debility, difficulty walking, history of falls, muscle wasting and/or weakness, decubitus ulcers, altered mental status or dementia, and use of durable medical equipment (DME).

With funding from multiple sources, Kristen Peck, Research Project Director for the Dartmouth Institute for Health Policy and Clinical Practice, created a lengthy report for the National Survey of Accountable Care Organizations (ACOs). In the report, titled "How ACOs Are Caring for People with Complex Needs," Peck along with her colleagues stated that people with complex needs account for nearly one fifth of healthcare spending even though this group is only 1% of patients (Peck et al., 2018). They further describe individuals with complex health needs as having multiple chronic conditions or functional limitations, the presence of significant nonmedical needs, and frail older adults (Peck et al., 2018). These individuals need care coordination with numerous providers, family and caregivers, and social service agencies to address mental health, physical health, and social needs (Peck et al., 2018).

Patients with a higher level of complexity obviously require more intensive support and resources. The need to provide complex care is emerging as the next best practice because of the focus on a patient-centered approach, but there is also an incentive to providers for providing high-quality care while controlling costs. This also supports the industry's shift from fee-for-service reimbursement to value-based payment to improve the quality of care while reducing costs, which are the goals of value-based care. Delivering value and the transformation of reimbursement have been and remain elusive goals (Bright & Balch, 2022). "Value over volume" has been prioritized but our healthcare system still struggles to deliver care based on value (Bright & Balch, 2022).

The delivery of care to individuals challenged with complexity requires a multidisciplinary approach by an integrated team of healthcare professionals. However, there should be an identified "lead" that is responsible and accountable for communication and completion of care coordination activities for the patient. The collaboration of professionals as part of an integrated team blends the expertise of each team member and ensures that the whole person and their concerns are addressed. The team lead for the patient makes sure the patient and family/caregiver are aware and understand any recommendations. The team lead asks for patient and family/caregiver feedback and then shares this with the team. This circular communication results in meeting the patient's needs, evaluation of the impact of care and treatment, involvement of family/caregiver, and feedback to the team of healthcare professionals informing of patient experience and satisfaction.

According to Tortajada et al. in an article published in the *International Journal of Integrated Care*, healthcare systems have been facing growing care demands related to the increasing number of chronic conditions (Tortajada et al., 2017). Internationally, case management has been recognized as an effective approach to the management of chronic disease, to improving individuals' health, and in addressing social needs (Tortajada et al., 2017). Case management, specifically ICM, has been shown to positively impact the lives of patients with multiple chronic conditions according to international studies (Tortajada et al., 2017). Defining ICM is as challenging as finding a consensus definition of complexity. An extensive literature search resulted in many definitions for ICM, but a consistent theme was discovered. ICM is a team-based, patient-centered model that addresses physical, mental, and social issues that result in poor health and well-being. The Case Management Society of America's (CMSA) ICM model encourages case managers to improve engagement and communication skills to assist the complex patient in achieving self-management and improved health outcomes by identifying and prioritizing risk. Risk is systematically assessed in four domains of health: biological, psychological, social, and health system. Once risk is assessed and prioritized, a targeted care plan is developed to reduce or eliminate risk. Assessment of the four domains is based on the case manager's worldview: the patient's challenges and opportunities and how best to assist the patient.

Individuals with complex medical conditions are typically a small percentage of a population but are responsible for using the majority of healthcare resources. Case management is a strategy implemented to improve access to care and quality of life while reducing the use of healthcare resources. CMSA's ICM model requires more intensive and time-dedicated interventions.

Patients best suited for ICM are identified and stratified to benefit from case management intervention. Case management is a relatively intensive and costly service; ICM is even more intensive. Offering case management to patients who are not expected to be high utilizers of hospital, specialty, and emergency department care would not reduce costs. Similarly, case management for patients with illnesses or conditions for which there is no hope of improvement or for whom there are no alternative treatment options typically would not benefit from this intense level of intervention. Examples are patients on dialysis without plans for a kidney transplant, or the patient at end of life receiving hospice care, but care coordination activities are certainly appropriate for these patients. The integrated model would only be appropriate for a patient with one of these or similar conditions whereby nonadherence is impacting health stability, costs are beyond what is expected, or the patient has significant social determinants that are preventing access to needed care and services.

Criteria for patients that will benefit from an integrated approach include the following:

- Poorly managed chronic medical conditions
- Acute medical conditions that result in decreased physical function and or with persistent physical symptoms
- Poorly managed mental health conditions
- Two or more hospital admissions in the last 6 months
- Two or more emergency department visits in the last 3 months
- Polypharmacy (eight or more medications)
- Multiple specialty providers with or without a primary care physician (PCP)
- Lack of social support
- Lack of access to trusted providers
- The uninsured or underinsured with chronic or acute conditions
- High deductible health coverage or high pharmacy co-pays
- Geographic isolation from providers
- Lack of transportation to medical or mental health appointments
- Poor health literacy that results in nonadherence
- Any other external factors that result in nonadherence
- Unsafe environment or living arrangements

This is not an exhaustive list and most often a combination of these factors are present resulting in complexity.

Medical conditions are more easily diagnosed than behavioral disorders. Behavioral/mental conditions cannot be diagnosed with traditional testing like blood tests, x-rays, and scans. There is no HgA1c to diagnose a mental illness. Mental conditions are typically diagnosed by patient self-report, health utilization data (claims for emergency department use and admissions and other outpatient access in the medical system), symptoms observed and reported, clinical interviews, and criteria-based scales.

A review of resource utilization will capture those with a mental health diagnosis. Reported symptoms and clinical assessments capture those who meet criteria for a mental disorder regardless of receiving a diagnosis or treatment. Of concern is that less than one third of individuals meeting criteria for a mental health disorder will actually receive condition-changing treatment. The prevalence of mental disorders must include the lifetime experiences of the individual.

> *"The United States spends more on healthcare than any other industrialized nation and much that spending is concentrated on a small percentage of the population from whom behavioral health and social needs are major contributors to poor health outcomes." (Humowiecki et al., 2018)*

The presence of comorbidities between mental and medical conditions is more common than not. Conditions such as diabetes, heart disease, cancer, arthritis, and dementia are often complicated by mood disorders (WEbMD, 2021). Mental health conditions can make dealing with a chronic condition more difficult. The mortality rate from cancer and heart disease is higher among people with depression and other mental conditions (WEbMD, 2021).

Consequently, the presence of medical and/or mental health conditions can be further complicated by social and health system deterrents. These issues are what creates risk for worsening health, and reducing that risk is goal of an ICM approach.

With every chronic medical condition, the likelihood of developing a comorbid depressive disorder increases. Subsequently, poor mental health can lead to poor physical health or harmful behaviors (WebMD, 2021).

The Integrated Case Management Process

The ICM process follows CMSA's *Standards of Practice* for guidance and accountability in case management practice and is designed to impact individuals with health complexity by a single point of contact, or primary case manager. Just as with any patient, the assessment identifies the patient's needs in four primary domains: biological (medical), psychological (behavioral/mental), social, and health system. However, what should be the priority is the development of a trusting relationship with the patient. The integrated case manager is asking the patient to share with them the most intimate details of their life. The patient must feel they can trust their case manager and believe that the case manager is genuinely empathetic to and concerned for their well-being.

To begin working with patients in this manner, the case management approach should not be robotic or indifferent. The integrated case manager should begin a conversation that establishes who the case manager is and their purpose for contact. The relationship between patient and case manager should be one of advocacy and support. Rather than jumping right in and interrogating patients about their diabetes or asthma, start the encounter by asking what is most important to them, what are their concerns, what worries do they have, what do they need help with, or simply ask, "So, how can I best help you?"

Individuals with health complexity typically have a long history of health and social challenges. Their experiences with the healthcare system may be less than satisfactory. Gaining patients' trust is the only way they will be willing to share the intimate details of their lives and health.

CMSA's ICM model incorporates the comprehensive assessment that an organization already uses. Then, the model recommends undertaking an investigation into the history, current state, and future risk. For adults, the last 5 years are assessed in history (except for mental health history), the current state examines the last 30 days, and future risk requires the case manager to consider history, the current state, in the absence of case management intervention to determine the potential risk in the next 3 to 6 months. History cannot be changed but may be a predictor of future risk. In the biological, social, and health system domains, the focus is on only the past 5 years for the adult and lifetime for the child/adolescent—what conditions and symptoms have been present during this time. An appendectomy or admission for pneumonia greater than 5 years ago really has no impact on the patient's current health; however, the presence of hypertension or diabetes will have an effect, regardless of when the conditions were diagnosed. For example, if a patient was diagnosed with type 2 diabetes 12 years ago, the condition is recorded in history. Conversely, if a patient was diagnosed with type 2 diabetes 6 months ago, it is also recognized in history. The history of medical conditions can impact the level of risk to which a patient is exposed in the future.

In the psychological domain, the patient's entire life is assessed for history of mental illness. Even if, at present, the patient is not having mental illness symptoms or receiving treatment, any diagnosed or treated mental illness regardless of when, is recognized. A past history of a mental health condition places an individual at risk for recurrence or the development of a different mental health condition. For example, a 45-year-old woman who suffered from severe postpartum depression at age 26 is at risk for depression throughout her life. All other elements in this domain follow the rules for time frames.

From the social perspective, examined are past disruptions in relationships, work history, residential stability, and presence of support. The last 5 years of health system history include a patient's access to care and relationships with providers. For the patient's current state, one assesses their ability and logistics of accessing care.

Assessing the level of risk in each domain allows the case manager to determine the greatest contributors to poor health. This prioritization of risk facilitates the development of a targeted care plan with interventions that will result in reduced risk. The CMSA's ICM model uses an assessment tool, the Integrated Case Management Complexity Assessment Grid (ICM-CAG) or the Pediatric Integrated Management Complexity Assessment Grid (PIM-CAG), which assists the case manager and patient in prioritizing risk. The tool walks us through the four domains, time frames, and guidelines for scoring the level of risk assessed. More detail is forthcoming on how to use the tool but to introduce the concepts, risk is scored as follows:

- Score of zero: no risk
- Score of one: requires monitoring
- Score of two: attention required
- Score of three: immediate intervention required

Individuals with health complexities may have multiple needs. The results of a case manager's comprehensive assessment may reveal many areas of risk and the ICM-CAG helps to recognize and prioritize that risk. Addressing all the immediate risks at one time may be overwhelming, not only to the case manager but also to the patient. Prioritization of the immediate risks using good clinical judgment is required to develop a care plan that will result in success for the patient and for the case manager. The presence of multiple risks may also require that the care plan and work with the patient be conducted in incremental steps. For example, a patient with uncontrolled diabetes, chronic obstructive pulmonary disease (COPD), and who is living in an abusive environment has multiple risk factors.

So, where to start?

The case manager cannot expect this patient to take medications, follow a diet, quit smoking, and move from the abuse all at one time.

So, what needs to happen first?

This is discussed and negotiated with the patient: "What do you think needs to happen first?" Likely helping the patient feel safe would be the primary concern; assisting the patient find a safe place to live will hopefully reduce fear, anxiety, and stress, thereby allowing for more of a focus on personal health. The full ICM process is discussed in detail using case studies later in the manual.

Qualifications and Practice Models

Case managers are licensed healthcare professionals or those who hold advanced degrees in health and human services (HHS). Experienced case managers are familiar with the processes related to assessment, care planning, advocacy, facilitation, and care coordination.

Traditional Practice Model

Traditionally, case managers practice within the discipline with which they are most familiar or for which their clinical practice was focused. For example, a medical case manager with a strong background in maternal/child health works with women who experience high-risk pregnancies. But if the pregnant patient is currently using heroin, the medical case manager will refer the patient to a behavioral health case manager to address the patient's addiction. This means that two case managers are outreaching the patient instead of one single point of contact with whom the patient can develop a trusted relationship. Coincidentally, a behavioral health case manager is working with a patient who has had multiple admissions for psychotic breaks. The patient has not been taking medications as prescribed to manage schizophrenia. The lack of schizophrenic symptom management has also resulted in the patient developing a wound from uncontrolled diabetes. Typically, the issue of uncontrolled diabetes and the wound would be addressed by a medical case manager, again, disallowing a single point of contact for the patient.

Integrated Case Management Model

In contrast, the ICM model requires case managers, regardless of background, to address all conditions and needs of a patient and be willing to be the primary facilitator for the patient's care. That means all communication to the patient and family comes from the primary case manager. Responsibility and accountability for meeting the needs of the patient starts and stops with the primary case manager. This does not mean you have to literally coordinate every care need, but it does mean that you are accountable for the completion of care coordination activity. Many case managers feel uncomfortable addressing conditions with which they are unfamiliar or do not routinely address. ***First and foremost, case managers must understand that they do not diagnose and do not treat.*** While it is understandable that a case manager may feel less than confident in addressing an unfamiliar condition, it is expected when practicing an integrated approach that the case manager takes the initiative to understand all the patient's conditions. This is part of the case manager's professional growth and stewardship required to be an effective advocate and support.

Learning Strategies

Learning about conditions is not the only strategy for being better prepared to support your patients. Consultations with peers or team members who may have experience in the area where you do not can be most valuable. Your peers can share their experiences to help you better understand the patient's conditions and suggest strategies that have worked. Consulting with medical directors will also result in guidance.

Case managers assist patients and their support system in managing both behavioral and medical conditions through care coordination, support, advocacy, and mitigation of barriers. Ideally, case managers with experience will be better prepared for the challenges of multidimensional support of complex patients. Experience is an asset, but additional training is also needed. Training should include:

- Motivational interviewing training to assist the patient in conversations about change
- Cross-disciplinary exposure to medical and behavioral conditions and an understanding of how conditions interact to cause complexity
- Relationship development for improved patient engagement

- An understanding of emotional intelligence
- The ability to advocate for shared decision-making

Clinical Versus Nonclinical Roles

Not every member of a health population will require case management. As discussed earlier, only a small percentage of a population will experience complexity. However, some others may need some level of health or social support, health coaching, or short-term care coordination from nonclinical care coordinators. In this manual, the focus is on the most complex individuals of a population.

Of added importance is the triage process which is essential to ensuring the complex patient is assigned the most appropriate primary case manager. This triage process should be based on the patient's risk. Where does the greatest risk lie? In the behavioral domain or the medical domain? The primary diagnosis that is causing the greatest risk should guide the assignment of the primary case manager.

CASE STUDY 1

Julia is a 44-year-old with uncontrolled diabetes, daily blood sugars fluctuating between 50 before breakfast and 300 after dinner, a nonhealing wound on her left foot, and chronic depression.

Should the primary case manager have a medical background or a behavioral background? The greatest risk lies with the patient's uncontrolled blood sugars. Severe fluctuations in blood sugar put the patient at risk of hospital admission and worsening of the wound. However, the patient's depression is likely contributing to her poor control. The case manager must work with the patient to discover how best to address her depression so that she can focus on diabetes management. In this instance, the primary case manager should have a strong medical background but focus on the patient's depression. Focusing on self-management at this point will not result in success.

CASE STUDY 2

Roger has been admitted for heroin overdose three times in the last 6 months. He also has been diagnosed with COPD and has been to the emergency department for shortness of breath four times in the last year because he continues to smoke and does not use the long-acting inhaler prescribed by his PCP. Should the primary case manager have a medical background or a behavioral background? The greatest risk lies with a potential for death from overdose. Roger has already had three heroin overdoses in the last 6 months. If his substance abuse is not addressed, the next overdose could be fatal, so his primary case manager should be a behavioral health case manager. Addressing his smoking and medication nonadherence is important but unless he stops heroin use, it is unlikely the COPD exacerbations will be controlled.

Cases such as these support the need for good triage practices that include critical thinking to make good clinical decisions. All primary case managers should also be supported by an interdisciplinary team. Case managers working with complex populations may be assigned very small caseloads as these patients take more time to engage. They have high needs across the domains and if the primary case manager is to meet all the patient's needs, a significant amount of time is required. The ICM model recommends that care teams be developed within the case management organization or place of practice. The care team is made up of both clinical and nonclinical staff. The nonclinical staff can assist the primary case manager's coordination of services like scheduling provider appointments, handling correspondence, and arranging for delivery of durable medical equipment or medical supplies. These tasks do not necessarily require patient contact but are essential for care coordination. To ensure effective use of resources, medical and behavioral case managers should spend their time working with clients and patients.

A suggested care team includes at minimum:

- Medical case managers
- Behavioral case managers
- Nonclinical support staff or case management extenders
- Community health workers
- Pharmacy staff
- Medical directors

The medical and behavioral case managers support each other with their respective expertise. The nonclinical staff assists with coordination activities that do not require clinical intervention. Pharmacy staff assist with medication review and reconciliation. Community health workers can be the eyes and ears of the case manager if only telephonic contact is the model and can become peer supports for the patients. Medical directors guide the case managers by advising on best practice and evidence-based practice, and can be a liaison with other providers. The members of the care team support each other while taking ownership of the patients they serve.

Mental Health Parity and Integrated Care Management

Historically, individuals with mental health conditions have been viewed as difficult to treat. Under the Affordable Care Act (ACA) passed in 2010, behavioral health services were included as one of the 10 essential benefits, meaning that insurers were required to cover mental health services equally to that of medical services. The Mental Health Parity and Addiction Equity Act of 2008 required most health plans or health insurers that offer coverage for mental health conditions or substance use disorders to make these benefits comparable to those offered for medical and surgical benefits. Unfortunately, payers have continued to fall short of the requirements, so the Department of Health and Human Services and the Department of Labor have produced informational resources for Americans to know and understand their rights. The Substance Abuse and Mental Health Services Administration have these resources available on their website.

Prevalence and Rates of Treatment

Nearly one in five Americans is living with a mental illness which include many different types of illnesses varying in severity (National Institutes of Health [NIH], 2022). These illnesses are often listed in one of two broad categories: Any Mental Illness (AMI) or Serious Mental Illness (SMI; NIH, 2022). AMI is defined as a mental, behavioral, or emotional disorder that can vary from mild to severe. SMI is defined as a mental, behavioral, or emotional disorder that results in serious functional impairment which interferes with one or more major life activities (NIH, 2022). Figures 2.1 through 2.4 illustrate the prevalence of mental illness and rates of treatment.

Of concern are the ratios of individuals with mental illness that report receiving treatment. Of the 52.9 million adults with AMI, only 46%, or 24.3 million, received any mental health treatment (NIH, 2022). In 2020, 14.2 million adults (over the age of 18 years) were reported to have an SMI, with 64.5% or 9.1 million receiving treatment. The percentage of adults who do not receive treatment for either category is of significant concern.

FIGURE 2.1 Past-year prevalence of any mental illness among U.S. Adults (2020).

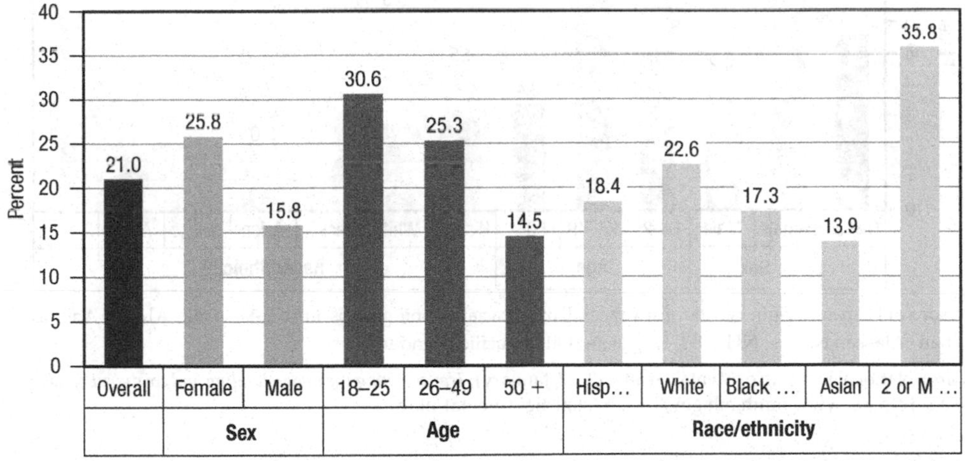

Persons of Hispanic origin may be of any race; all other racial/ethnic groups are non-Hispanic. Note: Estimates for Native Hawaiian/Other Pacific Islander, and American Indian/Alaskan Native groups are not reported due to low precision of data collection in 2020.

Source: National Institute of Mental Health. (2022, January). *Transforming the understanding and treatment of mental illness.* https://www.nimh.nih.gov/health/statistics/mental-illness

FIGURE 2.2 Mental health services received in the past year among U.S. adults with any mental illness (2020).

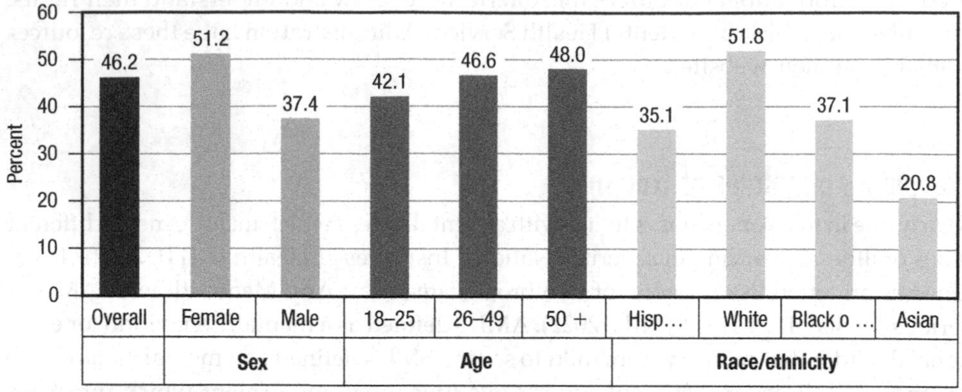

Persons of Hispanic origin may be of any race; all other racial/ethnic groups are non-Hispanic. Note: Estimates for Native Hawaiian/Other Pacific Islander, American Indian/Alaskan Native, and two or more race groups are not reported figure due to low precision of data collection in 2020.

Source: National Institute of Mental Health. (2022, January). *Transforming the understanding and treatment of mental illness*. https://www.nimh.nih.gov/health/statistics/mental-illness.

FIGURE 2.3 Past-year prevalence of serious mental illness among U.S. adults (2020).

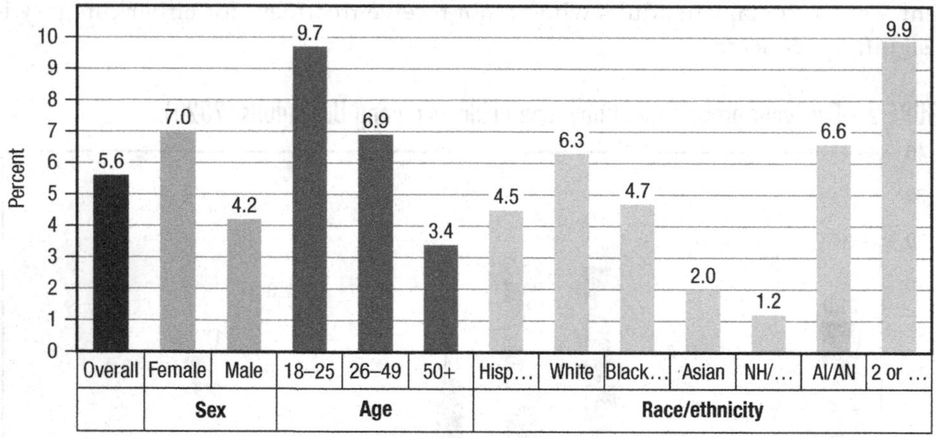

Persons of Hispanic origin may be of any race; all other racial/ethnic groups are non-Hispanic. AIAN = American Indian/Alaskan Native; NH/OPI, Hawaiian/Other Pacific Islander.

Source: National Institute of Mental Health. (2022, January). *Transforming the understanding and treatment of mental illness*. https://www.nimh.nih.gov/health/statistics/mental-illness.

The reasons individuals do not seek mental healthcare and services are varied. What is likely the primary contributor is the shortage of behavioral health providers. If a person is having a mental health crisis or has an urgent need, it may be weeks before an appointment can be secured. Telehealth has helped somewhat with making and arranging

FIGURE 2.4 Mental health services received in the past year among U.S. adults with serious mental illness (2020).

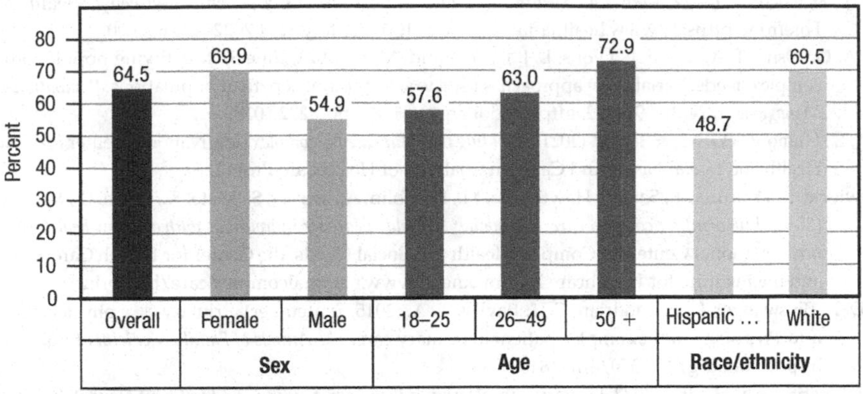

Persons of Hispanic origin may be of any race; all other racial/ethnic groups are non-Hispanic. AI/AN = American Indian/Alaskan Native; NH/OPI = Native Hawaiian/Other Pacific Islander. Note: Estimates for Black or African American, Asian, Native Hawaiian/Other Pacific Islander, American Indian/Alaskan Native, and two or more race groups are not reported due to low precision.

Source: National Institute of Mental Health. (2022, January). *Transforming the understanding and treatment of mental illness*. https://www.nimh.nih.gov/health/statistics/mental-illness.

appointments, but the number of needed providers is still lacking. The integration of mental health with primary care is fast becoming a desirable solution, especially in large ACOs and patient-centered medical homes, common in urban areas. The co-location of both medical and behavioral health professionals in clinics and primary care practices allows the patient to address all their needs in one visit rather than seeing multiple providers in multiple locations.

Another concern has been reimbursement because many insurers have traditionally contracted out behavioral services and employers have independently contracted with separate companies for these services. Mental health utilization practices may be more stringent and coordination and collaboration with the medical sector is absent. These types of contractual arrangements threaten the ability to integrate care. Mental health specialist groups and independent companies are not working with primary care, especially for the Medicaid population. Individual case managers are challenged with helping many patients access needed behavioral services in a timely manner and within close geographic proximity. Attempts to integrate care may become the responsibility of the case manager to facilitate and coordinate care between providers.

The needs related to physical medical conditions are not forgotten and are addressed in more detail later in the manual. Access and coordination of mental and behavioral health services continue to be challenging, more so than access to care for medical conditions. Setting the example for integrated care may fall to the integrated case manager.

REFERENCES

Bright, J., & Balch, A. (2022, March 4). *Health care value through the lens of patients' well-being*. Health Affairs Forefront. https://www.healthaffairs.org/do/10.1377/forefront.20220228.656900

Davis, A. O., Osuji, T. A., Chen, J., Lyons, L. J. L., & Gould, M. K. (2021, June 8). Identifying populations with complex needs: Variation in approaches used to select complex patient populations. *Population Health Management*, *24*(3), 393–402. https://doi.org/10.1089/pop.2020.0153

Hardin, L., Humowiecki, M., & Sale, V. (2021). *Building the value case for complex care*. National Center for Complex Health and Social Needs and Camden Coalition of Healthcare Providers.

Humowiecki, M., Kuruna, T., Sax, R., Hawthorne, M., Hamblin, A., Turner, S., Mate, K., Sevin, C., & Cullen, K. (2018). *Blueprint for complex care: Advancing the field of care for individuals with complex health and social needs*. National Center for Complex Health and Social Needs, the Center for Health Care Strategies, and the Institute for Healthcare Improvement. www.nationalcomplex.care/blueprint

Loeb, D. F., Binswanger, I. A., Candrian, C., & Bayliss, E. A. (2015, September). Primary care physician insights into a typology of the complex patient in primary care. *The Annals of Family Medicine*, *13*(5), 451–455. https://doi.org/10.1370/afm.1840

National Institutes of Health. (2022, January). *Transforming the understanding and treatment of mental illness*. https://www.nimh.nih.gov/health/statistics/mental-illness

Peck, K. A., Usadi, B., Mainor, A., Newton, H., & Meara, E. (2018). *How ACOs are caring for people with complex needs*. The Dartmouth Institute for Health Policy and Clinical Practice.

Tortajada, S., Giménez-Campos, M. S., Villar-López, J., Faubel-Cava, R., Donat-Castelló, L., Valdivieso-Martínez, B., Soriano-Melchor, E., Bahamontes-Mulió, A., & García-Gómez, J. M. (2017). Case management for patients with complex multimorbidity: Development and validation of a coordinated intervention between primary and hospital care. *International Journal of Integrated Care*, *17*(2), 1–8. https://doi.org/10.5334/ijic.2493

WEbMD. (2021, March 29). *How does mental health affect physical health*. https://www.webmd.com/mental-health/how-does-mental-health-affect-physical-health

CHAPTER 3

The Interaction of Medical and Behavioral Conditions

Rebecca Perez

OBJECTIVES

- Comprehend cross-disciplinary roles for an integrated approach
- Explore the roles and collaborative relationships needed for successful interdisciplinary teams.
- Define an integrated case manager
- Explore the collaboration of interdisciplinary teams
- Discover the impact of comorbid medical and mental health conditions

Introduction

For case managers to function as integrated case managers, they must be able to address all the patient's conditions. This requires the case manager to have a general understanding of medical and behavioral conditions. For some, this may be uncomfortable or even a bit overwhelming as conditions that are unfamiliar to the individual will require additional attention and intervention. The case manager must be willing to learn about less familiar conditions so that they can support condition-changing treatment. In addition to broadening their knowledge base, the case manager will have the support of an interdisciplinary team whose members may have experience that the case manager lacks. Of course, any case manager can draw upon their own experiences and consult with those who have knowledge in areas that they do not for effective patient support.

Cross-Disciplinary Roles

Integrated case management is a process in which a single case manager works with a patient to address all health concerns: medical, behavioral, social, and access to care. The assignment of a case manager should be based on the primary risk factors of the patient. The primary case manager should have expertise in those areas of risk. However, the expectation is that the primary case manager also works with the patient in all areas that impact health, even if the case manager lacks specific experience with all the patient's conditions. In order to assist a patient to regain health, we encourage case managers to become familiar with conditions less familiar. These may include the common conditions discussed in this chapter, or the patient may be challenged with less familiar conditions. Regardless, the case manager has a professional obligation to better understand the conditions, appropriate treatment, and associated challenges that may be faced.

To effectively function as an integrated case manager, it is not necessary to be an expert in the disciplines with which they are less familiar. Case managers coming from a physical medicine background do not need to know every medication prescribed for every mental health condition, nor should the case manager coming from a behavioral health background need to know every medication prescribed for every physical health condition. Case managers assist patients in accessing needed care and support adherence. That requires that we understand the treatment direction in which to guide a patient and that we support the treatment prescribed by a physician. Case managers do not diagnose nor prescribe treatment, unless you are a physician, physician assistant, or nurse practitioner. If we have a basic understanding of evidence-based treatments and have the support of a care team and physician advisor, we can be effective in helping a patient move toward improved health. This basic understanding of illnesses and conditions provides the ability to assist in removing barriers to access care that will result in illness improvement.

Guidelines for a basic understanding of illness:

- Recognize core signs and symptoms of the diagnosed condition(s).
- Know the common classes of medications used to treat a condition.
- Know the resources needed to gain additional information about medications.
- Understand the types of therapies that may be prescribed:
  - Psychotherapy (behavioral or cognitive)
  - Physical therapy for orthopedic conditions
  - Occupational therapies for stroke, cerebral palsy, developmental delays, or other cognitive issues
  - Speech/language therapies for communication and cognitive disorders

- Know how a patient should be monitored for their condition
- Know what constitutes a good response to treatment or what to look for if the patient is not responding to treatment
- Know how to document progress or lack of progress
- Know when improvement should be expected once treatment has been initiated
- Know when, what, and to whom to report if a patient is not making progress

Collaborating With an Interdisciplinary Team

For individuals with high-risk and serious illness, poorly integrated care leads to hospitalizations, increased physician visits, and increased costs. The presence of social determinants like food insecurity, an unsafe environment, or lack of social support push the level of complexity and increase health risks. The development of integrated teams that include physicians, nurses, social workers, pharmacists, and other allied health professionals increases the potential for successful care coordination and a connection to needed social services.

Another important component to the integrated team is the availability of mental health and behavioral healthcare from trained professionals. Patients with physical health conditions, especially those with multimorbidity, often deal with psychosocial needs that are intertwined with physical health conditions (National Academies of Science, Engineering, and Medicine [NASEM], 2022). Social workers are key to ensuring these services are included in a plan of care. Social workers and mental health professionals play an important role in helping other team members build the competencies needed to eliminate disparities and break down structural barriers, especially for people of color (NASEM, 2022). Social workers may sometimes be the forgotten team member because they work quietly in the background unlike physicians or nurses who often take the lead in managing the complex patient. They are also well equipped at providing culturally based care and can support team members in achieving cultural awareness.

Additional team members can include nutritionists or dieticians, physical, occupational, or speech therapists, certified specialty durable medical equipment providers such as seating specialists, respiratory therapists, community health workers, and nonclinical support staff. The contributions of these team members should be valued as highly as the core members of the team. Any input that results in improved care coordination, communication, access, and satisfaction should be embraced and included in the plan of care.

Current healthcare professional education is not geared to team learning (Dow et al., 2021). Interprofessional education should focus on identity and collaboration. The increasing demands on healthcare professionals come from complex care needs that require the knowledge, skills, and values to support interprofessional care and collaboration (Dow et al., 2021).

Improving interprofessional education prior to graduation of licensure is the mission of the Interprofessional Education Collaborative. However, for case managers currently in practice, a review of the core competencies for interprofessional practice can provide insight and direction for pursuit of additional training. These are the core competencies as outlined in the Interprofessional Education Collaborative in 2016 (Interprofessional Education Collaborative, 2016):

- **Competency 1:**
  Work with individuals of other professions to maintain a climate of mutual respect and shared values (Values/Ethics for Interprofessional Practice).
- **Competency 2:**
  Use the knowledge of one's own role and those of other professions to appropriately assess and address the healthcare needs of patients and to promote and advance the health of populations (Roles/Responsibilities).
- **Competency 3:**
  Communicate with patients, families, communities, and professionals in health and other fields in a responsive and responsible manner that supports a team approach to the promotion and maintenance of health and the prevention and treatment of disease (Interprofessional Communication).
- **Competency 4:**
  Apply relationship-building values and the principles of team dynamics to perform effectively in different team roles to plan, deliver, and evaluate patient/population-centered care and population health programs and policies that are safe, timely, efficient, effective, and equitable (Teams and Teamwork).

Case managers need to continue to develop skills and knowledge for successful collaborative relationships with other healthcare professionals, patients, families, and caregivers. These relationships will support a better understanding of the interaction of medical and behavioral health disorders and conditions.

Goals of Integrated Case Management

1. Have one primary case manager to address the conditions, health concerns, social concerns, and barriers to improvement experienced by the patient.
2. Case managers will familiarize themselves with the patient's conditions, prescribed treatment, and ability to follow the prescribed treatment plan.
3. Case managers will collaborate with the patient's clinicians and other treatment team members to support the prescribed treatment.
4. Case managers will report to the clinicians any concerns related to complications, new symptoms, and the patient's ability to adhere to prescribed treatment.

5. Case managers will assist the patient and family/caregiver in understanding their illness to support self-management.
6. Case managers will assist the patient and family/caregiver in the removal of barriers preventing a return to health.
7. Case managers will encourage healthy behaviors and initiate conversations about change.
8. Case managers will report unnecessary or harmful care.

Case managers whose careers have focused primarily in one discipline may experience concern when asked to address a patient's issues in multiple domains. Supports need to be put in place so that all integrated case managers know where and how to get the information needed to be effective. Interdisciplinary team members should include:

- Medical case managers
- Behavioral case managers
- Nonclinical case manager extenders or support staff
- Pharmacists
- Community health workers/peer supports/community supports
- Medical director/physician advisor
- Social workers
- Other allied health professionals; that is, dietician, physical/occupational/speech/respiratory therapists, palliative care, hospice, home care, and so on

The care team takes ownership of assigned patients. While there is one primary case manager working with a patient, the team is there to aid and support. We have mentioned the professional responsibility of case managers to learn about unfamiliar conditions, but the experience of team members will also result in a widened knowledge base and comfort level. Interdisciplinary rounds are an excellent conduit for advice and recommendations as the team comes together to learn how patients are progressing. Rounds are a perfect venue for discussion of challenges as well as successes.

CASE STUDY

George has a long history of chronic obstructive pulmonary disease (COPD) and until recently managed his symptoms well. In the last 6 months, George has been in the emergency department four times and had a lengthy admission for pneumonia and respiratory distress. Callie, his case manager, reviewed his pharmacy utilization only to find that it appears George has not been filling his medications in a timely way. When she talks with George, he is less than forthcoming about why he has not been filling his prescriptions. George tells Callie he just forgets to take his medicines sometimes and forgets to refill them. Callie is concerned because this is unusual for George. She brings George's case to interdisciplinary rounds. Callie's behavioral health team member Dan asks if Callie has screened George for depression. She had not, so Dan coaches Callie on how to begin the conversation to assess George for depression and recommends conducting the Patient Health Questionnaire (PHQ-9). During Callie's next encounter with George, she begins to ask about George himself and does not talk about his COPD. She learns that George's grandson was killed 8 months ago while serving oversees. George admits he is devastated by the loss. Callie's work with George now takes a different focus and she works with her team to offer George services and resources that may assist with his grief and subsequent depression. There is an expectation that George will once again be able to self-manage his COPD once his grief and depression are actively being addressed. Repeated assessments using the PHQ-9 will provide data to demonstrate if strategies implemented to address George's grief and depression have been effective.

Important Issues Related to the Interaction of Medical and Mental Health Conditions

According to a study by Lauders et al., individuals with serious mental illness (SMI) have more medical comorbidities and poorer health outcomes than the general population (Launders et al., 2022). Medical comorbidities often lead to decreased quality of life and increase the incidence of mortality in individuals with SMI. Individuals with SMI are at a higher risk of admission and 30-day readmission, and those with comorbid medical conditions are at a higher risk of psychiatric admission (Launders et al., 2022). The presence of these interacting conditions results in poor medication adherence, polypharmacy, poor care coordination, and unsatisfactory patient experiences (Launders et al., 2022).

The most common physical illnesses that interact with SMI are cardiovascular disease, COPD, diabetes, and liver disease (Launders et al., 2022). The SMI with the highest rate of hospitalization is schizophrenia (Launders et al., 2022).

Lauders et al. (2022) concluded that while hospitalizations are higher in individuals with chronic medical conditions and SMI, more education and research are needed to better understand certain conditions and their impact on the development of targeted interventions to reduce admissions.

When examining the considerations that professionals from either the medical or mental health disciplines may encounter, there are some significant differences, especially for mental health. Rarely is treatment for medical conditions forced. The exception is the presence of communicable diseases or when there is a community health threat. Individuals with severe psychiatric illness may be examined for competency or dangerous behaviors for involuntary commitment via court-ordered action. Forced admission or detention occurs when an individual's judgment is impaired to the point of risk, or they are a physical threat to self or others. Examples of conditions that can escalate these risks are dementia, substance abuse, eating disorders, or psychosis. Case managers are typically not involved in the legal process but should understand the process. The role of the case manager in these situations is to provide support to the patient and the patient's support system, and to assist in the coordination of care and services at the conclusion of the commitment or detention. Laws related to competency and commitment vary from state to state, and case managers must familiarize themselves with the process in their local jurisdictions.

Patients who verbalize suicidal or homicidal thoughts are at significant risk. Case managers from a medical background may find this expression frightening. When a patient expresses such thoughts, the case manager must be proactive and determine the level of intent. There are ways to determine how to escalate the intervention: Have discussions with your behavioral health team members and ask them to share some of their real-life experiences and how they have handled such crises. More detail regarding the management of medical and mental health conditions will be shared in Section III: Addressing Complex Patient Populations Using an Integrated Case Management Approach of this manual.

REFERENCES

Dow, A., Pfeifle, A., Blue, A., Jensen, G. M., & Lamb, G. (2021). Do we need signature pedagogy for interprofessional education? *Journal of Interprofessional Care, 35*(5), 649–653.

Interprofessional Education Collaborative. (2016). *Core competencies for interprofessional collaborative practice: 2016 update.* Inter p rofessional Education Collaborative.

Launders, N., Dotsikas, K., Marston, L., Price, G., Osborn, D. P. J., & Hayes, J. F. (2022). The impact of comorbid severe mental illness and common chronic physical health conditions on hospitalisation: A systematic review and meta-analysis. *PLoS ONE, 17*, e0272498. https://doi.org/10.1371/journal.pone.0272498

National Academies of Science, Engineering, and Medicine. (2022). *Integrating serious illness care into primary care delivery: Proceedings of a workshop.* The National Academies Press. https://nap.nationalacademies.org/catalog/26411/integrating-serious-illness-care-into-primary-care-delivery-proceedings-of

SECTION II

Strategies for Patient Engagement and Retention

CHAPTER 4

Communication Methods and Techniques

Rebecca Perez

"Therapeutic engagement is a prerequisite for everything that follows."

—Miller and Rollnick (2013)

OBJECTIVES

- Explore how communication impacts patient engagement and retention
- Define the principles of motivational interviewing and coaching
- Relate patient engagement and adherence to motivational coaching
- Comprehend how patient-centered preferences influence engagement and shared decision-making

Introduction

For patient engagement to occur, the effort to establish a trusted relationship must be a priority. Patient/clinician relationships are necessary, regardless of the presence of or absence of complexity. Every patient wants to be heard and understood, treated with dignity and respect, and have control over their health and well-being. Effective communication is key to the development of relationships. Patient-centered communication is not necessarily a skill acquired with professional education to achieve licensure or certification. While patient-centeredness is promoted in all factions of healthcare, there is little evidence that healthcare professionals are prepared to implement it. More detail on the development of relationships are discussed in Chapter 5. This chapter explores methods of communication that will assist in attaining the goal of patient-centeredness.

Patient Engagement

How case managers and their professional colleagues interact with patients will determine the patient's level of engagement. This also means "meeting patients where they are." And what exactly does that mean? It means that a case manager's initial encounters with a patient are to determine their current experience with health and care, their ability to manage their conditions, and the barriers preventing positive health outcomes. Early encounters need to include inquiries as to: What is concerning the patient most right now? What immediate needs are present? And how can the case manager help? Common patient responses include difficulty paying for medications, inability to get convenient medical appointments, lack of clarity regarding why certain medications have been ordered, and, in general, a lack of understanding regarding their health condition(s). The needs and concerns of the patient experiencing complexity are exponentially more serious and difficult to solve.

Complex patients do not always seem to make good decisions about their health, from the healthcare professional's point of view. Health behaviors such as treatment adherence and healthy choices can help to improve disease and condition burden and quality of life, if the patient makes good choices. Although one would expect a person to stop smoking after a diagnosis of heart failure, 16% of heart failure patients continue to smoke anyway (Son, 2020). This behavior increases mortality by 38.4% and readmission by 44.8% (Son, 2020). Case managers are positioned to support patients in making health behavior changes. To support treatment adherence, behavior change, and participation in shared decision-making, trusted relationships must first be developed. These relationships need to be fostered by all members of the patient's care team, and then extended to the patient's family, caregiver, or support system.

Communication as Customer Service

Before learning better ways to communicate, the case manager must first take time for self-examination. There has been a growing consumer movement among patients demanding more information and customer service when receiving healthcare services. This movement means healthcare is moving away from medical paternalism, (i.e., "the doctor knows best") to patients taking a more active role in their health (Hahn, 2017). Patients taking a more active role in their health means the case manager can no longer tell them what to do but instead inquire as to what is most important to them, what do they know, and what do they want to know. Information from the healthcare professional should be imparted with the patient's permission. Immediately launching into diabetic education for the individual with a 20-year history of type 2 diabetes and recent uncontrolled blood pressure will most likely result in the information falling on deaf ears. A better way to approach this patient can include questions such as:

- Tell me how things have been going?
- Do you have any concerns right now?

- You have always managed your blood sugar well. Why do you think it has been difficult to keep your blood sugar under control recently?
- How best can I help you?

These questions encourage conversation and help the case manager better understand the patient's challenges. These questions also promote collaboration. The case manager is demonstrating to the patient their desire to collaborate in problem-solving.

Emotional Intelligence

Now back to self-examination. Every person has opinions, biases, and even prejudices. Everyone is entitled to these, but personal feelings and opinions have no place in the care of others. Any bias, opinion, or prejudice must be separated from the professional development of patient–family–caregiver–case manager relationships. To accomplish this goal, the case manager must be willing to examine their own emotions and turn intent into action. Discovering and boosting one's emotional intelligence is a solution. Emotional intelligence helps to build stronger relationships professionally and personally. There are four attributes of emotional intelligence; resultant expectations are oulined in the following (HelpGuide, 2022):

1. *Self-management:* the ability to control impulsive feelings and behaviors, manage emotions in a healthy way, take initiative, follow through with commitments, and adapt to change.
2. *Self-awareness:* the ability to recognize one's own emotions and how they affect an individual's thoughts and behavior. A person should take the time to know their strengths and weaknesses and build their self-confidence.
3. *Social awareness:* an individual has empathy; is able to recognize and understand the emotions, needs, and concerns of others; is able to notice emotional cues, and recognize the power of group dynamics.
4. *Relationship management:* one can communicate clearly, inspire others, work as part of a team, manage conflict, develop, and maintain good relationships.

At one point or another, everyone has met individuals who are academically brilliant but are socially inept. This type of person often is unsuccessful in collaborating with a team and fostering personal relationships. In healthcare, often those who are admired are colleagues and other professionals who are talented and intellectually above others due to their expertise and clinical skills. But intellectual ability is not enough to truly be successful in one's career and in life (HelpGuide, 2022).

Gaining emotional intelligence will help an individual navigate the social complexities of the workplace, lead, and motivate others (HelpGuide, 2022). When communicating with patients, managing one's emotions is important to stress prevention. Furthermore, placing importance on stress prevention will help to prevent health problems. Uncontrolled emotions can lead to mental health problems like depression and anxiety. And uncontrolled emotions can leave one isolated, negatively impacting relationships and further exacerbating mental health problems (HelpGuide, 2022). Becoming emotionally intelligent helps an individual to remain calm in a crisis, read and respond to the emotions of others, inspire others to act, have strong relationships and be resilient when faced with adversity. Readers can explore their own emotional intelligence by taking the Emotional Intelligence Quiz found in the appendices.

Motivational Interviewing

Learning more about one's strengths, weaknesses, and emotional intelligence will prepare an individual for an enhanced ability to build strong relationships and gain the trust of others. Case managers collaborate with patients, families, and caregivers to improve health and well-being. To accomplish this, change is often required, especially when complexity has created multiple challenges for the patient, family, or caregiver. Change, sometimes significant change, is required to reduce complexity and risk. Case managers do not change individuals nor are they responsible for change. However, case managers can support their patients in deciding when and how to make changes.

How a case manager communicates with patients, families, and caregivers will have an impact on the decision to make changes. A proven method for communication is motivational interviewing (MI), a well-studied behavioral approach primarily known for its efficacy in the treatment of addiction. However, the principles and methodology have been integrated into medical practices to promote adherence and healthy behavior changes. MI has key qualities that guide communication by effectively listening and provides advice and information to empower individuals to make changes. MI is a conversation about change. A case manager cannot force an individual to change and case managers cannot "fix" them. Patient's are not cars, and case managers are not mechanics.

MI is a communication method that has a unique skill set that optimizes the possibility that a patient will consider making a change and then implement that change (Figure 4.1). According to Dr. Bruce Berger, MI requires a caring, nonthreatening, nonjudgmental way to understand and explore how patients make sense of health and illness (Berger & Villaume, 2020). MI provides a patient-centered approach that promotes honoring a patient's right to decide what is right, discovering what is important and what information they desire. Dr. Berger also reminds case managers that they cannot provide patient-centered care with provider-centered communication; the skills needed to be successful at MI need to be learned and incorporated into daily practice (Berger & Villaume, 2020).

Based on the development of a trusted relationship, the case manager guides the patient to share their perspective on current health problems and health behaviors. The patient and the case manager discover together what changes need to be made, what the patient is willing to change, and when and how to get started.

FIGURE 4.1 The spirit of motivational interviewing.

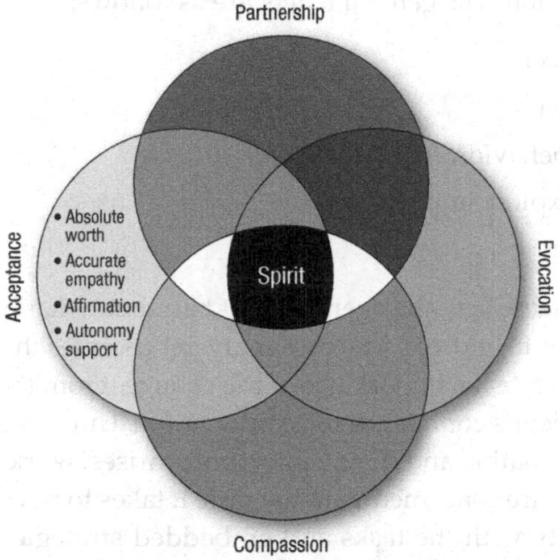

Source: PA Juvenile Justice System. (n.d.). *Motivational interviewing coaches' manual*. Pennsylvania Juvenile Justice System.

The need for behavioral change may be obvious to case managers but may or may not be clear to patients, families, or caregivers. The patients who recognize this need may be ready to change, while others may feel ambivalent or resistant. Those that recognize the need for change are motivated, whereas those ambivalent or resistant may be regarded as lacking motivation. However, all these individuals have potential for change-thinking and would benefit from a case manager skilled in MI.

Establishing Rapport

MI practice requires that rapport be established.

This syncs with one of the foundational tenets of integrated case management, which is to develop a trusted patient/case manager relationship. As the case manager collaborates with the patient and learns what behavior changes are needed and what the patient is willing to address, an agenda needs to be set. For example, the patient expresses a desire to quit smoking, they would like to increase their activity, or decide they will eat less fatty food. Once identified, the patient's feelings about the change need to be determined: Is this change important to the patient and do they have the confidence to make the change?

Collaborating with patients on behavior change requires a collection of strategies. The case manager's use of these strategies must be individualized. Talking about change is not a rote process of step one, step two, then step three. The framework for discussions about change are outlined in Rollnick, Mason, and Butler's book, *Health Behavior Change: A Guide for Practitioners*, published in 1999. Stephen Rollnick was one of the authors of early texts on MI. The framework is one that flows and can and should adapt to the patient and their situation. The general tenets are as follows:

- Establish rapport
- Set the agenda
- Identity the behavior(s)
- Assess and explore importance
- Build confidence

Once rapport is established, the agenda is set based on what behavior or behaviors the patient has decided to address. The case manager assesses the patient's confidence and asks the patient to rate the importance of the change. From there, the case manager helps to build the patient's confidence to be successful. Throughout this process there is an exchange of information and if the opportunity arises, work to reduce resistance.

Many practitioners are concerned with the time it takes to have conversations about change. The familiarity with the tasks and embedded strategies related to a change conversation will help estimate the time needed. The skills required include (Figure 4.2):

- Listening
- Reflective listening
- Use of open-ended questions
- Summarizing

Advice-giving should be avoided. If telling patients what to do was effective, communication methods like MI would not be necessary. Unless there is a safety concern, advice-giving will most likely result in the patient no longer listening or participating.

FIGURE 4.2 Motivational interviewing framework.

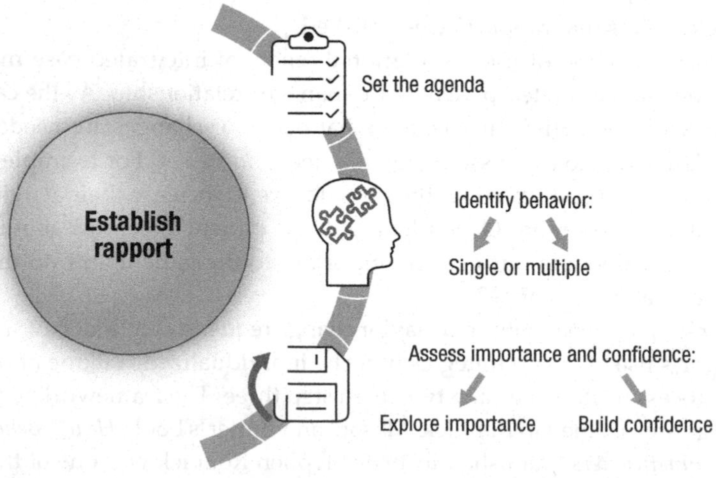

Source: PA Juvenile Justice System. (n.d.). *Motivational interviewing coaches' manual*. Pennsylvania Juvenile Justice System.

Telling patients what to do often makes them feel unheard and devalued. Advice-giving also has a fear component, as exemplified in this sample conversation between case manager and patient:

"You need to stop eating high fat foods."

"Yes, I know, but my kids are so picky, and those are the foods they like."

"So, I guess you're okay having a heart attack and your kids not having a mom?"

MI is a patient-centered method to encourage conversations about change. Being patient-centered involves more than just being nice; it requires careful listening (Rollnick, 1999). The patient's perspective is important to understand their ability to share in healthcare decisions about treatment and attitudes regarding behavior change.

The content provided here is not intended to be comprehensive MI training. If anything, the intent is to encourage participation in formal training. Resources and trainings are available to bring case managers closer to understanding and demonstrating the spirit of MI. To effectively engage with individuals challenged with complexity and the need for behavior change, the case manager should invest in formal MI training. See the appendices for additional resources for MI training.

The Essence of Motivational Interviewing

"I often hear people say that they 'do' motivational interviewing (MI) and they may refer to the many micro skills involved. Others may say that motivational interviewing is a 'technique.' While this is somewhat true, it short-changes MI. MI is a patient-centered approach for exploring a patient's motivation about a behavior (taking a med, losing weight, quitting smoking). It was developed for patients who are ambivalent or resistant to change. But, more than anything, MI is about connection. The micro skills are used to explore that ambivalence or resistance with the patient in a way that says, 'How you see the world . . . how you make sense of things is important and valuable to me. I would like to explore those things with you in a way that honors your decisions with the understanding that you ultimately decide.' This is called the spirit of MI. MI also operates effectively if we understand that we owe the patient everything. They owe us nothing. We are there for them and not the reverse. This is often very uncomfortable for healthcare professionals, especially when they have been trained that they are the expert, and they are 'in charge.' Nothing could be further from the truth. Ultimately, patients decide whether to treat an illness, lose weight, etc. We can certainly influence that decision through care, concern, and good information. However, trying to motivate, convince or persuade a patient to do anything does not work, especially when a patient is ambivalent or resistant. Persuasion and paternalism force the patient to defend their position. Want to make sure someone doesn't quit smoking? Spend your time persuading them to quit. Not only will they not quit, but they also won't want to talk with you about it. The greater danger is if the patient has a chronic illness, they won't want to talk with you about that either if they don't like how you talk with them about their smoking. Are you willing to open yourself up to really see and understand the patient? Without this understanding, MI is NOT MI and real care is compromised." —Bruce Berger, PhD; LinkedIn post; retrieved on 8/18/2022

The Patient's Voice

Even though patient-centered care is the model everyone professes to practice, patients still have little influence in the healthcare decisions most important to them. Listening to the patient's voice is becoming a catch phrase for improving autonomy. But what does that mean? According to Kate Niehaus, an advocate for the Patient Family Advisory Council for Quality at Memorial Sloan Kettering Cancer Center in New York City, the patient's voice provides a unique perspective and can point out existing gaps in healthcare systems (Niehaus et al., 2021). However, in order to listen to patients' voices, the effort must be embedded in an organization's processes and systems. Without it, one voice here and there might be heard, but not enough to impact change. One method of incorporating the patient's voice into systems and processes is to use validated patient-reported outcomes measures (PROMs) that allow patients to report their symptoms and functions. According to the *New England Journal of Medicine's* (*NEJM*) Catalyst Insights Council, 60% of members report PROMs as an effective way to evaluate the patient's experience. However, only 38% of the council members report their organization currently uses PROMs (Niehaus et al., 2021).

The Centers for Medicare & Medicaid Services (CMS) defines PROMs as tools that measure the patient and family/caregiver perspective on the quality of and satisfaction with the care received (CMS, 2022). The data collected from these tools are used to meet quality measures. Patient-reported outcomes report the status of a patient's health condition or health behavior. PROMS are the tools that gather this information and patient-reported outcome based performance measures (PRO-PMS) aggregate the data into a reliable measure of performance (CMS, 2022). Most of these measures are proprietary but a comprehensive list of available tools can be found on the CMS Measures Management System Hub.

Fee-for-service models have been a contributor to poor patient-reported outcomes. For physicians to score high for patient satisfaction, they must spend more time with a patient. However, when a patient has multiple chronic conditions, only one issue can be addressed during a visit, so traditionally, primary care physicians (PCP) have referred their patients to specialists because they cannot be reimbursed for the time needed to treat multiple problems. This is known to lead to miscommunication, overprescribing, and adverse events that result in hospital admissions. A primary care–based, patient-centered, community-based model does align with the time needed to spend with patients and aligns with improved care outcomes (Niehaus et al., 2021). For example, the Villages Health in Florida allow new patients 1 hour with their new PCP, and 30 minutes if they are an established patient, allowing patients to tell their stories and better connect with physicians (Niehaus et al., 2021). According to Niehaus et al., this type of model moves care delivery from "no money, no mission," to "no outcome, no income."

Jonathan David, a cardiac rehabilitation nurse coordinator at Stanford Health Care, and contributor to *NEJM* Catalyst's "The Power of the Patient Voice," related that "our systems are often so complex and fast-paced that we do not take the time to understand our patient enough." This lack of time with the patient is one of the major contributors to hospital admissions (Niehaus et al., 2021). Dr. Rene Crichlow, also a contributor, shared the story of the need to admit a patient who was a farmer. He refused the admission because if he did not work, he could lose his farm. He proposed coming to the clinic every day for treatment and kept his word. Dr. Crichlow shared, "You cannot assume every patient has the needed resources to participate in the care you order; instead you need to listen to needs and values and meet them where they are" (Niehaus et al., 2021).

Understanding and addressing social determinants of health (SDH) can improve patient satisfaction and experience. SDH are defined by the Centers for Disease Control and Prevention as the nonmedical factors that influence health outcomes. They are the conditions in which people are born, grow, work, live, and age, and the wider set of forces and systems shaping the conditions of daily life. There are many assessments for SDH; some may require licensure. Following are three assessments that are often used by the American Academy of Family Physicians:

- Protocol for Responding to and Assessing Patients' Assets, Risks, and Experiences (PRAPARE)
  - https://prapare.org/
  - https://www.aafp.org/family-physician/patient-care/the-everyone-project.html
- The Accountable Health Communities Health-Related Social Needs Screening Tool
  - https://innovation.cms.gov/files/worksheets/ahcm-screeningtool.pdf

The three most common social challenges that impact health are food insecurity, lack of safe housing, and transportation, especially to medical appointments. To address these and other determinants, case managers should create a list of resources available, while establishing relationships with the entities in their region that should be developed and maintained. Eliminating the barriers that contribute to poor health also aid in reducing admissions and readmissions. "The Power of the Patient Voice" also reminds case managers that if they are going to assess for SDoH, then they had better be prepared with resources to address them (Niehaus et al., 2021).

Communication Skills for Healthcare Professionals

Encounters between healthcare professionals and patients involve various aspects. These include for the patient:

- The patient's needs
- Suffering manifested
- The patient's perceived failures in communication (Mata et al., 2021)

Expressing Emotion

The professional's emotional availability does not predict the patient's lived experiences to justify communication about health as a priority. Patients often complain that healthcare professionals inadequately express a sense of caring which is needed to convey encouragement and support. Emotion is important for communication with patients but the skills to effectively communicate using emotion are often lost or missing altogether.

Communication Training

Communication training for healthcare professionals can have a beneficial effect on improving services and minimizing errors (Mata et al, 2021). Clinical training of illnesses, treatment, and health conditions does not guarantee the skills to establish patient–professional relationships based on empathy, support, and comfort. These skills require the professional to self-reflect, using methods like Emotional Intelligence, and collaborate with interdisciplinary colleagues to improve more than just the clinical experience.

There are multiple communication training approaches for healthcare professionals. Each have advantages but the major differences include the length of training. Those programs include multiple learning exercises like role-play, video representation, types of listening, spoken and written communication demonstrating support and understanding (Mata et al., 2021). The length of training impacted the sustainability of improved healthcare professional communication. According to Mata et al., the following trainings were noted to show communication improvements and included a representation of the learning exercises mentioned above (Mata et al., 2021):

1. AFLS (awareness, feelings, listen, solve).
   a. The AFLS is designed to be an easy-to-use assessment tool for parents, educators, professional staff, and other caregivers. The AFLS as aforementioned can be used from 2 years of age right throughout the life span.
   b. Training is completed after two 3.5-hour sessions repeated over 1 to 2 weeks.
2. Method identified by Maguire et al. in 1997.
   a. Maguire's research demonstrated how the hippocampus plays an important role in the laying down of new memories. It is found inside each hemisphere of the brain and is thought to play an important role in facilitating spatial memory and navigation. The study focused on how an environment can impact memory-changing from temporary to spatial memory.
   b. This involves two sessions, one, 3 days in length and one, 2 days in length with a period of 4 weeks separating the two sessions.
3. Integrated Communication Skills Training-Professional (ICSTP):
   a. Incorporated cross-cultural training to improve interpersonal skills.
   b. Training includes three, 7-hour per day sessions delivered over 3 weeks.

All three of these examples provide patient-centered communication instruction using multiple learning methods that include role-play, video, assignments, and group discussions.

Communication Technologies

In the last several years, there has been a shift in how most patients communicate with their providers. The COVID-19 pandemic required that healthcare rethink and rework patient and family communication. Preferences for communicating with providers and about health concerns may be dependent on the patient's concerns. According to Alexander et al., when patients experience cardiac or gastrointestinal symptoms, they are more likely to access emergent care, even if given self-management instructions via telehealth or instruction using a patient portal (Alexander et al., 2021). But for routine concerns or milder symptoms, using information and communication technologies (ICT) such as telehealth and patient portals show an increase in preference (Alexander et al., 2021).

ICT are a part of daily life for the majority of the world's population. However, there are still those without access to broadband, satellite, or cable connectivity, and areas where poverty is significant and access to any digital technology is not an option. For those with access, there has been an emergence in the use of telehealth, remote monitoring, video conferencing, patient portals, and text messaging as methods to communicate with healthcare providers and a trend of increasing participation in one's health.

- **Telehealth:**
  - Telephonic consultation
  - Secured texting and email communications with providers using a patient portal
- **Remote monitoring:**
  - Use of "smart scales" for heart failure monitoring
  - Use of "wearables" to download activity, diet, and so on for reporting to providers
  - Use of Bluetooth or other technology to report metrics like blood sugar
- **Video conferencing:**
  - Use of platforms for video consultations, therapeutic visits, physician visits, and other consultations
- **Patient portals:**
  - Used for direct email communication with providers, wellness reminders, managing appointments, medications, test results, and clinical history
  - Gives the patient the ability to better know and understand their health and health conditions

- **Text messaging:**
  - At one time, text messaging was anticipated to a be a meaningful change in digital communication but concerns regarding privacy have limited its use
  - Text messaging is still valuable for appointment and wellness reminders, but no direct health information is included in messaging

The use of PROMs in each of these communication methods allows the patient to communicate with providers regarding their symptoms and monitoring for condition changes.

Digital technologies use is expected to only increase as it allows patients to manage their health from the comfort of their home or office. Healthcare professionals should be collecting from patients their preferences for communication: whether that is to embrace all forms of digital communication, select methods, or no digital communication. Many patients who did not immediately embrace communication technology were pleasantly surprised by its ease and convenience when it was the only option available during the pandemic.

Alexander et al. conducted surveys of individuals arriving for a planned admission to determine their technology use and preferences. The survey participants were evenly divided between male 50.6% and female 49.4% (Alexander et al., 2021). The majority of the patients were between 51 and 80 years of age, and were admitted for orthopedic, gastrointestinal, or cardiac surgery (Alexander et al., 2021). The survey also assessed the patients' use of technology in general and in managing health. Eighty-nine percent of respondents reported using a laptop or desktop computer in general daily activities and 74% currently use these to manage health (Alexander et al., 2021). For those who use a tablet, 75.5% use it for general daily activities and 56.4% to manage health (Alexander et al., 2021). For those that use email, 93% use it for general daily activities, and 77.6% for health management (Alexander et al., 2021). The survey also looked at mobile phones, text messaging, mobile phone applications, online social networking, and tele/video conferencing. All of these technologies are used in daily activities between 97% and 48% and between 82% and 21% use for health management (Alexander et al., 2021). When asked about their preferences for post-discharge follow-up, the overwhelming preference was telephone, followed by in-person, and third, email. For reporting of symptoms, the preferred method was in-person, followed by telephone, and then email (Alexander et al., 2021).

Patients are under increasing pressure to adopt technology because of the efficiencies demonstrated, especially during COVID-19, but it is more important to offer patients multiple communication options. The potential for efficiencies using technology are expected to result in improved service delivery and patient satisfaction, but of equal importance is to allow patients to delineate their preferred communication methods (Alexander et al., 2021).

Interpersonal Communication

Regardless of the communication tools used, healthcare communication is interpersonal communication. Interpersonal communication, or inter-human communication, was the first tool of the socialization process (Chichirez & Purcărea, 2018). Interpersonal communication can be defined as the communication that occurs between two people in the context of their relationship and as it evolves the relationship is defined (Chichirez & Purcărea, 2018). The efficiency of communication is dependent on the type of relationship established and the type of relationship depends on the personality of each person. For healthcare professionals, communication needs to be a therapeutic technique that creates a fundamental relationship between the professional and patient that results in benefits to the patient and others involved with the patient.

Early in the 12th century, Spanish professor Bernardo Masci developed rules for medical ethics and deontology that are still truly relevant today (Chichirez & Purcărea, 2018):

- Honor your patient regardless of age.
- Offer the same gratitude and attention to the poor as to the rich.
- Respect your noble mission, beginning with your very own person.
- Let your fatigue be enlightened by faith and love.
- Never humiliate the sick, who are so humiliated by their illness.
- Never forget that the secret entrusted to you about a disease is something holy that cannot be betrayed, offered to another person.
- Do not see in your patients' worries a burden, a chore.
- Never show incongruence at the success of the treatment on a sick person.
- Not only benevolence but also science is required in the care of the sick.
- Do not discuss medical prescriptions with the patient and never contradict them. You take away their confidence in medicine; you destroy their hope of healing.

REFERENCES

Alexander, K., Ogle, T., Hoberg, H., Linley, L., & Bradford, N. (2021). Patient preferences for using technology in communication about symptoms post hospital discharge. *BMC Health Services Research, 21*(141). https://doi.org/10.1186/s12913-021-06119-7

Berger, B. A., & Villaume, W. A. (2020). *Motivational interviewing for health care professionals: A sensible approach,* (2nd ed.). American Pharmacists Association.

Centers for Disease Control and Prevention. (2022, November 4). *Fetal alcohol syndrome disorders*. Author. https://www.cdc.gov/ncbddd/fasd/facts.html#:~:text=Fetal%20alcohol%20spectrum%20disorders%20(FASDs)%20are%20a%20group%20of%20conditions,a%20mix%20of%20these%20problems

Chichirez, C. A., & Purcărea, V. L. (2018). Interpersonal communication in healthcare. *Journal of Medicine and Life, 11*(2), 119–122.

Hahn, D. H. (2017). Tokenism in patient engagement. *Family Practice*, *34*(3), 290–295. https://doi.org/10.1093/fampra/cmw097

HelpGuide. (2022, October). *Improving emotional intelligence*. Author. https://www.helpguide.org/articles/mental-health/emotional-intelligence-eq.htm#:~:text=Emotional%20intelligence%20(otherwise%20known%20as,overcome%20challenges%20and%20defuse%20conflict

Mata, Á. D., de Azevedo, K. P. M., Braga, L. P., de Medeiros, G. C. B. S., de Oliveira Segundo, V. H., Bezerra, I. N. M.., Pimenta, I. D. S. F., Nicolás, I. M., & Piuvezam, G. (2021). Training in communication skills for self-efficacy of health professionals: A systematic review. *Human Resources for Health*, *19*(30), 1–9. https://doi.org/10.1186/s12960-021-00574-3

Niehaus, K., Macrae, C., LowenKron, J., Crichlow, R., David, J., & O'Connor, M. A. (2021). *The power of the patient voice: How health care organizations empower patients and improve care delivery*. http://catalyst.nejm.org/

PA Juvenile Justice System. (n.d.). *Motivational interviewing coaches' manual*. Author.

Rollnick, S. M. (1999). *Health behavior change: A guide for practitioners*. Churchill Livingstone.

Son, Y. J. (2020, January). Association between persistent smoking after a diagnosis of heart failure and adverse health outcomes: A systematic review and meta-analysis. *Tobacco Induced Diseases*, *18*(5). https://doi.org/10.18332/tid/116411. PMID: 31997987

CHAPTER 5

Building Relationships

Rebecca Perez

OBJECTIVES

- Define the attributes needed to build trusted relationships
- Compare patient relationships to customer service

Introduction

Throughout Section II: Strategies for Patient Engagement and Retention, concepts and methods are presented to improve patient engagement and retention. This brief chapter will reinforce why relationships in healthcare are important, and provide tips on how to establish those relationships. The patient/healthcare professional relationship facilitates mutual collaboration and trust so that patients can improve their health and well-being. Once again, communication is central to achieving a relationship.

Caring Behaviors

Management of health conditions occurs primarily in the outpatient setting. Caring for patients in acute care settings are often brief, not allowing for long-lasting, trusted relationships to develop. However, research in diabetes and cancer has shown that relationships with healthcare professionals is essential to the ability of patients to cope with their disease (Prip et al., 2018). After a review of qualitative and quantitative studies by Prip et al. (2018), patient responses to caring behaviors by healthcare professionals created an atmosphere in which treatment was simplified, patients felt better because of the support, and their bodies could heal without concerns about the prescribed treatment. The caring behaviors were valued above the actual treatment.

Relationship Building

Case managers are in a position to initiate and strengthen relationships with patients because of the role they play in care coordination, advocacy, and education. The skills needed for relationship building may or may not be inherent. They include:

- **Interpersonal skills**
  - Relationships are people-centered
  - Being able to understand another person's perspective, showing respect or showing compassion
- **Nonverbal communication skills**
  - Learning how to read body language can help the case manager pick up on other people's emotions
  - Being aware of the clinician's own body language
- **Verbal communication skills**
  - Include opportunities to contribute ideas and ask questions
  - Demonstrate personal interest in and open to hearing the case management team's ideas as well as becoming motivated to contribute personal thoughts
- **Listening skills**
  - Active listening is an essential part of communication
  - Active listening encompasses making eye contact, being aware of nonverbal cues, and asking questions that show that the listener is invested in the conversation
- **Empathy**
  - Seek to understand the emotions and feelings of others
- **Emotional intelligence**
  - Being emotionally intelligent can mean that an individual observes the dynamics of those around them for understanding and conflict resolution
- **Networking skills**
  - The ability to exchange ideas, to offer assistance, and to increase one's ability to make and maintain professional relationships
- **Team-building skills**
  - Requires effective relationship building
  - Show respect for the ideas and preferences of others
  - Contribute and assist when and where needed

These skills are honed by training and experience. Patient-centered communication, which focuses on the needs and preferences of patients, are discussed throughout this section as well as suggestions for how to communicate in a patient-centered manner. Physicians and other healthcare professionals are now expected to adopt patient-centered communication to develop trusted relationships.

The once paternalistic practice of medicine saw physicians as the receptacle of all medical knowledge used in the management of patients (Chandra et al., 2018). Medical knowledge is now expected to be shared between patient and doctor with care customized to the patient. The famous Canadian physician, Sir William Olsen, said, "a good physician treats the disease, and a great physician treats the patient." And in the movie, "Patch Adams," Robin Williams quotes Dr. Hunter Patch Adams when he said, "You treat a disease, you win, you lose. You treat a person, I guarantee you, you'll win, no matter what the outcome." These are important sentiments that should remind anyone working in healthcare that the development of a trusted relationship is not automatic and should not be expected if the sole focus is on treating someone's disease.

Relationship Building Tips

Following are seven tips for building positive relationships in healthcare from Dr. David Brown, Medical Director and Executive Director of the Great Lakes Surgery Center and Ambulatory Surgical Center in Michigan:

1. **Be friendly.** Show interest in people by asking them things outside of the original goal of conversation. For healthcare encounters, that means asking them what is important, ask them to tell you about a typical day, or what they know and want to know about their health.
2. **Practice humility.** Recognize and acknowledge the value and worth of everyone you encounter. Be willing to do whatever it takes to relieve suffering and meet the needs of those we serve.
3. **Be kind.** Remember, you always attract more flies with honey than vinegar. And kindness doesn't cost a thing.
4. **Enjoy humor.** Everyone likes to laugh. Sometimes it makes difficult things a bit easier.
5. **Be an active listener.** Active listening is demonstrated by reflective listening—make sure you correctly hear what is said. Repeat back what you heard to be certain. Reflecting back what you heard also gives you time to think about what was said and allows improved perception.
6. **Keep calm.** Conflict cannot always be avoided, nor can urgent or concerning situations. Pay attention to your emotions and put them in check if you find yourself becoming irritated or angry and take a deep breath before overreacting.
7. **Be empathetic.** Try to understand a situation from another's perspective; try to appreciate alternative views or thinking. These can create opportunities for learning and growth. (Brown, n.d.)

Cultivating trusted patient relationships is also good customer service. Patients are now consumers of healthcare; with rising medical costs and health plans with higher premiums, deductibles, and copays, patients are looking for quality healthcare services, competitive pricing, and excellent customer service delivered by physicians and healthcare organizations. Healthcare organizations recognize this and are identifying opportunities to attract and retain patients or healthcare consumers for life.

Role of the Primary Case Manager

A true integrated case management model includes the assignment of a primary case manager. This case manager is "where the buck stops" and is accountable for the coordination and delivery of a patient's needed care. That is not to say that the case manager literally or physically delivers all of the care a patient needs, but they are responsible to oversee the timely delivery of care and evaluate its effectiveness and the patient's satisfaction. Trusted relationships take time, focus, and patience. Relationships are more likely to develop when one case manager is the primary contact for the patient and family/caregiver. When multiple team members are reaching out to a patient, communication is inconsistent, even with the best of intentions to be consistent. Multiple contacts are confusing for a patient and family/caregiver. They become unsure of who to call for what. There will be times when another team member needs to communicate with a patient, but this interaction should be initiated by the primary case manager, with patient permission granted, and reassurance that the case manager is aware of and will ensure consistency in communication.

CASE STUDY

Cami is a 22-year-old female that was transported to the hospital by ambulance after collapsing while waiting for a bus. She was on her way to work as a waitress when she fell ill. In the emergency department, Cami was diagnosed with severe dehydration, electrolyte imbalance, malnourishment, and first trimester pregnancy. Cami is mostly noncommunicative, only answering compelled questions. The hospital social work case manager, Sharon, decides to try and draw Cami into a conversation. She will probably be discharged in 24 to 48 hours and Sharon is concerned about how well Cami will manage once discharged.

Cami is hesitant to answer more questions; she appears to Sharon to be distrustful. Sharon begins to engage with Cami by asking her if she is feeling any better, and what could Sharon do for her right now. Cami looks a bit surprised by the question, is unsure how to answer. Sharon continues to share with Cami that she would like to make sure Cami has everything she needs once discharged but needs to know what is most important. The conversation is not easy, but after about 30 minutes, Sharon learns that Cami lives in an apartment with two other girls and feels relatively safe. She has no health insurance, and while she works full time as a waitress, she barely makes ends meet. She suspected that she was pregnant because she has been unable to eat and has vomited three to four times a day for the last 4 weeks.

Sharon tried to reassure Cami that she would do her best to coordinate whatever Cami needs before she goes home. She promised to come back in a couple of hours, and asked Cami to think about what she would like to know and what she may need.

Sharon's approach was one of creating trust, not telling the patient what she needed or what needed to be done. Once Sharon understands Cami's needs, she can work with her colleagues to coordinate care and services to meet those needs. Helping Cami enroll in Medicaid will provide some reassurance that she will have access to care.

REFERENCES

Brown, D. (n.d.). *7 tips for productive working relationships in healthcare.* University of Southern California. https://healthadministrationdegree.usc.edu/blog/productive-healthcare-relationships/

Chandra, S., Mohammadnezhad, M., & Ward, P. R. (2018). Trust and communication in Doctor-Patient Relationship: A literature review. *Journal of Health Communication, 3*(3:36), 1–6. https://doi.org/10.4172/2472-1654.100146

Prip, A., Møller, K. A., Nielsen, D. L., Jarden, M., Olsen, M.-H., & Danielsen, A. K. (2018). The patient–healthcare professional relationship and communication in the oncology outpatient setting: A systematic review. *Cancer Nursin g, 41*(5), E11–E22. https://doi.org/10.1097/NCC.0000000000000533

CHAPTER 6

Patient/Person-Centered Care

Rebecca Perez

OBJECTIVES

- Define person-centered care (PCC)
- Compare PCC communication models
- Comprehend the need for advanced communications skills in the delivery of PCC

Introduction

Patient-centered care or person-centered care (PCC) is a part of everyone's vocabulary in healthcare. Those with many years of experience ask, "If patient-centered care is so important now, what were we doing 10 years ago, 20 years ago? Was the care we tried our best to deliver not patient-centered?" Most healthcare professionals have always tried to make the patient a priority, but many of our health systems have not. This chapter defines PCC, compares PCC communication models, and explores the need for communication skills in the delivery of PCC.

Definition of Patient-Centered Care

PCC requires a holistic approach oriented around an individual's goals and preferences and is essential to the delivery of high-quality care. During the COVID-19 pandemic, the organizations able to sustain their ability to provide service to others relied on these principles to survive. In a report funded by the SCAN Foundation, Tavares, Hwang, and Cohen shared the results of their review of the literature as it pertains to PCC (Tavares, 2021).

Patient-centered care or person-centered care seems not to have one universal definition, but a search revealed that all the of the definitions include components related to:

- Patient participation in care
- An individual's specific healthcare needs and desired health outcomes are the driving force
- Respectful care that is responsive to the needs and values of each individual
- Care that is comprehensive and coordinated for continuity
- Provision of education and information
- Ensuring access to care
- Provision of support to relieve fear, anxiety, and suffering

Figure 6.1 was located on a case management website in the United Kingdom and was developed based on content found on the *British Medical Journal* website (ajcasemanagement, 2018). Tavares (2021) provided some interesting information as a result of their research. Lower-income level households are associated with higher chances of individual preferences being ignored. Those receiving Medicaid reported their needs

FIGURE 6.1 The four principles of person-centered care.

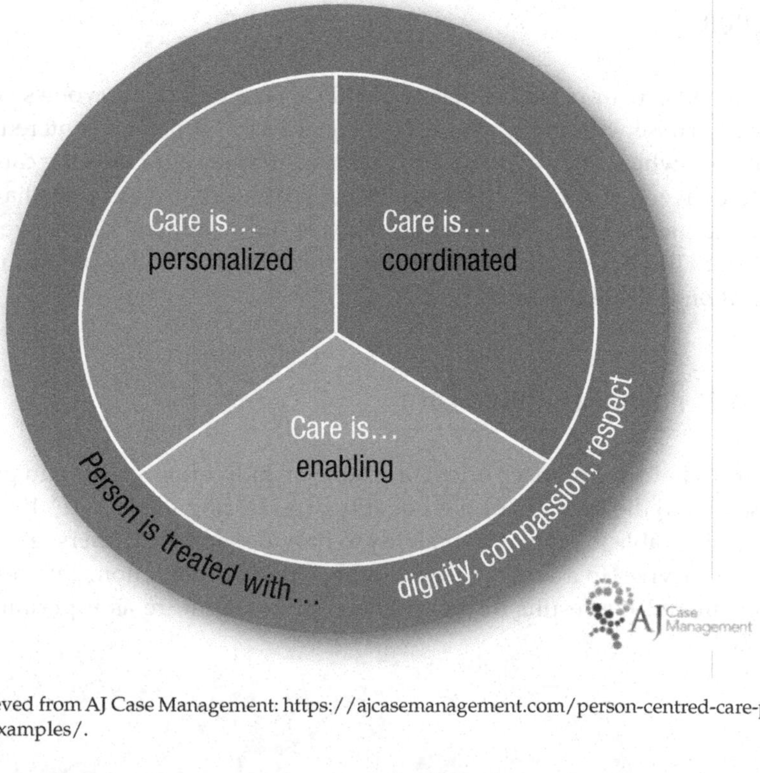

Source: Retrieved from AJ Case Management: https://ajcasemanagement.com/person-centred-care-principles-definitions-examples/.

were only sometimes or never met. However, the opposite was found among Medicare recipients; Taveras (2021) reported healthcare systems always consider their preferences. Those with dual coverage, Medicare, and Medicaid, reported similar experiences to those with Medicaid only (Tavares, 2021).

For those who report satisfaction with their care, consideration of their preferences was 1.25 times more likely to occur. When examining race and ethnicity, minorities were 1.9 to 2.4 times less likely to have their preferences included in care (ajcasemanagement, 2018; Tavares, 2021). In most cases, when poor health status is reported, there is a lower likelihood that preferences are considered (Tavares, 2021). A study to compare the effects of preference inclusion in years 2014 and 2016 revealed that those whose preferences were not considered in 2014were less likely to access care and services in 2016 (Tavares, 2021).

The shortcomings of our healthcare system became glaringly apparent during the pandemic. Of concern were the vast racial and ethnic disparities in health outcomes and quality. The analysis by Tavares demonstrates this deep divide; consideration of patient preferences is almost absent for racial and ethnic minorities, those uninsured or underinsured, and those with limited income or wealth (Tavares, 2021). However, the message to take from this analysis reinforces the importance of PCC and making sure all patients' preferences are considered. See Figure 6.2 for an overview of the disparities associated with a lack of patient preference consideration. The infographic can also be located in the "Tracking Progress of Person-Centered Care for Older Adults: How Are We Doing?" published by the Center for Consumer Engagement and Health Innovation and LeadingAge LTSS Center @UMass Boston funded with a grant from the Scan Foundation.

The term "patient-centered care" is used interchangeably with "person-centered care" but regardless, the concept and objective are to implement shared decision-making by supporting autonomy (Gover et al., 2022). This concept is becoming more accepted as we move away from the historical paternalistic method of healthcare delivery. Where once considered only theory, PCC is now viewed as the strategy to deliver high-quality care to enhance patient satisfaction, admission and readmission reduction, and hospital lengths of stay (Gover et al., 2022). Providing care that respects and meets patients' and family/caregivers' needs is essential to the delivery of PCC. To be patient-centered, to deliver care that promotes autonomy, engagement, and satisfaction demands effective communication (Kwame & Petrucka, 2021). There are three dimensions of effective communication that should be adopted by healthcare professionals and emulated for patients, families, and caregivers (Kwame & Petrucka, 2021). The first dimension requires the healthcare professional to be welcoming to patients, families, and caregivers by listening to them, to their story, share information with consent only, and show respect. The second dimension requires that the healthcare professional be seen and respected as a person so that previous assumptions by patients are debunked. It is important that healthcare providers not overemphasize their expertise but demonstrate that experience has allowed them to better understand the challenges and needs of the patient. The third dimension requires the healthcare professional to cultivate a trusted relationship so that patients, families, and caregivers see the professional as a confidant and are comfortable engaging in conversations about their health, needs, challenges, and goals for health improvement (Kwame & Petrucka, 2021).

FIGURE 6.2 Person-centered infographic (Center for Consumer Engagement in Healthcare and Leading Age LTSS Center, UMass, Boston 2021).

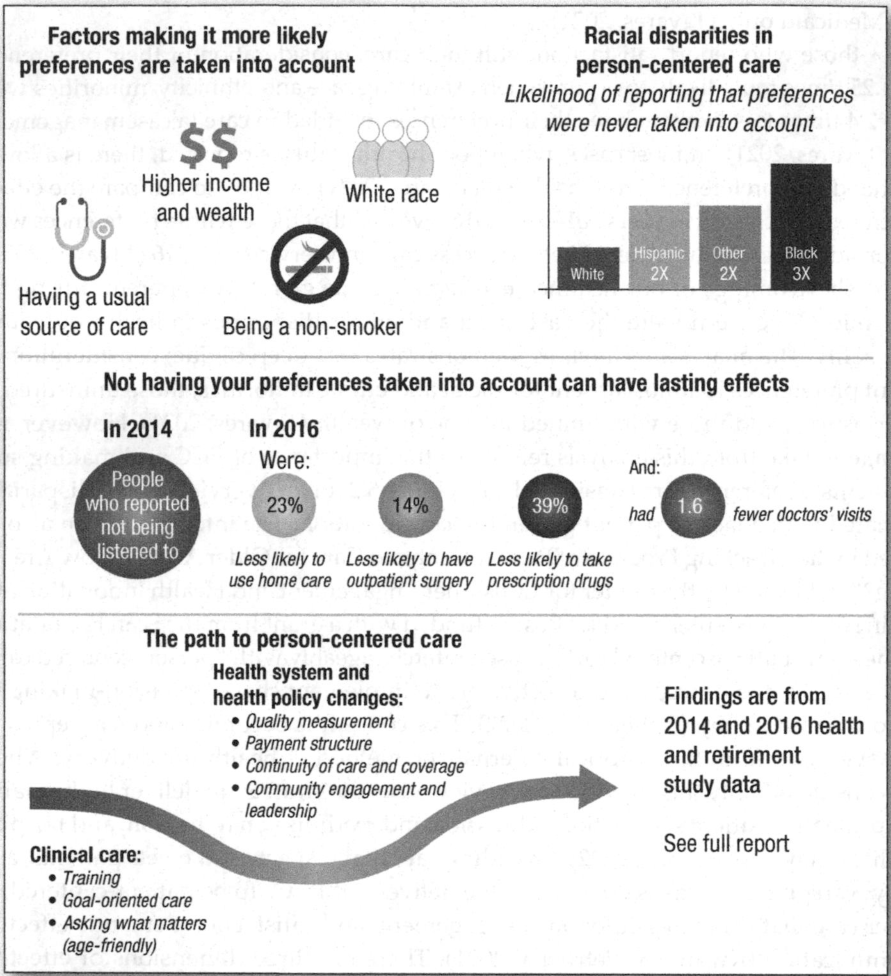

Source: Retrieved from: www.healthinnovation.org/resources/publications/body/Person-Centered-Care-Infographic_Jan-2021.pdf.

Read the full report: www.healthinnovation.org/resources/publications/body/Person-Centered-Care-Report_Jan-2021.pdf

Patient-Centered Communication Model: PC4

Kwame and Petrucka (2021) propose a PCC and communication continuum named PC4. This model or pathway assists with the practices needed for PCC communication. At the heart of this model, the person is emphasized rather than the patient, because there is a person who becomes a patient (Kwame & Petrucka, 2021). The model also applies to all persons associated with patient care, reinforcing respect and the dignity of the person (Kwame & Petrucka, 2021). The model describes three types of communications performed among care providers, patients, and family/caregiver (Kwame & Petrucka, 2021). The components are:

- **Task-centered communication.** The healthcare provider's role in the completion of tasks as fast as possible usually with little to no communication with the patient and family/caregiver. Patients and the family/caregiver are treated impersonally because the healthcare professional is focused on tasks that need to be completed such as assessments, ordering medical testing, reviewing results of testing, documentation, and medical prescription or order fulfillment. This low-end form of communication occurs when professionals have time limitations, high workloads, and are understaffed, pushing the professional to complete tasks on as many patients as possible. Patients and family/caregivers are often not allowed the time to ask questions, or their questions go unanswered, information received is brief or not understood, and no consideration of preferences is asked or answered.
- **Process-centered communication.** This is the intermediate stage of communication in which the healthcare professional may move from task-oriented to person-centered communication. The healthcare professional may ask the patient questions to better understand the conditions a patient has, but there is no effort to allow the patient to ask questions or express their thoughts or needs. Assessments are often conducted in this fashion. This form of communication is less authoritative, and information is shared unlike task-centered communication.
- **Person-centered communication.** This is the high end of the scale and is where all healthcare professionals need to be for the delivery of PCC. Communication at this stage of the continuum is mutually respectful and collaborative. Communication is both "personal and explanatory." The healthcare professional has created a trusted and meaningful relationship with the patient, family, and caregiver to understand better the patient's needs, concerns, and challenges using open-ended questions to encourage expression of thoughts and feelings. Communication at this level must also be flexible to meet the patient where they are; for example, if the patient is in the ICU, you will communicate with the patient and family/caregiver much differently that the patient who is post-op a total knee replacement. Communication with those that may have an impairment that interferes with communication, such as the individual with hearing loss, requires additional effort to ensure the individual comprehends the care they are receiving (Kwame & Petrucka, 2021).

A case manager must employ empathetic communication and conversation with individuals that may have challenges with expression or comprehension. Individuals should use any tools at their disposal to ensure medical information is heard and understood, like active listening, reflective listening, showing genuine interest in the patient and their situation, and showing warmth and respect. Different strategies may be used when establishing a trusted relationship. "Chit-chat," humor, and silence are things that enrich and enhance relationship-building and relationship-protection communication.

Healthcare professionals need to be cognizant of how their communications are oriented. Are they just completing tasks and following care processes? Or are they truly addressing patients' and family/caregivers' needs (Kwame & Petrucka, 2021)? Case managers must reflect on how they communicate and interact with patients and family/caregivers. Suggestions for restructuring questions include asking, "What is most important to you right now?" instead of, "What's the matter?" The preferred question immediately tells the patient that you are interested in them and gives them a voice to contribute to care needs (Kwame & Petrucka, 2021). When working in clinic or acute care settings, healthcare professionals should make sure to check on a patient who may have been in the waiting room for some time or a patient in the hospital waiting for a procedure or physician consult (Kwame & Petrucka, 2021).

Empowers Framework

Communication is multifaceted and requires a set of skills and strategies determined by the type of communication, the participants, and the context (Links et al., 2020). Communication curricula should be part of all healthcare education but can be a challenge because of a multitude of potential conversations by multiple professionals. But studies have shown that clinical communication skills have an impact on patient outcomes (Links et al., 2020).

In the development of the EMPOWERS Framework, Links et al. (2020) reviewed many communication frameworks and found many similarities. All conversations have a beginning, a middle, and an end. So, to structure a conversation, the healthcare professional must prepare, communicate, and then support action. Preparation is supported by establishing a clear purpose or goal. Action occurs through coaching for change management (Links et al., 2020).

As was shared earlier, how people communicate impacts the development of a trusted relationship. This is accomplished by displaying empathy and working to establish rapport. The middle of the conversation is to negotiate an understanding of the desired outcome or goals, understand what has happened, what it means, and what must be done by encouraging the patient to share in needed decisions (Links et al., 2020).

This is where consideration of the patient's preferences, values, and needs comes to play. At the end of the conversation, an agreement is reached on what actions will be taken. It is important to check understanding and provide additional explanations for less than clear concepts and general recall (Links et al., 2020). These strategies are summarized by the EMPOWERS framework (Links et al., 2020) in Figure 6.3.

FIGURE 6.3 EMPOWERS framework.

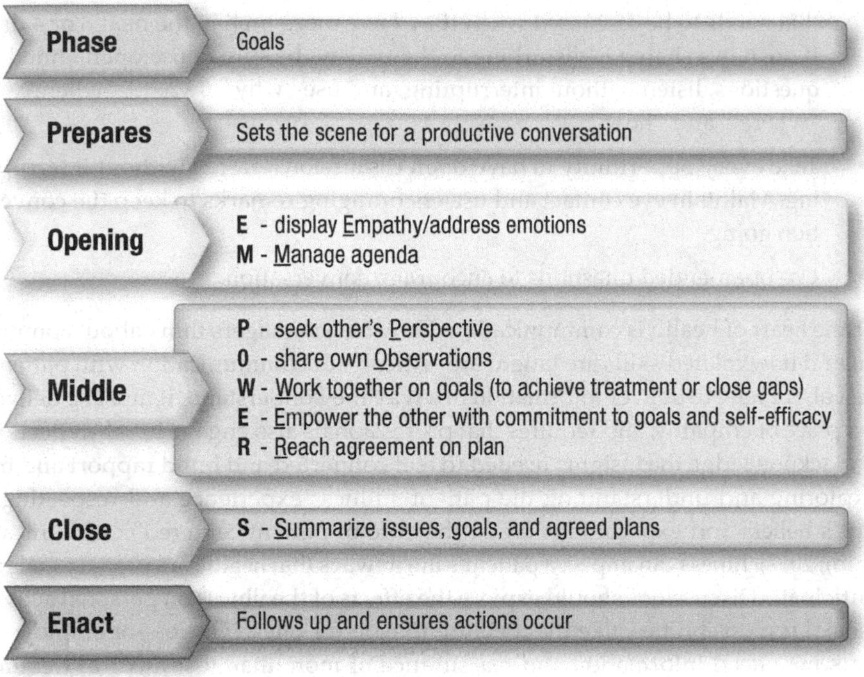
Phase
Goals
Prepares
Sets the scene for a productive conversation
Opening
E - display Empathy/address emotions
M - Manage agenda
Middle
P - seek other's Perspective
O - share own Observations
W - Work together on goals (to achieve treatment or close gaps)
E - Empower the other with commitment to goals and self-efficacy
R - Reach agreement on plan
Close
S - Summarize issues, goals, and agreed plans
Enact
Follows up and ensures actions occur

Professional communication training requires a multidisciplinary perspective of patient care to improve teamwork and PCC. The following are suggestions for improving communications with patients (Ahern, 2019).

- Timing and location are important. Make sure the patient is at a place where they can thoughtfully engage with the case manager. If not, the encounter will be less than productive. Meeting face to face is always best, but if by telephone is the only option, the healthcare professional will need to work a bit harder for engagement.
- Be relaxed and conversational. Case managers should start their encounters with a conversation other than questions about the patient's health. Ask how their day has been going, what is most important to them today. If some rapport has already been established, ask after family, children, hobbies, or other things known to be of interest to the patient.
- Make sure the environment is conducive to conversation. Do not try to engage the patient if the area is noisy or busy.
- Turn off personal cell phone or other electronic devices (if not being used to converse with the patient). Do not answer personal calls, e-mails, or text messages while engaging with a patient,

- If an important topic needs to be discussed, but there are distractions that may interfere with the encounter, vaguely mention that there is something that needs to be discussed when they have more time in the next 3 or 4 days. If the news shared is disturbing to the patient, be sure to use open-ended questions, listen without interrupting, and use "why," "what," "when," "where," and "how."
- Take every opportunity to have open discussions. Listen without interrupting. Maintain eye contact and use encouraging remarks to keep the conversation going.
- Use open-ended questions to encourage conversation.

At the heart of health is communication. How case managers think about communication and how related skills are taught are critical. But communication with patients is not just about how to deliver information in a way they understand, it must be delivered from a place of empathy, and requires that professionals also engage in self-reflection to gain or acknowledge the insights needed to feel connected and build rapport and trust.

Exploring and understanding the patient's illness experience and respecting the patient's beliefs and expectations are at the core of patient-centered communication (Hashim, 2017). Illness can impact a patient's life in ways that healthcare professionals may not anticipate. Discussions should explore the effects of the illness on personal activities and social responsibilities, like the inability to care for oneself or loss of employment. Patients may need information and reassurance of more than just medical treatment. PCC respects the patient's preferences and expectations which may require exploration to discover underlying concerns and questions. Table 6.1 provides examples of phrasing that will assist in these discussions (Hashim, 2017).

TABLE 6.1 Recommended Sequence for Patient-Centered Interviewing and Communication

Communication Goal	Suggested Phrases or Comments
Introduction and build rapport	All persons present during the initial encounter should be introduced. If the encounter is not urgent, generalities can be exchanged such as the weather, current events, or nonspecific observations, like "I love that color you are wearing," "Your daughter looks just like you," "That is a beautiful bracelet." These statements can help everyone feel relaxed and help to build rapport.
Elicit the patient's agenda	Avoid using the question: "How are you feeling?" or "How are you today?" as these questions may cause the patient to somatize or downplay physical symptoms. Instead, ask, "How best can I help you today?" or "What can I do for you today?" to bring focus to the encounter.
List all of the patient's agenda items	After reviewing the concerns shared by the patient and family, ask, "Is there anything else concerning you?" or "Is there anything else I can help with today?" until they answer in the negative.

(continued)

TABLE 6.1 Recommended Sequence for Patient-Centered Interviewing and Communication (*continued*)

Communication Goal	Suggested Phrases or Comments
Negotiate the agenda	To help the patient establish priorities, try using these phrases: • "Which of these concerns you the most?" • "I would also like to talk about _____today, would that be alright?" • "Because we have limited time, which of your concerns would you like to discuss today?" • "I know _____ concerns you, and I am concerned about _____. Could we start with _____?"
Begin discussing the patient's concerns using open-ended questions	Here are some suggested phrases/questions: • "Tell me more about _____" • "Would you like to talk about _____?" • "Can you tell me how _____ started?" • "Tell me what ____ was like?" • "Have you noticed anything else?"
Ask more direct questions to elicit details about the patient's chief concern: feelings, ideas, concerns, impact, and expectations	"How did that make you feel?" "Tell me what is worrying you." "What would you say is worrying you most?" "What do you think is the cause of ____ ?" "Is there something you worry might happen?" "How has your illness affected your daily life?" "What difficulties do you face?" "What more can I do for you today?"
Empathize	"I can see this makes you feel ____ " "I can understand how this might upset you." "I cannot imagine what that must feel like." "This has been a hard time for you." "I respect your courage to keep a positive attitude in spite of your difficulties." "You have been through a lot." "I am here to help you in any way I can." "What has happened since last we met/talked?" "Tell me more about what happened when you were sick."
Summarize	"So, from what you have told me so far, you ____ " "You have told me a lot today; let's go over everything to make sure I didn't miss anything."
Transition	"Now, if you agree, I would like to ask you some additional questions about your health."
Additional data	Elicit information about medications, allergies, medical history, social and family histories including social support, hobbies, interests, work, and spirituality.

Source: Adapted from Hashim, M. J. (2017, January 1). Patient-centered communication: Basic skills. *American Family Physicians, 95*(1), 29–34. https://www.aafp.org/pubs/afp/issues/2017/0101/p29.html

REFERENCES

Ahern, G. (2019, July 2019). *Communication skills in healthcare*. https://www.ausmed.com/cpd/guides/communication-skills

ajcasemanagement. (2018, September 28). *What is person centred care? Principles, definitions & examples*. https://ajcasemanagement.com/person-centred-care-principles-definitions-examples/

Gover, S. E., Fitzpatrick, A., Azim, F. T., Ariza-Vega, P., Bellwood, P., Burns, J., Burton, E., Fleig, L., Clemson, L., Hoppmann, C. A., Madden, K. M., Price, M., Langford, D., & Ashe, M. C. (2022, July). Defining and implementing patient-centered care: An umbrella review. *Patient Education and Counseling, 105*(7), 1679–1688. https://doi.org/10.1016/j.pec.2021.11.004

Hashim, M. J. (2017, January 1). Patient-centered communication: Basic skills. *American Family Physicians, 95*(1), 29–34. https://www.aafp.org/pubs/afp/issues/2017/0101/p29.html

Kwame, A., & Petrucka, P. M. (2021). A literature-based study of patient-centered care and communication in nurse-patient interactions: Barriers, facilitators, and the way forward. *BMC Nursing, 20*(158). https://doi.org/10.1186/s12912-021-00684-2

Links, M. W., Watterson, L., Martin, P., O'Regan, S., & Molloy, E. (2020, February 11). Finding common ground: Meta-synthesis of communication frameworks found in patient communication, supervision and simulation literature. *BMC Medical Education, 20*(45). https://doi.org/10.1186/s12909-019-1922-2

Tavares, J. H. (2021). *Tracking progress on person-centered care for older adults: How are we doing*? Center for Consumer Engagement in Health Innovation and LeadingAge.

CHAPTER 7

Addressing Social Determinants of Health

Rebecca Perez

OBJECTIVES

- Describe the interaction of clinical and nonclinical issues impacting patient engagement and adherence
- Recognize the role of social issues in care and transition plan adherence
- Identify social determinants of health through the integrated case management process

Introduction

Individuals experiencing health complexity are often challenged by more than medical or mental health conditions. Social factors can sometimes be the primary driver of poor health. The Case Management Society of America's (CMSA) Integrated Case Management (ICM) method examined social factors long before the push to identify social determinants of health (SDH). In this chapter, recent efforts to address SDH are addressed while reinforcing how ICM supports those efforts.

Addressing Social Determinants of Health

The Centers for Medicare & Medicaid Services (CMS) and Institute for Healthcare Improvement's (IHI) Triple Aim recognize that social factors have a direct impact on an individual's ability to be healthy. The Triple Aim is a framework available to assist health systems optimize performance and is comprised of three dimensions: improving the patient experience of care, improving the health of populations, and reducing the per capita cost of healthcare (IHI, 2023). In most healthcare settings, no one entity is accountable for all three dimensions. The IHI recommends a change process that includes identification of

FIGURE 7.1 Design of a Triple Aim enterprise.

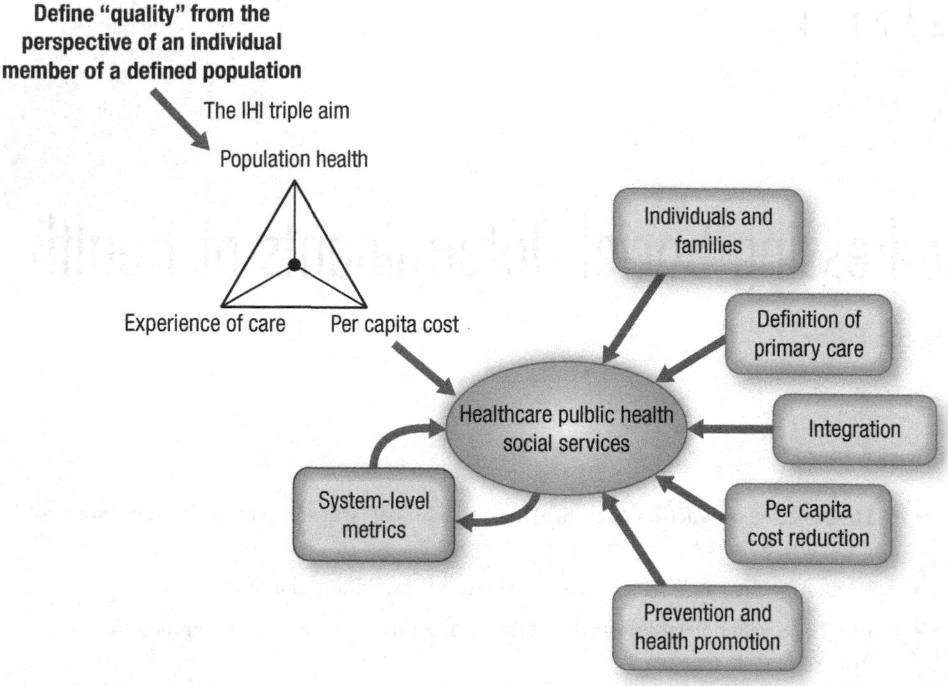

Source: Institute for Healthcare Improvement. (2023). *IHI Triple Aim Initiative*. https://www.ihi.org/Engage/Initiatives/TripleAim/Pages/default.aspx

target populations and defines systems of aims and measures, development of a strong portfolio of work that produces system-level results, and rapid testing and scales that adapt to local needs and conditions (IHI, 2023) (Figure 7.1).

Individuals with a low socioeconomic status are less healthy than those with a higher socioeconomic status. Addressing SDH must be addressed as a priority to impact the overall health of the patients served. The Triple Aim helps to define how to assess and address SDH.

According to *Healthy People 2030*, "Social determinants of health are the conditions in the environment where people are born, live, learn, work, play, worship, and age that affect a wide range of health, functioning, and quality of life outcomes and risks" (U.S. Department of Health and Human Services [DHHS], 2022). SDH may be grouped into five domains (DHHS, 2022):

1. **Economic stability**
   a. One in 10 people in the United States live in poverty.
   b. Healthy foods, healthcare, and housing may be unaffordable.
   c. People with steady employment are less likely to live in poverty.
   d. Employment programs, career counseling, and high-quality childcare opportunities can help more people find and keep jobs.

2. **Education access and quality**
    a. People with higher levels of education are more likely to be healthy and live longer.
    b. Children from low-income families, children with disabilities, and children who are routinely exposed to social discrimination, like bullying, are more likely to struggle with math and reading.
    c. Children living in areas with poorly performing schools and many families are unable to afford college.
    d. The stress of living in poverty can affect the brain development of children resulting in poor school performance.
3. **Healthcare access and quality**
    a. Approximately 1 in 10 people in the United States do not have health coverage.
    b. People without insurance are less likely to have a primary care provider and may not be able to afford medications.
    c. Without a primary care provider, important health screenings may not be ordered or completed.
4. **Neighborhood and built environment**
    a. Many people in the United States live in neighborhoods or communities with high rates of crime and violence, unsafe air or water, and other safety risks like secondhand smoke or loud noises.
5. **Social community context**
    a. Relationships and interactions with families, friends, coworkers, neighbors, and other community members can have a major impact on health and well-being.
    b. Positive relationships can help reduce the negative impacts experienced in the individual's environment (Figure 7.2).

These days, the term SDH seems to be on the lips of everyone in healthcare. There are multiple assessments for SDH, including now specifying Social Determinants of Mental Health (SDMH). Some organizations focus on just one or two identified social determinants, and yet it is still challenging to find the resources needed to address them.

Social Determinants of Health Assessment

Assessing for SDH is part of most comprehensive assessments regardless of practice setting. Organizations many have their own "home-grown" assessment methods and models that are meant to meet the needs of patients in a specific practice setting or may use a published screening tool. Two well-known examples of evidence-based assessments are Protocol for Responding to and Assessing Patients' Assets, Risks, and Experiences

FIGURE 7.2 Social determinants of health.

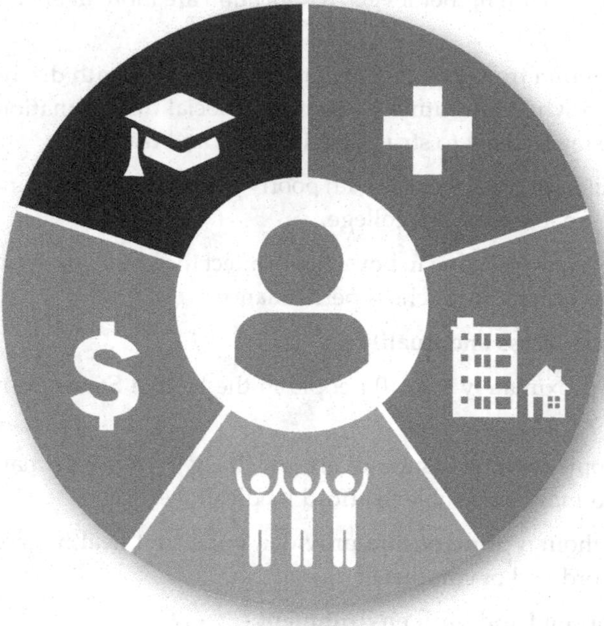

Source: Healthy People 2030. (2022, November 22). *Social Determinants of Health*. U.S. Department of Health and Human Services, Office of Disease Prevention and Health Promotion. https://health.gov/healthypeople/objectives-and-data/social-determinants-health.

(PRAPARE) and the Accountable Health Communities's (AHC) Health-Related Social Needs (HRSN) screening tool. The PRAPARE is a nationally recognized and standardized assessment for healthcare and community partners to better understand and act on the social drivers of their patients. PRAPARE helps providers address the needs of underserved populations by defining the complexity of patients, better target clinical care, enable services and community partnerships, enable providers to demonstrate the value they bring to patients, and advocate for change at the community and national levels (Figure 7.3).

The AHC's HRSN screening tool was developed by the CMS for the screening of health-related social needs across all communities. The 10-item tool assesses:

- Housing instability
- Food insecurity transportation problems
- Utility assistance
- Other financial strain
- Employment
- Family and community support

- Education
- Physical activity
- Substance use
- Mental health
- Disabilities

The Kaiser Permanente and the Robert Wood Johnson Foundation developed the Social Interventions Research and Evaluation Network (SIREN) which compiles several of the most widely used social health screening tools to facilitate comparison. The comparison evaluates the number of domains screened, intended population, number of questions, reading level, and domain-specific measures. The inclusion of tools did not automatically validate the tool nor does the comparison verify validity. SIREN continues to evaluate these tools as well as examining new tools (SIREN, 2019).

The body of evidence documenting the impacts of SDH outcomes continues to grow. And as such, organizations are increasingly evaluating their roles and responsibilities related to these determinants. Still being considered is the level of effort required to

FIGURE 7.3 Protocol for Responding to and Assessing Patients' Assets, Risks, and Experiences (PRAPARE) model.

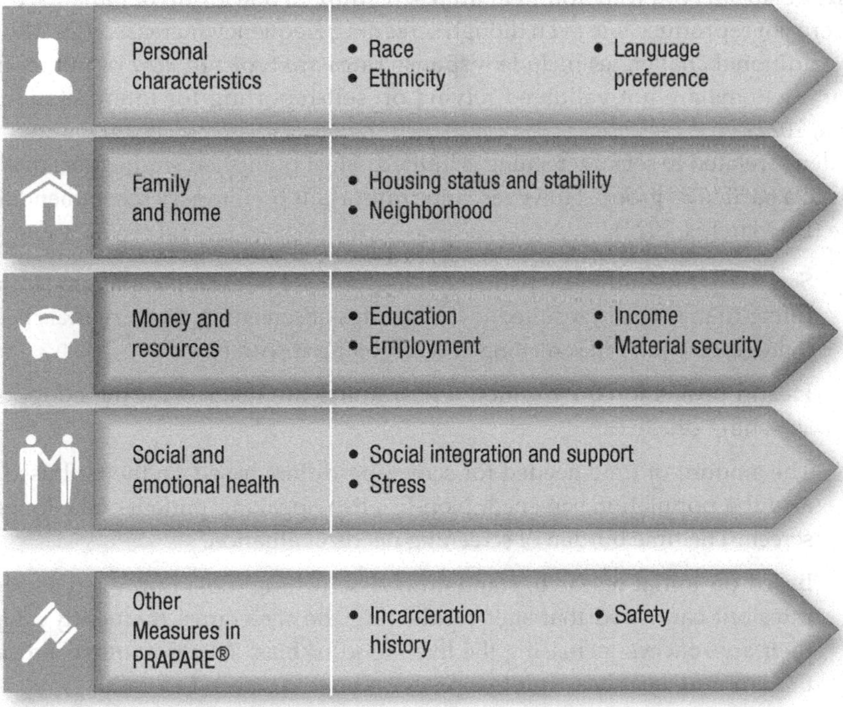

Personal characteristics
• Race
• Ethnicity
• Language preference
Family and home
• Housing status and stability
• Neighborhood
Money and resources
• Education
• Employment
• Income
• Material security
Social and emotional health
• Social integration and support
• Stress
Other Measures in PRAPARE®
• Incarceration history
• Safety

Source: NACHC and AAPCHO. (2022). *PRAPARE implementation and action toolkit*. https://prapare.org/prapare-toolkit/

identify social and economic risk factors which led to the National Academies of Science, Engineering and Medicine's 2019 report, "Integrating Social Care into the Delivery of Health Care to Improve the Nation's Health." The report prioritized efforts to identify patients' social risks and assets which was termed "awareness," action strategies identified as adjustment, assistance, alignment, and advocacy (De Marchis, 2022). A framework to address or mitigate the impacts of social adversity was adapted from these activities.

Awareness indicates patient-facing, point-of-care screening to identify a patient's social risks and assets, also known as social screening (De Marchis, 2022). The adoption of social screening tools has prompted the need to develop quality measures as activities related to awareness are evolving. A sufficient body of evidence demonstrates the need for screening and implementation of interventions and has garnered the attention of policy makers and payers. But how are health systems implementing screening? How do patients feel about the screening? Are health systems capturing and using social data? If screening alone is performed without any intervention, could that result in negative patient experiences?

In 2021, the Kaiser Family Foundation's Survey of Medicaid Officials reported almost one half of state Medicaid agencies required social needs screening in state-managed Medicaid contracts (De Marchis, 2022). However, it is not clear if screenings translated to changed practices in which data were not just collected but acted upon. Unfortunately, organizational surveys were found to limit screening to one group of patients, or surveys were not reproduceable even though screening frequency increased (De Marchis, 2022). Additional challenges include response rates are typically low or not reported and survey items are not validated relying on self-reporting for interpretation (De Marchis, 2022).

Evidence related to social screening is limited. Most published studies are small and specific to a particular group. However, some important preliminary recommendations include (De Marchis, 2022):

1. Screening rates differ by patient demographic. For example, patient language (other than English) resulted in lower rates of screening. More work is needed to increase equity in screening and screening research.
2. Health professional education and training are needed for the adoption of screening practices.
3. The amount of time needed for screening differs based on the tool used, but also the population screened. Non-English-speaking patients take longer to screen. The time burden of screening needs evaluation.
4. Based on initial research, standardized screening tools improved screening rates but cautioned that staff conducting the screenings frequently adapted their approaches increasing the likelihood of bias. This is another indication that training healthcare professionals on how to screen has value.
5. Initial research indicated that screening rates increased when conducted by community health workers rather than nurses.

6. Use of digital devices or other technologies for screening need to be further studied, especially with low literacy and in settings with limited staff capacity.

To summarize, suggested implementation guidelines for screening include preparation that engages key internal stakeholders, continuous evaluation of screening programs for flaws and barriers, and staff and clinician training on screening practices (De Marchis, 2022).

Integrating Social Services With Healthcare

No nation has a truly integrated a system of healthcare and social services, but many nations, other than the United States, invest more heavily in social services even though the United States spends more per capita on healthcare than any other nation. Researchers and policy makers in the United States have been discussing the integration of care and social services for some time as integration is seen as a way to improve the quality and outcomes of healthcare and a way to control overall costs (National Academies of Science Engineering and Medicine [NASEM], 2019). In 2018, the NASEM conducted a workshop to discuss the integration of healthcare and social issues. The following are some of the recommendations from that workshop (NASEM, 2019):

1. **For physician offices/practices:**
   a. Ensure social service resources are available to staff to assist patients and families to find the supportive services they need.
   b. These resources should also include support for new parents of children with chronic illness.
2. **Within hospital and health systems:**
   a. Create a role/position that can assist patients and families in the submission of waivers and applications for chronic illness support.
   b. Invest in hiring and training staff to be person- and family-centered.
   c. Ensure electronic health records (EHRs) complement a patient- and family-centered approach.
3. Develop and implement a standardized assessment for caregiver depression, anxiety, and overall health.
4. Improve the resources available to caregivers, especially bereavement. And improve training to staff on collaborating with caregivers.
5. Ensure all patients with serious illness and their families have case management services available to them.
6. Understand caregiving is a longitudinal experience that changes over time and remember that all caregivers do not need coordinated healthcare.
7. Interventions for serious illness need to be tailored to the individual patient, be comprehensive, and sensitive to the family member's preferences.

8. Caregiver assessments should be conversations about preferences, needs, specific challenges, and love.
9. Strengthen, clarify, and legitimize the role of the family caregiver by assessing and respecting their capacity for a truly active role in the patient's care.
10. Look for ways to partner, promote, establish, and fund approaches that will integrate healthcare and social issues.

Funding for Social or Nonmedical Services

Healthcare in the United States is more reactionary than preventive. If someone is sick, the healthcare system knows how to come in and rescue that person, and usually will spare no expense in doing so. However, if the goal is to prevent that same person from getting any worse, the overall strategy is not very robust. Social services should be viewed as the upstream prevention needed, and not just when illness manifests. When social spending occurs in higher ratios to healthcare spending, the outcomes are lower rates of infant mortality, fewer premature deaths in adults, longer life expectancy, fewer low birth weight babies, and reductions in adult obesity, asthma, lung cancer, acute myocardial infarction, and type 2 diabetes (NASEM, 2019).

Policy makers need to adopt a broader view that goes beyond hospital, clinic, and healthcare spending to focus on social needs. So much is spent on healthcare in the United States that there are few to no funds remaining to allocate to social services. When social issues are not addressed, more healthcare is required, resulting in more spending. Not addressing social issues results in a sicker population.

The NASEM workshop identified three areas that held the strongest evidence of health impacts (NASEM, 2019):

1. **Housing**
   a. Particularly for the unhoused, especially families
2. **Nutrition**
   a. For example, the Women, Infants, and Children (WIC) program
   b. Home-delivered meals for the elderly
   c. Access to healthy foods
3. **Case management**
   a. Home visitation
   b. Facilitation of resources, care coordination, and care transitions

The mitigation of social determinants does not fall to one person or group. Improving the health and well-being of all people requires a commitment from government, the healthcare industry, communities, and individuals. Case managers alone will not be able to address every challenge a patient or their family faces but can when resources are known and the there are means to access them. The following discusses areas that can be impacted by case managers.

Economic Stability

Through a network of available community resources, case managers can help patients connect with resources to assist with the acquisition of food; for example, application for food stamps or access to food pantries, payment of utilities, and affordable housing. For those individuals seeking employment assistance, the case manager can connect the patient to vocational resources. Reducing the stress of financial concerns allows the patient to better focus on health issues. Case managers should collaborate with team members and the community to develop a list of resources that can easily and quickly be referenced so that prompt assistance can be provided.

Education

Having resources available related to education can assist a patient in reaching a personal goal of advancing education. An individual's ability to advance their education may open the door for improving status in life by providing employment opportunities not previously available. This may mean achieving a general education diploma (GED) or entrance to community college, university, or trade school. Personal educational advancement may lead to improved financial stability and improved quality of life. Case managers need to determine the local and federal resources that may be available for an individual to pursue education and employment.

Social and Community Support

Patients with complex health needs require social support to better manage their health. Without social support, their health and ability to self-manage are at risk. For patients with family or other available social supports, case managers need to encourage the involvement and participation of these supports. Patients may refuse this involvement, but case managers can encourage the benefits of social support especially if the patient struggles to manage their conditions. The use of motivational interviewing skills may encourage the patient to begin thinking about the benefits of additional support. When a patient has no visible means of support and no family or dependable friends, make recommendations to participate in support groups, join community social groups, or faith-based communities. These can be highly effective at supplementing the absence of related social supports.

Health Status and Access to Healthcare

As case managers, assisting patients to get healthcare and services to improve their health is a priority. However, recognition of the barriers preventing stable health should lead to mitigation of the interference and risks related to poor health. The inability to access needed healthcare and services can be related, for example, to limited access to providers due to geographic reasons or language barriers; limited insurance benefits like high deductibles; lack of mental health coverage; lack of transportation to get to appointments; providers with limited appointment schedules or office hours; and of most concern, a patient's distrust of healthcare providers.

Case managers must diligently work to remove these barriers. The place of practice, health plan, insurance company, hospital, long-term care, independent practice, may limit what benefits and services are reimbursable or covered for the patient. Some managed Medicaid and Medicare plans see the value in providing services like nonemergent transportation to provider appointments. However, if nonemergent transportation is not a covered benefit for a patient, explore other resources that could assist the patient in keeping medical appointments. Another strategy could be assisting the patient to get an appointment time that would be more convenient for available transportation. Patients whose primary language is not English may need help in finding a physician who speaks their primary language or finding a medical translator to interpret provider visits. Patients who live in rural areas have an especially challenging time finding providers, most notably specialty and behavioral health providers. Case managers must provide the assistance to find providers and schedule appointments. When multiple appointments are needed, for example, coordinated appointments to see a physician and complete diagnostic tests, or a medical appointment and counseling appointment, every effort should be made to get these appointments scheduled to be completed on the same day so that the patient is not making multiple long trips to complete appointments.

During the assessment process, the patient's understanding of their conditions and prescribed treatment plan are determined. The patient's level of health literacy directly impacts this understanding. First, and foremost, determine what the patient knows and understands, what the physician has imparted, and then bring this all together to help the patient understand, using language that is easily comprehended. This means using nonmedical and simple terms, analogies, and visuals.

Stability of Neighborhood and Environment

Case managers do not typically "build" healthy environments but can certainly support what a community may offer. Access to healthy foods may mean guiding the patient to shopping at a local farmer's market that accepts food stamps to purchase fresh, locally grown, and affordable fruits and vegetables. If the patient is residing in housing that is in disrepair, infested with insects or vermin, is in a high crime area, or is a victim of abuse or neglect, the case manager has a responsibility to help the patient find safe housing. A safe environment reduces the risk of poor health, injury, and trauma.

Assessing the presence of social determinants and risk occurs as part of the integrated, comprehensive assessment. Social concerns are included in the four domains assessed when using CMSA's integrated approach. Case managers may find that a patient's health conditions are stable at present but may be at risk due to the presence of social determinants. Addressing the social concerns as a priority can result in continued health stabilization and prevention of complications.

The social concerns assessment for ICM using the Integrated Case Management Complexity Assessment Grid (ICM-CAG) tool reviews the history of a patient's ability to work or go to school. Source of income not from a job would also be included. Working includes being a stay-at-home partner who manages a household and/or children, or a caregiver. Social relationships encompass the quality and the presence of active engagement with family, friends, and coworkers. Also assessed are the presence and availability of a support system: family, friends, or others who are available to assist the patient when needed, and the environment in which they live safely. The safety of the environment includes the ability to pay for a mortgage or rent, utilities, food, medications, clothing, and the physical safety of the environment.

All healthcare organizations are focusing on SDH, but how data are gathered and used vary. Reporting of SDH and interventions to address them will be required reporting later in 2023, but how to synthesize what we know has yet to standardized. Another consideration of screening is what patients and families think of these practices. There is speculation that patients and families may distrust screening practices, furthering poor access and worsening experiences with healthcare systems (SIREN, 2019). Healthcare professionals, especially case managers, may have concerns with implementation of social screenings into busy schedules. Case managers would benefit from training in conducting assessments, helping create the workflows that will effectively allow for assessments, and to be prepared to address concerns expressed by patients and families. Assessments without resources to address the challenges discovered makes the process an ineffective use of time. Having a resource guide or database at the ready to address patients' needs is paramount to reducing health inequities and poor health outcomes.

CASE STUDY 1

Cassie is a 6-year-old girl living in subsidized housing with her grandmother and brother Sam. The apartment building was built in the early 1960s, is in disrepair, and cockroach infestations are frequent. Mold is visible in the building hallways due to leaking pipes in the ceiling. Cassie has asthma, is in the emergency department at least once per month with exacerbations, and often misses school.

Which intervention is most important to reduce Cassie's visits to the emergency department?

a. Notify the local division of family services
b. With the permission of Cassie's grandmother, notify the local housing authority regarding the unsafe housing
c. With the permission of Cassie's grandmother, look for emergency temporary housing
d. Schedule an appointment with Cassie's pediatrician

CASE STUDY 2

Brittany is a 32-year-old woman who is in the emergency department three to four times per month on average with complaints of abdominal pain. Brittany currently lives with her boyfriend who has a violent temper and physically assaults her. The hospital emergency department has referred Brittany to a social worker, but Brittany has never contacted the social worker.

Which intervention might be appropriate for Brittany to reduce her risk of injury?

a. Make another appointment for Brittany to see a social worker
b. Make a referral for Brittany to see a gastrointestinal specialist
c. Contact Brittany to determine if she feels safe; provide options to change her living arrangements
d. Provide Brittany with an emergency hotline number for domestic violence

CASE STUDY 3

George is a 72-year-old gentleman living alone since his wife Sarah passed away 2 years ago. George has diabetes but the co-pay for his medications and testing supplies forces him to choose between getting his medications and supplies or paying for utilities and groceries. George will buy his testing supplies every other month and buy only canned soup at the grocery store to be able to meet all his expenses.

Which intervention should be implemented first to assist George?

a. Provide the names and locations of food pantries
b. Provide George with written education regarding the importance of regularly checking his blood sugar
c. Collaborate with a pharmacist to locate discounts on medications and glucose testing supplies
d. Locate community resources to assist with the cost of utilities

Think about how you would address the needs of these three patients in your current practice setting. Are you aware of resources that would help? Do you know how to find resources that would help? How would you advocate for the implementation of these resources? This may have been more of a challenge than anticipated. For these case studies, all of the choices provided could be appropriate, but the correct choice would be to choose the intervention that would address the patient's greatest risk. The facilitation of the remaining interventions follow.

- **For Cassie**: Work with her grandmother to explore emergency housing. If that is not a viable option for a particular location, the next best intervention would be to schedule an appointment with her pediatrician.

- **For Brittany**: The need to determine if she feels safe is imperative. She may or may not be ready to discuss domestic violence, but your concern for her safety will begin the development of a trusted relationship.
- **For George**: Locating resources to help with the cost of medications and testing supplies will help the patient to adhere to diabetes management.

As has been reinforced in this manual, social challenges may be the greatest interference to achieve health improvements. Case managers are on the frontline of assessing and mitigating these challenges. Take an active role in your organization's SDH processes for the best patient care and outcomes.

REFERENCES

De Marchis, E. H., Brown, E., Aceves, B. A., Loomba, V., Molina, M., Cartier, Y., Wing, H., & Gottlieb, L. M. (2022). *State of the science of screening in healthcare settings*, Social Interventions Research & Evaluation Network.

Institute for Healthcare Improvement. (2023). *IHI triple aim initiative*. Author. https://www.ihi.org/Engage/Initiatives/TripleAim/Pages/default.aspx

NACHC AND AAPCHO. (2022). *PRAPARE implementation and action toolkit*. https://prapare.org/prapare-toolkit/

National Academies of Science Engineering and Medicine. (2019). *Integrating health care and social services for people with serious illness: Proceedings of a workshop*. Author.

Social Intervention Research and Evaluation Network. (2019). *Social needs screening tool comparison table*. University of San Francisco. https://sirenetwork.ucsf.edu/tools-resources/resources/screening-tools-comparison

U.S. Department of Health and Human Services. (2022). *Healthy people 2030*. Author. https://health.gov/healthypeople/priority-areas/social-determinants-health

CHAPTER 8

Addressing Health Inequities

Rebecca Perez

OBJECTIVES

- Define health inequity
- Identify the groups most impacted by health inequities
- Discover frameworks and interventions for the elimination of health inequities

Introduction

Health inequity is not a new problem. However, recent events in the United States have increased awareness among historically and predominantly White healthcare leaders and organizations of the pervasiveness of racism and other causes of health inequity. The social and structural drivers of inequity include healthcare access, treatment, and outcomes, as well as policies and practices of some healthcare institutions contributing to poor health outcomes for some communities, especially communities of color (Reid, 2022).

The existing concerns with health inequity were magnified by the most devasting health event in more than 100 years: the COVID-19 pandemic. At the time of this writing, globally,nearly 3 million people had died and more than 135 million were sickened by the virus (National Academies of Science, Engineering, and Medicine [NASEM], 2021). The COVID-19 pandemic brought to light the mistrust that many ethnic groups have of healthcare systems and providers. The tragic Tuskegee Syphilis Study conducted between 1932 and 1972 continues to impact how African Americans view the medical establishment. Hispanics and Native Americans experience poverty, language, and cultural barriers, and for Native Americans, a separate healthcare system that may or may not be adequately funded. Health inequities and health outcomes are closely related to the social determinants of health (SDH) as they relate to the importance of health and all aspects of life. This chapter provides a definition of health inequity, identities the groups most impacted, and illustrates frameworks and interventions for the elimination of health inequities.

Defining Health Inequities

According to a report from NASEM on the future of nursing, health inequities are defined as the "systemic differences in the opportunities that groups have to achieve optimal health, leading to unfair and avoidable differences in health outcomes" (NASEM, 2021). These inordinately impact people of color, the LGBTQ+ community, people with disabilities, those with low income, or those living in rural areas. The evidence clearly indicates these groups have poor access to care which is connected to SDH. Other determinants connected to these groups' poor access to care originate with employment, education, housing, income, public safety, and social environments (NASEM, 2021). Those with higher education and income levels will fare better, while others without these positive determinants will fare poorly.

As mentioned throughout this text, the United States has overinvested in the treatment of disease and not the causes of illness. If we, as a country, hope to improve the lives and well-being of our citizens, we must address poverty, racism, and discrimination, and all healthcare professionals can play a role in contributing to the reduction of these inequities.

The Starting Point

Creating a workforce that is grounded and built with a strong and shared foundation for health equity is a place to start. That means that organizations and institutions must examine their history, and from there, begin to create learning models around consistent language, frameworks, and acceptance of values and norms that support equity. Institutions and organizations need to support learning about what it means to have equity in healthcare and what inequity looks like. As suggested by Reid et al. (2022), one should consider these three activities to prevent a rush to solutions that may result in unintended consequences:

1. Build a supportive and healing environment for exploration and collaboration.
2. Understand and share the history of inequities and racism as they pertain to one's specific environment.
3. Assess the current state of health equity in one's organization.

These activities require the ability to explicitly name and acknowledge structural inequities and practices. This can begin by establishing a diverse, multistakeholder group that can evaluate from perspectives of experience and levels of power (Reid et al., 2022). The team to examine health inequities requires diversity, which will lead to accurate information, decision-making, and better outcomes. This group must be willing and open to discussing potentially uncomfortable topics, engage in nonthreatening conflict, question long-standing norms or practices, and yet be able to work together to establish new practices that will change the current culture for the benefit of all.

Moving toward health equity will take time but once the group feels their foundation is strong, next steps include agreeing on shared definitions, especially for terms like "racism," health "equity," and health "inequity." Resources for building individual knowledge is next. These can include recommended books, articles, documentaries, and training in structural racism and racial justice to perpetuate not only individual learning but for reflection and discussion to build a base from which all team members can operate. Team members should be able to share personal stories of inequities or lack of experience of inequities so that all can learn from each other. To build a culture of equity requires a better understanding of those most affected.

Populations Affected by Health Inequity

All people of color, those with low income, the LGBTQ+ population, and those living in rural and prairie areas of the United States have been subject to some form of health inequity.

American Indians and Alaska Natives

Among all of these disparate populations, however, there is one group that has been the recipient of inequity far longer than even African Americans. American Indians and Alaska Natives (AIAN) have suffered since Europeans first landed on our shores. The Indigenous people of the United States have suffered from policies that called for genocide, acculturation, and domination (Aroumbola Solomon et al., 2022). Reichard Henry Pratt, an American Civil War soldier, fought many conflicts with Native Americans and believed they should receive an American education and be absorbed into American society. He is famously, or infamously, known for saying "kill the Indian and save the man," meaning acculturation and American education would "save" Native Americans from themselves.

Much like Africans forced and sold into slavery in the United States, the practices and policies forced on Native Americans resulted in intergenerational effects that marginalized AIAN access to healthcare and health outcomes. These effects crumbled the value systems of the AIAN whose beliefs are based in community and the sanctity of all creation (Aroumbola Solomon et al., 2022). It was not until June 2, 1924, that Native Americans were granted U.S. citizenship, but were not granted the right to vote until 1957. In 1866 and 1867, Congress passed the 14th and 15th Amendments allowing Black American men the right to vote. That is not to say that either group were welcomed with open arms at polling places.

LGBTQ+ Population

The LGBTQ+ population experiences health inequities due to preventable gaps in stigma, discrimination, and denied rights based on sexual orientation and gender identity. LGBTQ+ people are less likely to have a primary care provider. Lesbian and bisexual women have higher rates of breast cancer, and transgender people are at greater risk of the human papilloma virus (HPV) infection and related cervical or anal cancers. LGBTQ+ people of color will experience the highest rate of health disparities (Gillespie, 2022).

When compared to straight people, LGBTQ+ people experience different stressors. These include bullying, harassment, fear of rejection, internalized homophobia, body image distress, limited access to medical and mental health treatment, and violence (Gillespie, 2022). The seven major disparities affecting the LGBTQ+ community include (Gillespie, 2022):

1. **Sexually transmitted infections (STI)**
    a. Men who have sex with men are at the greatest risk.
        i. HIV
        ii. Syphilis
        iii. Chlamydia
        iv. Gonorrhea
2. **Violence**
    a. Evidence is mounting that transgender people experience higher rates of violence.
    b. Transgender women are more likely to live in poverty and experience higher rates of sexual assault and murder because poverty increases the risk of prostitution and imprisonment.
3. **Substance use**
    a. Smoking
    b. Alcohol abuse
    c. Methamphetamines and cocaine
4. **Mental health conditions**
    a. Transgender and gender nonconforming adolescents are more prone to attention deficit and depressive disorders.
    b. Anxiety
    c. Suicidality
    d. Eating disorders
5. **Obesity and eating disorders**
    a. Bisexual and lesbian women are more likely to be overweight or obese.
    b. Eating and body image disorders are contributors.
6. **Breast and cervical cancers**
    a. These appear to disproportionately impact the LGBTQ+ community.
    b. Bisexual and lesbian women are less likely to receive preventive screenings.
7. **Heart disease**
    a. The LGBTQ+ community has higher rates due to smoking.

Impact of the COVID-19 Pandemic

As mentioned earlier, the COVID-19 pandemic impacted people of color more than non-Hispanic Whites. According to a report by the Kaiser Family Foundation (KFF) in 2022, AIAN, Hispanic, and Black people experienced higher rates of death during the initial surge of the virus in the summer of 2020 (Hill & Artiga, 2022). Hispanic people were five times more likely to die, AIAN three times more likely to die, and Black people four times more likely to die of the virus (Hill & Artiga, 2022). Deaths peaked between December 2020 and January 2021 with AIAN and Hispanic peoples experiencing the highest rates of death (62.5 and 59.0 per 100,00 lives, respectively; Hill & Artiga, 2022). Then, during the Delta variant surge of late summer 2021, deaths were highest among the AIAN. As of January 2022, during the Omicron surge, Black, AIAN, and Hispanic people experienced the highest rates of death: 36.5, 33.1, and 29.4 per 100,00 population, respectively (Hill & Artiga, 2022).

Geographic Location

The presence and degree of health inequity varies by geographic location and the case manager's practice setting. The case manager working for a managed Medicaid payer in a large metropolitan area may be exposed to disparities based on income, education, and sexual orientation and preference, whereas the case manager working in Albuquerque for Indian Health Services will be working to eliminate the disparities of Native Americans which include finding a trusted provider, nutrition, substance use disorder, depression, preventive services, chronic disease management, and transportation. SDH are closely tied to health disparities. Working to find and offer needed resources for some of the social determinants can assist in reducing inequities.

Working Toward a Solution

Reducing health inequity cannot be achieved by a single individual, organization or community, nor do these have sole ownership, accountability, or capacity to sustain the health of a given population (Gomez et al., 2021). Interventions to address health inequity encompass structural and systemic solutions requiring short- and long-term actions (Gomez et al., 2021):

- Discover and address the root causes of inequity.
  - Identify the social and environmental determinants of health and healthcare.
- Identify and address groups that have faced major obstacles.
  - Determine socioeconomic disadvantages.
  - Determine historic and recent injustices.
- Promote equal opportunity for all people to be healthy and to seek the highest level of health and well-being.

- Make available and distribute socioeconomic resources needed to be healthy.
- Persist in the goal of equity by continuing efforts to eliminate health inequities.

As with any good case management process, monitoring and evaluation of the impact of interventions are required. Measures for improvement in health equity should evaluate if improvements in physical, social, and economic conditions have translated to improved health. Three components are suggested for evaluation (Gomez et al., 2021):

1. An indicator of modified health, such as access to care or improved living conditions
2. An indicator related to social position, such as gender, ethnicity, income, or education
3. A method to compare indicators for health or health determinants across various social positions

Health equity is achievable in the United States if evidence-based policy changes and processes result in all people achieving their health potential (Gomez et al., 2021). Case managers and case management organizations can lead in these efforts. Resources are available to provide frameworks to begin the work of improving and eventually achieving health equity. These frameworks can be accessed from two evidence-based sources: *Healthy People 2030* and the Institute for Healthcare Improvement.

Health equity is part of the larger framework of *Healthy People 2030*. For health equity, the Office of Disease Prevention and Health Promotion suggests the following to advance health equity:

- Identify priorities based upon identified leading indicators then compare progress to national targets. Throughout the life span, these include (Office of Disease Prevention and Health Promotion, n.d.):
  - Oral health, especially for children and adolescents
  - Consumption of calories from added sugars by persons aged 2 years and over (2+ years)
  - Drug overdose deaths
  - Exposure to unhealthy air
  - Homicides
  - Household food insecurity and hunger
  - Persons who are vaccinated annually against seasonal influenza
  - Persons who know their HIV status (13+ years)
  - Persons less than 65 years of age with medical insurance
  - Suicides
- Other age-related indicators (Figure 8.1).

FIGURE 8.1 ***Healthy People 2030*** **leading health indicators.**

LHIs by life stage

All ages*

Children, adolescents, and adults who use the oral health care system (2+ years)
Consumption of calories from added sugars by persons aged 2 years and over (2+ years)
Drug overdose deaths
Exposure to unhealthy air
Homicides
Household food insecurity and hunger
Persons who are vaccinated annually against seasonal influenza
Persons who know their HIV status (13+ years)
Persons with medical insurance (<65 years)
Suicides
***Except where otherwise noted**

Infants

Infant deaths

Children and adolescents

4th grade students whose reading skills are at or above the proficient achievement level for their grade

Adolescents with major depressive episodes (MDEs) who receive treatment

Children and adolescents with obesity

Current use of any tobacco products among adolescents

Adults and older adults

Adults engaging in binge drinking of alcoholic beverages during the past 30 days

Adults who meet current minimum guidelines for aerobic physical activity and muscle-strengthening activity

Adults who receive a colorectal cancer screening based on the most recent guidelines

Adults with hypertension whose blood pressure is under control

Cigarette smoking in adults

Employment among the working-age population

Maternal deaths

New cases of diagnosed diabetes in the population

Source: Office of Disease Prevention and Health Promotion. (n.d.). *Health equity in Healthy People 2030*. Healthy People 2030. https://health.gov/healthypeople/priority-areas/health-equity-healthy-people-2030

To achieve the Triple Aim as defined by the Institute for Healthcare Improvement (IHI), health equity must first be addressed. Figure 8.2 illustrates IHI's framework for developing health equity (IHI, 2016).

As integral members of healthcare interdisciplinary teams, case managers play a role in reducing health inequities by ensuring that patients whose primary language is not English can access a provider that speaks their primary language or, at the very least, has access to a medical translator; participation in organizational process improvement activities to reduce inequities and disparities; supporting partnerships with providers and community resources that are sensitive to the needs of underserved populations;

FIGURE 8.2 Institute for Healthcare Improvement's framework for developing health equity.

Make health equity a priority	• Demonstrate leadership commitment to improving equity at all levels of an organization • Secure sustainable funding through new payment models
Develop structure and processes to support health equity work	• Establish a governance structure to oversee and manage equity work across organizations • Dedicate budget resources to support equity work
Display specific strategies to address the multiple determinants of health on which healthcare organizations can have a direct impact	• Healthcare services • Socioeconomic status • Physical environment • Healthy behaviors
Decrease institutional racism within organizations	• Improve physical spaces: buildings and design • Health insurance plans accepted by organizations • Reduce implicit bias within organizational policies, structures and norms, and in patient care
Develop partnerships with community organizations	• Leverage community assets to work together on community issues related to improving health and equity

Source: Institute for Healthcare Improvement'. (2016). *Achieving health equity framework*. Institute for Healthcare Improvements. https://www.ihi.org/resources/Pages/IHIWhitePapers/Achieving-Health-Equity.aspx

examining yourself and your organization for the presence of bias; and, as a result of knowing the populations served, ensuring resources are compiled and at the ready to meet the needs of those you serve.

Reflection

In this chapter, examples of existing inequities experienced by several groups were highlighted. As the case manager, how would you begin to address some of the disparities experienced by these groups?

Black Americans

It is a well-known fact that Black Americans experience higher mortality rates from chronic illness. What are the challenges that lead to this disparity? The primary contributors are access to care and economics. For Black Americans living in rural areas, access to care can be nearly impossible due to the absence of facilities that offer high-quality healthcare services. For poor Black Americans living in urban areas, a lack of providers that accept Medicaid reimbursement results in a similar situation as those living in rural areas; that is, few options for accessing condition-changing care.

INTERVENTIONS

1. Help locate providers that accept Medicaid.
2. Call to make outpatient appointments for your patient—introduce yourself as the patient's case manager.
3. Facilitate telehealth visits for patients living remotely.
4. Coordinate community health events in rural areas: at churches, schools, community centers to reinforce good nutrition, medication management, and other health behaviors.

AMERICAN INDIAN AND ALASKA NATIVE PEOPLES

American Indian and Alaska Native (AIAN) peoples have been subject to heath and other inequities for multiple generations. AIAN peoples have a separate healthcare system known as Indian Health Services but may also have access to Medicare and Medicaid reimbursement. Living on a reservation often results in poor access if individuals live far from medical facilities. Many living remotely on reservations do not have running water, electricity, or broadband. Generational trauma has resulted in mental health concerns for which condition-changing care may or may not be available. Practitioners of Western medicine may not be sensitive to spiritual beliefs nor incorporate those beliefs into a treatment plan.

INTERVENTIONS

1. Support the integration of Native medicine and beliefs with Western medicine.
2. Display respect for Native beliefs and language.
3. Coordinate transportation to medical facilities for outpatient care.
4. Whenever possible, utilize peer support to reinforce access to care and healthy behaviors.
5. Determine how best to provide mental health support based on the patient's preferences.

LGBTQ+ Population

Individuals identifying with the LGBTQ+ population face discrimination on multiple fronts, whether it be employment or bias related to lifestyle. Mental health support seems to be one of the greatest challenges experienced.

INTERVENTIONS

1. Locate providers sensitive to the challenges of the LBGTQ+ population.
2. Coordinate mental health services whether in person or via remote access.
3. Encourage testing for sexually transmitted infections.
4. Engage peer support to reinforce healthy behaviors and prevention.

As a case manager, you will not solve all of the injustices these and other groups face, but one patient at a time, case managers can advocate for what each individual needs and deserves. If all case managers functioned in this advocacy role, disparities would be reduced, and the healthcare industry would take notice.

REFERENCES

Aroumbola Solomon, T. E., Starks, R. R. B., Attakai, A., Molina, F., Cordova-Marks, F., Kahn-John, M., Antone, C. L., Flores, M., Jr., & Garcia, F. (2022). The generational impact of racism on health: Voices from American Indian Communities. *Health Affairs, 41*(2), 281–288. https://doi.org/10.1377/hlthaff.2021.01419

Gillespie, C. (2022, November 23). *7 Major health disparities affecting the LGBTQ+ community*. Health. https://www.health.com/mind-body/lgbtq-health-disparities

Gomez, C. E., Kleinman, D. V., Pronk, N., Gordon, G. L. W., Ochiai, E., Blakey, C., Johnson, A., & Brewer, K.H. (2021, November/December). Addressing health equity and social determinants of health through healthy people 2030. *Journal of Public Health Management and Practice, 27*(6), S249–S257. https://doi.org/10.1097/PHH.0000000000001297

Hill, L. A., & Artiga, S. (2022, August 22). *COVID-19 cases and deaths by race/ethnicity: Current data and changes.* KFF. https://www.kff.org/coronavirus-covid-19/issue-brief/covid-19-cases-and-deaths-by-race-ethnicity-current-data-and-changes-over-time/

Institute for Healthcare Improvements. (2016). *Achieving health equity framework.* Author. https://www.ihi.org/resources/Pages/IHIWhitePapers/Achieving-Health-Equity.aspx

National Academies of Science, Engineering, and Medicine. (2021). *The Future of nursing 2020–2030: Charting a path to achieve health equity.* Author. The National Academies Press, Inc. https://doi.org/https://doi.org/10.17226/25982

Office of Disease Prevention and Health Promotion. (n.d.). *Health equity in healthy people 2030.* Health People 2030 https://health.gov/healthypeople/priority-areas/health-equity-healthy-people-2030

Reid, A. B.-M., Brandes, R., Butler-MacKay, D., Ortiz, A., Kramer, S., Sivashanker, K., & Mate, K. (2022, January). Getting grounded: Building a foundation for health equity and racial justice work in health care teams. *NEJM Catalyst, 3*(1), 1–13. https://doi.org/10.1056/CAT.21.0320

SECTION III

Addressing Complex Patient Populations Using an Integrated Case Management Approach

CHAPTER 9

Common Physical and Mental Health Conditions

Rebecca Perez

OBJECTIVES

- Review basic information for common adult mental health conditions
- Review basic information for common childhood and adolescent mental health conditions
- Review basic information for common chronic medical conditions: diabetes, heart failure, coronary artery disease, chronic obstructive pulmonary disease, asthma, and chronic kidney disease

Introduction

To function as integrated case managers, the case manager must be able to address all the patient's needs and conditions. This requires a general understanding of medical and behavioral conditions. For some, this may be uncomfortable or even a bit overwhelming as conditions that are unfamiliar will require an effort to understand. Case managers must be willing to learn about conditions that are less familiar so that condition-changing treatment can be supported. In addition to broadening the case manager's knowledge base, the support of an interdisciplinary team whose members may have experience in areas less familiar will be available for mentoring. The case manager draws upon gained experiences and seeks consultation for the less familiar. This chapter reviews basic information that case managers need to know on a variety of chronic medical and mental health conditions.

Cross-Disciplinary Roles

Integrated case management is a process in which a single case manager collaborates with a patient to address all health concerns: medical, behavioral, social, and access to care. The assignment of a case manager should be based on the primary risk factors of the patient. The primary case manager should have expertise in those areas of risk. However, the expectation is that the primary case manager also collaborates with all the team members in all areas that impact health, even if the case manager lacks specific experience with all the patient's conditions. In order to assist a patient to regain health, case managers are encouraged to become familiar with conditions that are less familiar to them. These may include the common conditions discussed in this chapter, or perhaps their patient is challenged with less familiar conditions. Regardless of condition, the case manager has a professional obligation to better understand the conditions, appropriate treatment, and associated challenges that may be faced.

To effectively function as an integrated case manager, it is not necessary to be an expert in every discipline, including those that may be less familiar. For example, case managers coming from a physical medicine background do not need to know every medication prescribed for every mental health condition, nor should the case manager coming from a behavioral health background need to know every medication prescribed for every physical health condition. Case managers assist patients in accessing needed care and services. That requires an understanding of the direction in which to guide a patient and providing support for the treatment prescribed by a physician. Case managers do not recommend treatment. If case managers have a basic understanding of evidence-based treatments and have the support of a care team and physician advisor, then case managers will be able to be effective in helping a patient move toward improved health. This basic understanding of illnesses and conditions provides a case manager with the ability to assist a patient to remove barriers and access care that will result in illness improvement.

Guidelines for a basic understanding of illness:

- Recognize core signs and symptoms of the diagnosed condition(s).
- Know the common classes of medications used to treat a condition.
- Know the resources needed to gain additional information about medications.
- Understand the types of therapies that may be prescribed:
    - Psychotherapy: behavioral or cognitive
    - Physical therapy for orthopedic conditions
    - Occupational therapies for stroke, cerebral palsy, developmental delays, or other cognitive issues
    - Speech/language therapies for communication disorders

- Know how a patient should be monitored for their condition.
- Know what constitutes a good response to treatment or what to look for if a patient is not responding to treatment.
- Know how to document progress or lack of progress.
- Know when improvement should be expected once treatment has been initiated.
- Know when and what to report if a patient is not making progress.

Goals of Integrated Case Management

1. Have one primary case manager to address all of a patient's conditions, health concerns, social concerns, and barriers to improvement.
2. Case managers will familiarize themselves with the patient's conditions, prescribed treatment, and ability to follow the prescribed treatment plan.
3. Case managers will collaborate with the patient's clinicians to support the prescribed treatment.
4. Case managers will report to the clinicians any concerns related to complications, new symptoms, and the patient's ability to adhere to prescribed treatment.
5. Case managers will assist the patient in understanding their illness and how to eventually self-manage.
6. Case managers will assist the patient in removal of barriers that prevent a return to health.
7. Case managers will encourage healthy behaviors and initiate conversations about change.
8. Case managers will report unnecessary or harmful care.

Case managers whose careers have focused primarily in one discipline may experience concern when asked to address a patient's issues in multiple domains. Supports need to be put in place so that all integrated case managers know where and how to get the information needed to be effective and take ownership of patients assigned.

The care team with which a case manager works can be a resource for less familiar experience and knowledge. While there is one primary case manager collaborating with a team member, the team is there to aid and support. It has been mentioned that the professional responsibility of case managers is to learn about unfamiliar conditions, but the experience of team members will also result in a widened knowledge base and comfort level. Interdisciplinary rounds are an excellent conduit for advice and recommendations as the team comes together to learn how patients are progressing. Rounds are a perfect venue for discussion of challenges as well as successes.

How Case Managers Talk to Patients About Unhealthy Behaviors

Medical professionals are often uncomfortable asking questions about a patient's behavioral conditions, ability to cope, or unhealthy behaviors. Everyone knows that "life happens" and the way an individual reacts to what comes their way differs from person to person. For the patient with complex conditions, the challenges of life can affect their ability to self-manage. Asking questions about a patient's emotional state is as important as understanding what physical symptoms the patient is experiencing. Overcoming this discomfort can be achieved by working with behavioral health team members and colleagues and using scripting until the conversations become comfortable. The connection between physical concerns and emotional/behavioral responses leads to impairment in everyday functioning.

How Mental Health Professionals Address General Medical Disorders

Mental health professionals have traditionally avoided and been discouraged from addressing an individual's medical concerns. They have been taught that the mind and body are not connected, which is contrary to the beliefs of many ancient cultures and to holistic practice. Avoidance of addressing physical concerns along with behavioral concerns was thought to result in a transference of behaviors to physical symptoms. The lack of confidence in addressing medical concerns also leads to avoidance. For mental health professionals to become effective integrated case managers, they must be willing to address medical issues.

Regardless of primary discipline, much can be learned through conversation and use of open-ended questions. Through conversation, and not interrogation, much can be learned from the patient about their health, feelings, concerns, and hopes. These conversations also build trust with the patient and promote engagement.

Suggested Assessment Questions for Both Physical and Behavioral Case Managers

General Life Questions	• "Hello Ms./Mr. ______, my name is _______ and I am a nurse/social worker from your benefit plan ______. I am reaching out as it appears you have been having some health problems lately. I would very much like to assist you in any way needed. Would it be alright if I ask you a few questions?" • "Can you tell me what health problems concern you the most?" • "How has ______ affected your everyday life?"
Physical Health	• "How have you been managing your _________?" • "What worries you the most right now?" • "Can you tell me what you see as challenges to managing your _____?" • "How often do you see your doctor?"

Emotional Health	• "How does your health affect you emotionally?" • "Are you feeling worried, anxious, sad?" • "How many days do you feel worried, anxious, sad?" • "Do you have trouble remembering things?" • "If so, what things are hard to remember?"
Relationships With Providers	"Whom do you see for your health problems?" "Do you feel as though you have a good relationship with Dr. ______?"
Access to Care	"Are you able to get appointments with your doctor when needed?" "If not, what do you see as the problem?" "When you have appointments, do you have any problems getting there?" "Do your health benefits adequately cover the care you need (prescriptions, co-pays)?"
Social Issues	• "Who is available to help you when you need it?" • "Do you feel safe where you live?" • "If no, what are your safety concerns?" • "Do you have a job?" "What kind of work do you do?" "What are your current responsibilities?" (Includes full-time homemaker, children, school) • "Are you able to meet your financial obligations?" • "If no, what financial challenges do you face?"
Additional Information	• "Right now, what is your greatest concern?" • "What would you like to work on?" • "What things did I not ask that you like for me to know?"

Important Issues Related to Medical and Mental Healthcare

When examining the considerations that professionals from either the medical or mental health disciplines require, there are some significant differences, especially for mental health (Table 9.1).

"Mental illness is like any other medical illness." A passionate debate regarding to the truth of this statement has been going on since the time of Hippocrates (Malla, 2015). The definitions and causes of mental health have ranged from imbalances of bodily humors to brain illnesses. The statement implies that mental illness has a biological basis and should be treated as a biological illness. The following compares treatment of diabetes to treatment of a mental illness (Malla, 2015).

Type 2 diabetes is the result of dysfunctional glucose metabolism due to the insufficiency of the pancreas to produce insulin. Causes of diabetes can range from an endocrine dysfunction or poor personal choices in diet and activity. Diagnosis is confirmed by elevated serum glucose and other glucose metabolic markers. The illness cascade impacts other systems such as the cardiovascular and central nervous systems. Glucose levels can be controlled and complications avoided or minimized with changes in habit and medication.

TABLE 9.1 Differences Between Medical and Mental Health Conditions

Medical Conditions	Mental Conditions
Biological origin	Origin can be genetic, increased by psychological deprivation and trauma, isolation, poverty, and poor family environment
Manifests biological complications	Manifests primarily through altered thinking, perceptions and consciousness of self, others, and the world
Response to treatment is improved biological complications	Response to treatment is positive changes and interactions with the environment, feelings, self-esteem, mood, perceptions, thoughts, and actions

Source: Adapted from Malla, A. R. (2015, May). Mental illness is like any other medical illness: A critical examination of the statement and its impact on patient care and society. *Journal of Psychiatry and Neuroscience, 40*(3), 147–150. https://doi.org/10.1503%2Fjpn.150099

Mental health disorders impact individuals through a range of experiences that vary in severity that alter thinking, perceptions and consciousness of self, others, and the world. These experiences are more severe in psychoses and bipolar disorder and less severe in anxiety, mood, and eating disorders. The factors that increase the risk for developing mental health disorders are genetic, psychological deprivation and trauma, isolation, poverty, and poor family environments.

Therapeutic interventions are meant to help the patient feel better and to positively interact with their environment. While medical conditions require psychological attention, mental health interventions focus primarily on achieving positive change in feelings, thoughts, self-esteem, mood, perceptions, thoughts, and actions. Treatment usually involves psychological therapies and medication. Advances in neuroscience have delivered better biological explanations for cognitive, emotional, and cognitive functions like memory, thinking, perception, mood, and action. These advances indicate that many mental illnesses derive their vulnerability from underlying biological variations, but there is still much work to do.

The statement, "Mental illness is like any other medical illness" oversimplifies a complex problem and at worst does not serve patients and their families. It is necessary to continue social and professional conversations to determine where neurobiology, social, cultural and environmental factors, personal histories and individual uniqueness to understand, explain, and treat mental disorders (Malla, 2015).

Rarely is treatment for medical conditions forced. The exception is the presence of communicable diseases. However, individuals with severe psychiatric illness may be examined for competency or involuntary commitment via court-ordered action. Forced admission or detention occurs when an individual's judgment is impaired to the point of risk, or they are a physical threat to self or others. Examples of conditions that can escalate these risks are dementia, substance abuse, eating disorders, or psychosis. Case managers are typically not involved in the legal process but should understand the basics. The role of the case manager in these situations is to provide support to the patient and their support system, as well as to assist in the coordination of care and services at the conclusion of the commitment or detention. Laws related to competency and commitment vary from state to state, and case managers must familiarize themselves with the process in their local jurisdictions.

Patients who verbalize suicidal or homicidal thoughts are at significant risk. Case managers coming from a medical background may find this expression frightening. When a patient expresses such thoughts, the case manager must be proactive and determine the level of intent. There are ways to determine how to escalate intervention. A case manager can engage in discussions with their behavioral health team members. The case manager can ask the team members to share some real-life experiences and how they have managed such crises.

Understanding Mental Health and Behavioral Disorders

The terms "mental" and "behavioral" are often used interchangeably but it is important to understand that there is a difference between mental/psychiatric illness and behavioral disorder. Mental disorders or mental illness are defined as conditions that effect mood, thinking, feeling, and behavior (Medicine, 2020). These conditions can sometimes become chronic and significantly effect function. Examples of mental disorders or illnesses include:

- Anxiety disorders
- Depression, bipolar disorder, or other mood disorders
- Eating disorders
- Personality disorders
- Posttraumatic stress disorder (PTSD)
- Psychotic disorders including schizophrenia

The American Psychological Association (APA) defines behavioral disorders as "any persistent pattern of behavior that violates societal norms or rules, seriously impairs a person's functioning, or creates distress in others" (APA, 2022). The term is used to cover a wide range of disorders or syndromes (APA, 2022). Examples of behavioral disorders include:

- Attention-deficit/hyperactivity disorder (ADHD)
- Autism spectrum disorder
- Eating disorders
- Learning disorders

- Obsessive-compulsive disorder
- Obstructive sleep apnea
- Panic disorder

Genetics and environment play a role in the heritability of mental health and behavioral disorders. Table 9.2 provides examples of potentially inheritable disorders and the associated risk level (Tracy, 2019).

The difference between a behavior disorder and a mental or psychiatric disorder is choice. Mental or psychiatric disorders are considered to be involuntary while, in behavioral disorders, choice is available (Tracy, 2019). Some behavioral disorders have a physical source, but most are rooted in the choice to behave in a certain way or to control behaviors.

Behavioral disorders are most often seen in children. All children act out from time to time, but when their conduct becomes extreme, it may be considered pathological. These behaviors are always present in the child's home setting and may or may not be present in the community or school. The two most common pediatric behavioral disorders are oppositional defiant disorder and conduct disorder (Tracy, 2019).

OPPOSITIONAL DEFIANT DISORDER

Oppositional defiant disorder is a recurring pattern of anger and irritable mood, argumentative and defiant behavior, or vindictive behavior that lasts more than 6 months (Tracy, 2019). The specifics of these behaviors are as follows (Tracy, 2019).

TABLE 9.2 Inheritable Disorders and Associated Risk Levels

Disorder Type	Risk Level
Bipolar disorder	85%
Schizophrenia	81%
Alzheimer's disease	75%
Cocaine use disorder	72%
Anorexia nervosa	60%
Alcohol dependence	56%
Sedative use disorder	51%
Cannabis use disorder	48%
Panic disorder	43%
Stimulant use disorder	40%
Major depressive disorder	37%
Generalized anxiety disorder	28%

Behavior Type	Characteristics
Angry/irritable mood	• Loses temper often • "Touchy" or easily annoyed • Often angry or resentful
Argumentative/defiant behavior	• Argues with parent or authority figure • Actively defies or refuses to follow instructions or comply with requests, especially from an authority figure • Deliberately annoys others • Blames others for their mistakes
Vindictiveness	• Spiteful or vindictive to others at least twice in the last 6 months

CONDUCT DISORDER

This disorder is considered one of the most difficult to treat and involves troubling behaviors like oppositional and defiant behaviors as well as other behaviors such as lying or stealing (Tracy, 2019). The *DSM-5* defines conduct disorder as behavior that violates the basic rights of others or major societal age-appropriate norms (Tracy, 2019). These behaviors must cause clinically significant impairment in social, academic, or occupational functioning (i.e., school attendance). These behaviors in those 18 years or older will be evaluated for antisocial personality disorder. The presence of at least three of the following criteria determines the diagnosis of the disorder (Tracy, 2019):

Behavior Type	Characteristics
Aggression to people and animals	• Bullies or threatened others • Initiates fights • Has used a weapon that can cause serious harm (bat, brick/rock, broken bottle, knife, gun) • Has been physically cruel to people • Has been physically cruel to animals • Has stolen while confronting a victim (mugging, purse snatching, extortion, armed robbery) • Forced sexual activity on another
Destruction of property	• Deliberately engages in setting fires with the intention to do harm or cause damage • Deliberately destroys another property by means other than fire
Deceitfulness or theft	• Broken into someone else's home, car, or building • Lies to obtain goods or favors to avoid obligations, "cons" others • Stolen items of nontrivial value without confronting the victim, i.e., shoplifting

Behavior Type	Characteristics
Serious violations of rules	• May stay out at night despite parental rules to the contrary, usually starting before the age of 13 years • Has run away from home at least overnight at least twice while living with parents or guardians or without returning for a lengthy period • Often truant from school beginning before age 13 years

Behavioral Health

Behavioral health is the connection between behaviors and the health and well-being of the body, mind, and spirit (Alvernia University, 2022). However, behavioral health was also related to the prevention of illness and promotion of health. The discipline of behavioral health may include both mental health and substance use to encompass the continuum of prevention, intervention, treatment, and recovery support services (Alvernia University, 2022).

SUBSTANCE USE DISORDER

According to the American Psychiatric Association, substance use disorder (SUD) is "a complex condition in which there is uncontrolled use of a substance despite harmful consequences such as alcohol, tobacco, or illicit drugs, to the point where the person's ability to function in day-to-day life becomes impaired" (American Psychiatric Association, 2022). Use of the substance continues despite the person knowing the harm it causes.

Changes in the structure and function of the brain are the cause of cravings, changes in personality, abnormal movements, and other behaviors. SUD causes changes in the areas of the brain that relate to judgment, decision-making, learning, memory, and behavioral control can be seen on brain imaging studies (American Psychiatric Association, 2022). Tolerance to the substance occurs with prolonged use resulting in dependence and increased use. Individuals begin taking drugs for a variety of reasons, including:

- To feel good, feel pleasure;
- To feel better, forget troubles, relieve stress, relieve pain;
- To do better, enhance performance, improve thinking; and
- Curiosity, peer pressure, or desire to experiment.

SUD is one of the disorders that crosses between a behavioral disorder and one that has physical roots (American Psychiatric Association, 2022).

GENERAL PROCEDURES FOR HANDLING SUICIDAL THOUGHTS/EXPRESSIONS

Addressing suicidal ideation can be one of the most challenging, and even frightening, encounters for the case manager. A patient expressing thoughts of self-harm requires the case manager to listen carefully and clarify intent. Suicide was the 12th leading cause of death in the United States in 2020, claiming the lives of 50,000 people. While complicated and tragic, suicide can be prevented if warning signs are observed and knowing where and how to get help (National Institutes of Mental Health [NIMH], 2022). NIMH, a division of the National Institutes of Health (NIH), instructs clinicians to avoid using the terms, "committing suicide," "successful suicide," or "failed suicide," because they carry negative connotations (Medicine, 2020).

Suicide is when people harm themselves with the intent to end their life and their own death results. A suicide attempt is when an individual harms themselves, but death is not the result. Suicidal thoughts or actions are not a normal way to respond to stress. Suicidal thoughts or actions should never be ignored.

Warning signs include:

- Talking about dying or wanting to kill themselves
- Talking about feeling empty, hopeless, or having no reason to live
- Talking about feeling trapped or feeling problems have no solutions
- Feeling unbearable emotional or physical pain
- Talking about being a burden to others
- Withdrawing from family or friends
- Giving away important possessions
- Saying good-bye to family and friends
- Putting affairs in order, making a will
- Risk-taking behaviors that could lead to death
- Talking or thinking about death often (NIMH, 2022)

Other behaviors that may be warning signs:

- Extreme mood swings, changing from incredibly sad to very calm or happy
- Planning, searching for lethal methods online, stockpiling pills, or buying a gun
- Talking about feeling significant guilt or shame
- Using alcohol or drugs more often
- Acting anxious or agitated
- Changes in sleep and eating habits
- Displaying rage or talking about getting revenge (NIMH, 2022)

Regular screening for thoughts of self-harm are now incorporated into all places of medical practice. Regular screening began in emergency departments with the Patient Safety Screener (PSS-3), developed by a suicide prevention steering committee at the University of Massachusetts Medical School (PSMJ, 2018). Suicide screenings are commonly included in most assessments regardless of care delivery site. The following are the questions included in the PSS-3 (PSMJ, 2018):

1. Over the past 2 weeks, have you felt down, depressed, or hopeless?
   a. An answer of "yes" indicates depression.
2. Over the past 2 weeks, have you had thoughts of killing or harming yourself?
   a. An answer of "yes" indicates suicide risk.
3. Have you ever attempted to kill yourself?
   a. If the person answers "yes" to item 3, then you follow up by asking them when the suicide attempt took place.
   b. An elevated level of risk is indicated.

Simply completing a screening does not conclude the clinician's responsibilities. Clinicians need to know what to do should their patient express thoughts or a plan of self-harm. Table 9.3 outlines six things that clinicians should know about collaborating with a client at risk for suicide (Shumway, 2021) (Figure 9.1).

TABLE 9.3 What to Know When Collaborating With a Client at Risk of Suicide

Topic	What to Know
Laws and Protocols	• Learn state laws as they relate to suicidality. • Many states mandate that clinicians report suicidal behaviors regardless of confidentiality. • Trust and confidentiality are essential to patient/clinician relationships but not at the cost of the patient's safety.
How to Ask	• Determine intent (intent is the desire or motivation to carry through with suicidal thoughts). • Does the patient have a plan? If so, how do they plan to conduct suicide? • Ideation ■ Ask if the patient is having thoughts of suicide. ■ If "yes," ask "how often have you had these thoughts?" ■ "On a scale of 1 to 10, how intense are these thoughts?" Or, "how strong are these thoughts?" ■ "How serious do you feel about carrying out these thoughts?" "If you left here right now" or "If we hang up right now, how likely are you to go through with these thoughts of killing yourself?" ■ "Have you thought about how you will harm yourself?" ■ If yes, "tell me how you would do that."
Suicide vs. Self-Harm	• Understand the difference between suicidal and nonsuicidal self-directed violence. • Some patients may think about hurting themselves, but they do not want to die. • Suicidality may include elements of self-harm, like cutting wrists to bleed out or practicing behaviors to gain confidence to progress toward suicide. • For many, self-harm is a coping mechanism for stress and emotional pain. • Self-harm actions include: ■ Superficial cutting of the skin ■ Hitting/beating ■ Hair-puling ■ Burning ■ Initiating physical conflicts • In self-harm instances, do not discount suicide; patients may still be at risk for suicide when stressed or left untreated.

(continued)

TABLE 9.3 What to Know When Collaborating With a Client at Risk of Suicide (*continued*)

Topic	What to Know
Protective and Risk Factors	• Moderate to high-risk factors ■ Suicidality (ideation, intent, plan) ■ Rehearsal of an attempt ■ Previous or recent attempts (within the last 3 months) ■ Childhood trauma/abuse ■ Drug and alcohol use (intoxication increased the risk) ■ Mental health diagnosis of depression, bipolar disorder, and/or anxiety ■ Social isolation ■ Major life stressors or transitions ■ Having a plan with preparation ■ Access to a means of suicide: firearm • The following protective factors may reduce risk: ■ Support from family and friends ■ Religious beliefs ■ Family responsibilities ■ Coping skills ■ Having reasons to live ■ Employment
Available Resources	• Who? ■ Colleagues with more experience ■ Hospital emergency departments ■ Community/church ■ Case manager • What? ■ Acute psychiatric inpatient admissions ■ Subacute care ■ Respite care
What to Do	• Determine the patient's risk ■ Do not panic, stay calm; bring in a colleague or supervisor for support. ■ Know your organization's policy for collaborating with patients who are suicidal. ■ If the patient is at risk of harm to themselves, call 911 for transport to the closest emergency department. ■ If not at imminent risk, facilitate an appointment with a mental health professional as soon as possible; coordinate transportation if needed. ■ Follow-up with the patient and work with them to create a safety plan to recognize the warning signs, who to call for help and support. Include family members if possible. Work with the patient and family to remove access to anything that could be used in a suicide plan. ■ If the patient is unwilling to draft a safety plan, explore the reasons why and if necessary, alert local law enforcement to escort the client to the emergency department or a provider appointment. ■ Commit to thorough documentation of your actions, the rationale and the patient's response. ■ Monitor interventions and response to interventions regularly.

Source: Adapted from Shumway, K. (2021, September 22). Working with suicidal clients: 6 things you should know. *Time2Track*. https://blog.time2track.com/working-with-suicidal-clients-6-things-you-should-know

FIGURE 9.1 #BeThe1: To help someone in emotional pain.

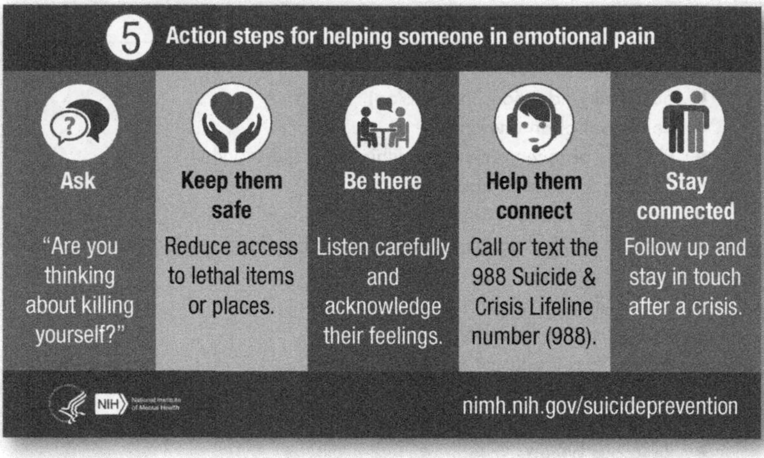
5 Action steps for helping someone in emotional pain
Ask
"Are you thinking about killing yourself?"
Keep them safe
Reduce access to lethal items or places.
Be there
Listen carefully and acknowledge their feelings.
Help them connect
Call or text the 988 Suicide & Crisis Lifeline number (988).
Stay connected
Follow up and stay in touch after a crisis.
NIH
nimh.nih.gov/suicideprevention

Source: Retrieved from National Institutes of Mental Health. (2022, August). *Suicide prevention*. Author. https://www.nimh.nih.gov/health/topics/suicide-prevention

RESOURCES TO SHARE WITH NONCLINICAL COLLEAGUES, FRIENDS, AND FAMILY

Table 9.4 provides a list of resources for substance use, mental health, and co-occurring disorders that can be shared with your patients, family/caregiver, and colleagues. These resources would be valuable for all case managers working with patients and family/caregivers challenged with substance use and/or mental health conditions. One very valuable resource is specifically for adolescents and young adults.

TABLE 9.4 Substance Abuse and Mental Health Resources

Organization	Description	URL
Substance Abuse and Mental Health Services Administration	In 2020, Congress designated the new 988 dialing code to be operated through the existing National Suicide Prevention Lifeline. SAMHSA sees 988 as a first step toward a transformed crisis care system in America	https://www.samhsa.gov/find-help/988
FindTreatment.gov (SAMHSA)	FindTreatment.gov is a confidential and anonymous resource for persons seeking treatment for mental and substance use disorders in the United States and its territories	https://findtreatment.gov/

(*continued*)

TABLE 9.4 Substance Abuse and Mental Health Resources (*continued*)

Organization	Description	URL
SAMHSA's National Helpline	SAMHSA's National Helpline is a free, confidential, 24/7, 365-day-a-year treatment referral and information service (in English and in Spanish) for individuals and families facing mental and/or substance use disorders. 1-800-662-HELP (4357)	https://www.samhsa.gov/find-help/national-helpline
MentalHealth.gov	MentalHealth.gov provides resources on suicide prevention, disaster distress, and coping with COVID-19. Resources for veterans are also available In addition to reinforcing the resources available through SAMHSA, the site shares information on behavioral health equity and parity, and fact sheets on mental illness and substance use	https://www.mentalhealth.gov/
National Institute of Mental Health: Substance Use and Co-Occurring Mental Disorders	Substance use disorders and other mental health disorders commonly co-occur. This site provides guidance to the healthcare professional on diagnosis and treatment, where to find help, and opportunities to join clinical trials	https://www.nimh.nih.gov/health/topics/substance-use-and-mental-health
Society for Adolescent Health and Medicine: Substance Use Resources for Adolescents and Young Adults	Resources are made available to healthcare professionals serving youth that include online resources, support groups treatment service locations, peer networks, helplines, and advocacy opportunities	https://www.adolescenthealth.org/Resources/Clinical-Care-Resources/Substance-Use/Substance-Use-Resources-For-Adolesc.aspx

SAMHSA, Substance Abuse and Mental Health Services Administration.

Behavioral Health Case Managers Addressing Physical Health

Just as the medical case manager may be hesitant to address mental and behavioral health issues, so the mental health case manager may feel the same about medical/physical illnesses and conditions. In this section, responding to medical emergencies is discussed.

Addressing Medical Emergencies

Case managers who do not come from a medical background also need to know what to do in a medical emergency. Knowing what to do in every emergency is not feasible, but with medical emergencies the best strategy is common sense. Case managers must always err on the side of caution, keeping the patient's safety as the priority. That may mean conducting a three-way call with the treating physician, sending the patient to the emergency department, or calling emergency responders. Conditions that indicate a medical emergency may be occurring include, but are not limited to, the following:

- Chest pain
- Shortness of breath
- Severe diaphoresis (perspiring, feeling clammy)
- Severe weakness
- Gastrointestinal (GI) bleeding (vomiting blood or dark vomit, bleeding from the rectum)
- Severe headache
- Weakness on one side of the body
- Confusion
- Loss of vision
- Any combination of the above symptoms

Pediatric Emergencies

Reacting to pediatric medical or behavioral emergencies is subject to the same guidelines as adults. Case managers working with pediatric populations are also challenged with knowing and understanding local legislation as it pertains to the age of consent. Depending on their local jurisdiction, adolescents may have a voice in the consent to release information or share protected health information. Case managers must also be aware of legislation related to the reporting of child abuse and neglect; laws may differ from state to state. The child's safety and well-being must be the priority and the case manager must always act in the child's best interest. However, always remember that the child or adolescent must remain safe. **Do not hesitate to act on a threat to a child's safety.**

Child abuse and neglect are defined as any type of cruel act inflicted on a child including physical harm, emotional abuse, neglect in care like isolation or withholding food, or sexual abuse and exploitation. **Known or suspected child abuse and neglect are subject to mandatory reporting.** Failure to report known or suspected abuse and neglect to protective agencies may be subject to criminal prosecution. If a case manager is unsure of the presence of abuse and neglect, they should consult with their supervisor or medical director. **Again, the welfare and safety of the child is paramount.**

Common Medical Conditions

This section examines some of the common medical, mental/psychiatric, and behavioral conditions that case managers may encounter in their practice. This is not a comprehensive list of diseases or conditions. Case managers have a responsibility to know and better understand disease processes and conditions of their patients.

Diabetes Mellitus

Diabetes is an endocrine disorder in which insulin, the hormone that transfers sugar from the blood to cells (for energy) during food digestion, is either not produced by the pancreas or the insulin that is produced is of inferior quality.

TYPES OF DIABETES

- Type 1; type 2; gestational

EPIDEMIOLOGY

- Diabetes mellitus is the most common form of diabetes, the one with which most are familiar. Diabetes insipidus is a different condition and is much less common and treated differently.
- Type 1 diabetes is an autoimmune destruction of the pancreatic beta cells leading to absolute insulin deficiency. In other words, the pancreas produces little to no insulin so it must be replaced by insulin injections or continuous infusion via a pump. Type 1 diabetes can be diagnosed in childhood or adulthood.
- In type 2 diabetes, the pancreas ineffectively produces insulin; either it is not strong enough to achieve its function, or it is ineffectively used by the body. This can occur as a progressive loss of insulin secretion.
- Gestational diabetes is the development of diabetes during pregnancy. Babies are often larger than normal and may have hypoglycemia after birth. Gestational Diabetes often dissipates in the mother after pregnancy but leaves her at risk of developing diabetes later in life.

CLINICAL PRESENTATION (SIGNS AND SYMPTOMS)

- Type 2 diabetes
  - Polyuria: Increased urination
  - Polydipsia: Abnormal or increased thirst

  - Nocturia: Frequent nighttime urination
  - Blurred vision
  - Weight loss
- Type 1 diabetes: Diabetic ketoacidosis is often the diagnosing factor. Children experience a rapid loss of insulin secretion whereas adults experience a less rapid loss. Adults will experience the symptoms as outlined for type 2 diabetes.

COMPLICATIONS OF POOR CONTROL

- Elevated blood glucose (hyperglycemia)
- Hyperglycemia over time will damage eyes, kidneys, and nerves.
- Heart disease
- Peripheral vasculr disease: amputations, poorly healing wounds
- Regardless of the type of diabetes, untreated hyperglycemia will result in these conditions, especially over time. Often the most damaging is severe fluctuations in high versus low blood sugar.

DIAGNOSIS

- Hemoglobin A1c: 6.5% or higher may indicate diabetes
- Fasting plasma glucose (FPG): 126 mg/dL or higher (fasting is defined as no caloric intake for at least 8 hours)
- Two-hour plasma glucose: 200 mg/dL or higher (performed with a glucose load)

DIABETES MANAGEMENT: TYPE 1

- Diet
- Exercise
- Medication
- Regardless of the type of diabetes, these are the standard treatment approaches. In type 2 it is possible for patients to manage their diabetes with diet and exercise alone!
- Insulin replacement
- Regular monitoring of blood sugar
- Dietary modifications: Balance of carbohydrates and proteins
- Exercise
- Regular monitoring of blood sugar, kidney function, blood pressure, lipids, vision, skin
- Physician follow-up: Primary care physician (PCP) quarterly; endocrinologist at least annually unless complications are present, then increased visits to an endocrinologist may be necessary.

DIABETES MANAGEMENT: TYPE 2

- Goal of treatment: Blood sugar control; prevent complications such as heart attack, stroke, kidney failure, peripheral vascular disease, and neuropathies.
- Dietary changes: Balance of carbohydrates, proteins, and fats
- Exercise
- Medications
- Weight loss
- Abstain from smoking

DIABETES SURVEILLANCE

- Hemoglobin A1c: 2 to 4 times per year
- Self-monitoring of glucose: Per MD orders
- Annual exams: Eye, kidney, serum cholesterol, blood pressure if no hypertension

RESOURCES

- American Diabetes Association (www.diabetes.org)
- National Libraries of Medicine (www.nlm.nih.gov/medline/diabetes)

HEART FAILURE

Heart failure (HF) is a cardiac clinical syndrome caused by a variety of cardiac diseases. The heart cannot pump enough blood to the body to meet its needs. It can result from any structural or functional cardiac disorder that impairs the left ventricle to fill with or eject blood.

EPIDEMIOLOGY

HF is the resulting condition with dysfunction of either ventricle or heart valves. Right-sided HF is caused by pulmonary HTN, pulmonic or mitral valve dysfunction. Left-sided HF is caused by mitral or aortic valve dysfunctions and is a common cause of right-sided HF.

CLINICAL PRESENTATION (SIGNS AND SYMPTOMS)

- Exertional angina
- Dyspnea
- Fatigue
- Fluid retention

CLASSIFICATION OF HEART FAILURE SEVERITY

- Class I: Heart disease without limitation of physical activity
- Class II: Slight limitations in physical activity
- Class III: Marked limitations in physical activity
- Class IV: Inability to continue any physical activity without discomfort

STAGES IN THE DEVELOPMENT OF HEART FAILURE

- Stage A: High risk for HF without structural heart disease or symptoms
- Stage B: Structural heart disease without symptoms
- Stage C: Structural disease with symptoms
- Stage D: Refractory HF requires specialized interventions

DIAGNOSTIC TESTS

- EKG
- Complete blood count (CBC)
- Serum electrolytes
- Liver function tests

- Fasting blood sugar
- Thyroid stimulating hormone
- Echocardiogram
- Exercise testing (measurement of maximal oxygen uptake VO_{2max}); (6-minute "walk test")
- Thallium perfusion imaging, PET scan or dobutamine echo
- Echocardiography
- Stress test
- Coronary arteriography

HEART FAILURE MANAGEMENT GUIDELINES

The therapies listed are not inclusive. Patients may be prescribed other treatments based on symptoms and cardiac structural complications.

- Stage A: At risk; lifestyle management
- Stage B: Angiotensin-converting-enzyme inhibitors (ACEi), angiotensin receptor blockers (ARB), beta-blocker, implantable cardioverter defibrillators (ICD) recommended for primary prevention of sudden cardiac death if postmotivational interviewing (MI) with LEVF 30% or less
- Stage C: Diuretics; ACEi; ARB; angiotensin receptor/neprilysin inhibitor (ARNi)
- Stage D: Determine patient's goals of care and severity of symptoms; inotropic support (milrinone, dobutamine, digoxin, levosimendan, pimobendane); left ventricular-assist device (LVAD); cardiac transplantation; palliative care

HEART FAILURE RISK FACTORS

- Past medical history of heart disease (coronary artery disease [CAD])
- Family history of heart failure
- History of a heart attack
- Poorly managed CAD and HTN will result in weaker heart function resulting in heart failure. History of a heart attack or family history of heart failure also increase risks.

GOALS OF TREATMENT

- Treat underlying conditions (CAD, HTN, disease management [DM]).
- Decrease signs and symptoms.
- Prevent further progression.
- Improve quality of life and life expectancy.
- Early diagnosis and treatment help people with heart failure to live longer and more active lives. Treatment depends on the severity of the failure.

CONSERVATIVE TREATMENT OPTIONS

- Smoking cessation
- Healthy diet
- Fluid intake
- Weight loss
- Physician-advised activity level
- Changes in habits or choices like quitting smoking, eating a healthy diet, modifying fluid intake as prescribed, losing weight, following a physician-prescribed activity level can result in decreased heart failure symptoms.

SURGICAL/PROCEDURAL INTERVENTIONS

- Implantable defibrillator (also known as cardiac resynchronization therapy)
- Pacemaker
- LVAD
- Heart transplant
- For more serious heart failure, more aggressive therapies are required. Implantable devises may be required to help the heartbeat.
  - For poor contractibility, a pacemaker will help the heart beat regularly.
  - If there is a threat that the heart could stop beating, an implantable defibrillator will jump-start the heart.
  - When the heart cannot pump enough blood to sustain life, the LVAD will be implanted to take over and assist the heart. While this device can be used long term, you typically see it before a transplant.
- A heart transplant is a life-saving intervention and listing will occur when there is little or no hope that other treatments can sustain life indefinitely.

IMPORTANT SELF-CARE

- Making and keeping regular appointments with physicians.
- Reporting weight gain over short periods of time; for example, 3 lbs or more in 24 hours.
- Controlling other conditions.
- Avoiding respiratory infections.
- These areas are where the case manager can have the most impact. These interventions require adherence on the part of the member. Promoting that adherence and self-care can make all the difference in how well the member's heart failure is managed.

RESOURCE

- 2022 AHA/ACC HFSA Guideline for the Management of Heart Failure https://doi.org/10.1016/j.jacc.2021.12.012

KIDNEY DISEASE

The kidneys, located in the mid to lower back, are about the size of a human fist. Their role is to filter waste and excess fluid from the blood; this results in urine, which is then excreted. This filtering process also helps keep the body's chemical balance, helps control blood pressure, and makes hormones. Kidney disease occurs due to an "injury" to the kidney(s) from poor vascularization and circulation, physical injury, infection, certain drugs/medication, high blood pressure, and diabetes.

TYPES OF KIDNEY DISEASE

- Chronic kidney disease (CKD)
- Kidney failure

ETIOLOGY OF KIDNEY DISEASE

CKD means that one or both kidneys are damaged and cannot filter the wastes from the blood. Over time, if CKD is not controlled, the kidneys will fail. Once this happens, dialysis or kidney transplant is required.

CLINICAL PRESENTATION (SIGNS AND SYMPTOMS)

- Fatigue
- Weakness
- Loss of appetite
- Insomnia
- Unable to think clearly
- Swelling in feet and ankles

Unfortunately, most people do not notice symptoms when the disease is in its early stages. However, as the disease progresses, an individual can expect to experience these symptoms.

RISK FACTORS

- Congenital conditions;
- Diabetes;
- High blood pressure;
- Heart disease;
- Chronic urinary tract infections;
- Urinary blockages; and
- Obesity.

Conditions in which blood flow is compromised cause kidney disease. Diabetes, HTN, and heart disease are the most common causes of kidney disease. Chronic infections and blockages also result in destruction of the kidneys which results in failure.

DIAGNOSTIC AND MONITORING TESTS

- Glomerular filtration rate (GFR): Over 60 for 3 months or more;
- Blood pressure monitoring;
- Urine albumin: 30 or higher for 3 months or more;
- Serum creatinine; and
- Albumin-to-creatine ratio (ACR).

Routine screening for kidney disease is not recommended. If a member has chronic or poorly controlled diabetes, HTN, and/or heart disease, it would be important for the physician to order these tests.

GOALS OF TREATMENT

- Prevent progression of kidney disease to kidney failure

Kidney disease is usually rated by stages. Stages 4 and 5 mean dialysis or even a kidney transplant is indicated.

MANAGEMENT OF KIDNEY DISEASE

While kidney failure may or may not be completely preventable once advanced disease is present, efforts can continue to slow the progression.

- Healthy diet and exercise
- Control blood pressure and diabetes
- Smoking cessation

- Eat less protein
- Schedule and keep regular appointments
- Medications: Vitamin supplements, calcium reducer, diuretic, iron supplement, erythropoietin, or other bone marrow stimulant with dialysis
- Dialysis (hemo- or peritoneal)
- Kidney transplant

RESOURCES

- National Kidney Foundation: https://www.kidney.org/kidney-basics
- Kidney Disease: Improving Global Outcomes (KDIGO) 2022: https://kdigo.org/wp-content/uploads/2022/10/KDIGO-2022-Clinical-Practice-Guideline-for-Diabetes-Management-in-CKD.pdf

ASTHMA

Asthma is a chronic disease characterized by acute exacerbations caused by bronchial tube swelling and increased production of mucus. Unlike COPD, the individual with asthma will have symptom-free periods. Episodes of wheezing, breathlessness, chest tightness, or early morning coughing are common symptoms, which can be controlled with medication and by avoiding the triggers.

CLINICAL PRESENTATION (SIGNS AND SYMPTOMS)

- Shortness of breath
- Chest tightness
- Chronic coughing
- Wheezing
- Trouble sleeping linked to coughing and/or wheezing

RISK FACTORS

- Having a parent with asthma
- Past history of a severe respiratory infection (especially in children)
- Allergens
- Exposure to chemicals
- Occupational exposures related to pollutants, dust, particulates
- Smoke (of any kind)
- Emotional distress
- Exercise intolerance

DIAGNOSTIC TESTS

- None—asthma is diagnosed based on the first exacerbation.

MANAGEMENT OF ASTHMA

- Education
  - How to prevent exacerbations
  - Learn what triggers exacerbations

- Avoid asthma triggers
  - Control allergies
- Annual flu vaccination
- Improving coping skills
- Asthma action plan for home, school, work
  - What to do when symptoms start
  - When to go to the emergency department
- Adherence with physician follow-up and prescribed treatment
- Medications (not an inclusive list; see the table following this section):
  - Short-acting beta agonists (SABA)—albuterol
  - Long-acting bronchodilators
  - Systemic glucocorticoids
  - Inhaled glucocorticoids
  - Long-acting beta agonists (LABA)

RESOURCES

- Global Initiative for Asthma: https://ginasthma.org/severeasthma/
- American Academy of Pediatrics: https://publications.aap.org/pediatrics/article/148/5/e2021054270/181397/Biologics-for-Asthma-and-Allergic-Skin-Diseases-in?autologincheck=redirected
- American Academy of Allergy, Asthma, and Immunology: https://www.aaaai.org/

CHRONIC OBSTRUCTIVE PULMONARY DISEASE

COPD is a group of chronic inflammatory lung diseases characterized by persistent respiratory symptoms and airflow limitation due to airway and alveolar abnormalities caused by exposure to noxious particles or gases and influenced by factors that can result in abnormal lung development.

CLINICAL PRESENTATION (SIGNS AND SYMPTOMS)

- Shortness of breath;
- Wheezing;
- Chest tightness;
- Clearing throat of excess mucus;
- Chronic cough with or without mucus;
- Cyanosis of lips or fingertips;
- Frequent respiratory infections;
- Lack of energy;
- Unintended weight loss; and
- Swelling of lower extremities.

RISK FACTORS

- Tobacco smoking; and
- Inhalation of occupational pollutants.

DIAGNOSTIC TESTS

- Lung function tests;
- Chest x-ray;
- CT scan of the chest; and
- Arterial blood gases (typically done only in the acute care setting).

COPD MANAGEMENT

- Stop smoking tobacco;
- Medications;
  - Short-acting beta agonists (SABA)
  - Short-acting muscarinic antagonists (SAMA)
  - Short-acting combination (SABA + SAMA)
  - Long-acting beta agonists (LABA)
  - Long-acting muscarinic antagonists (LAMA)
  - Combination LABA + LAMA
  - Oral steroids for exacerbations
- Pulmonary rehabilitation
  - Improve lung function
  - Improve exercise/activity tolerance
- Oxygen therapy: When lung function has deteriorated to the point of ineffective oxygenation for the body.

RESOURCES

- Global Initiative for Chronic Obstructive Lung Disease (GOLD): https://goldcopd.org/2023-gold-report-2/#
- U.S. Preventive Services Task Force: COPD Screening https://www.uspreventiveservicestaskforce.org/uspstf/document/RecommendationStatementFinal/chronic-obstructive-pulmonary-disease-screening

ANXIETY DISORDERS

Generalized anxiety disorder (GAD) is one of the most common mental disorders and is twice as common in females. GAD is often a comorbidity of depression. Genetics predispose individuals and carries a heritability with major depression and with the personality trait of neuroticism. Evidence of neurotransmitter disturbances have not been replicated, but other data suggest that acid-sensing ion channels in the amygdala and elevated levels of C-reactive protein are potentially linked to the development of GAD. Evidence of changes in neuroimaging and brain metabolism have been demonstrated in individuals with GAD.

CLINICAL PRESENTATION (SIGNS AND SYMPTOMS)

- Excessive worry (health, work, interpersonal relationships, life events);
- Worries seem realistic;
- Distress resulting in impairment of psychological functioning; and
- Increased worries over minor matters (household chores, car repairs, being late for an appointment).

RISK FACTORS

- Average age of onset is 30 years;
- Being female;
- Exposures to stressful life events in childhood or adulthood;
- Family history;
- PTSD;
- Depression; and
- History of thyroid disease, cancer, cardiac disease, irritable bowel syndrome, migraine, mitral valve prolapse, vestibular disorders, allergic conditions, respiratory disease.

ANXIETY DISORDER MANAGEMENT

- Evaluation: Assessment of past psychiatric history, general medical history, history of substance use disorder, major life events, occupational and family histories, review of medications, past treatments, and review of systems.
- Evaluate the types and severity of physical or functional impairment and suicide risk.
- Establish treatment goals.
- Educate patient, family/caregiver.
- Coordinate care with the patient's other clinicians.
- Support treatment adherence.
- Define signs of early relapse.
- Initiate cognitive behavioral therapy (CBT). Settings: outpatient; telehealth; hospitalization for extreme cases.
- Medications:
    - Serotonin-norepinephrine reuptake inhibitor (SSNRI)
    - Selective serotonin reuptake inhibitor (SSRI)
    - Tricyclic antidepressants (TCA)
    - Benzodiazepines in the absence of co-occurring mood disorder

RESOURCES

- American Psychiatric Association: https://psychiatryonline.org/pb/assets/raw/sitewide/practice_guidelines/guidelines/panicdisorder-guide.pdf
- U.S. Department of Veterans Affairs: Management of Posttraumatic stress disorder and acute stress disorder: https://www.healthquality.va.gov/guidelines/MH/ptsd/VADoDPTSDCPGFinal012418.pdf

DEPRESSIVE DISORDERS

Depressive disorders are a group of mood disorders characterized by persistent feelings of sadness and loss of interest. Depression is the most common psychiatric disorder in the general population and the prevalence worldwide is increasing. In the United States, the lifetime prevalence of depression is 21%. In patients with chronic medical illness, the prevalence rate is approximately 25%. Conditions in which depression is particularly high are central nervous system disorders (stroke, traumatic brain injury, Parkinson's), cardiovascular disorders, cancer, and conditions involving immune and inflammatory mechanisms (systemic lupus, multiple sclerosis).

TYPES OF DEPRESSIVE DISORDERS

- Major depressive disorder (MDD);
- Persistent depressive disorder (PDD);
- Bipolar disorder;
- Seasonal affective disorder (SAD);
- Postpartum depression (PPD);
- Premenstrual dysphoric disorder (PMDD); and
- Atypical depression.

RISK FACTORS

Risk factors involve genetic, medical, environmental, and social influences.

- Family history;
- Younger age;
- Female sex;
- Childbirth;
- Childhood trauma;
- Lower income;
- Poor social support;
- Stressful life events;
- Serious medical illness; and
- Substance use disorder.

CLINICAL PRESENTATION (SIGNS AND SYMPTOMS)

- Feelings of sadness, tearfulness, emptiness, hopelessness;
- Angry outbursts, irritability;
- Loss of interest or pleasure;
- Sleep disturbances;
- Anxiety, restlessness, or agitation;
- Slowed thinking or movement;
- Difficulty thinking or concentrating;
- Unexplained physical problems; somatic complaints;
- Frequent or recurrent thoughts of death or suicide;
- Changes in appetite;
- Lack of energy; and
- Change in weight.

COMPLICATIONS OF DEPRESSION

- Weight gain or obesity;
- Reluctance to acknowledge symptoms of depression;
- Alcohol or substance misuse;
- Decreased quality of life;
- Increased mortality;
- Increased economic burden; and
- Suicidal feelings or attempts.

DEPRESSION SCREENINGS

- PHQ-9;
- PHQ-2;
- Beck Depression Inventory for Primary Care; and
- WHO-5.

DEPRESSION MANAGEMENT

- Therapy:
  - Cognitive behavioral therapy
  - Psychotherapy
  - Behaviorial therapy
- Antidepressants:
  - Selective serotonin reuptake inhibitor
  - Serotonin and norepinephrine reuptake inhibitors
  - Tricyclic antidepressant
  - Anxiolytics
  - Antipsychotics
  - Electroconvulsive therapy (ECT)
- Talking therapy

Talking therapies should be the first line of treatment with medication for support. Conditions like bipolar disorder will always require medication. ECT is an option when response to therapy and medication has been ineffective. However, some researchers argue ECT should be a first-line therapy in certain situations.

RESOURCES

- National Alliance on Mental Illness (www.nami.org)
- American Psychological Association (www.apa.org)

PSYCHOTIC DISORDERS

Psychotic disorders are a group of serious mental illnesses characterized by the individual losing touch with reality and experiencing a range of symptoms including hallucinations and delusions. The conditions listed are forms of serious mental illness (SMI) and serious persistent mental illness (SPMI). The incidence of psychosis worldwide is approximately 50 in 100,000 people and schizophrenia approximately 15 in 100,000. Psychosis is a feature of many psychiatric disorders but may also be a manifestation of substance use or underlying medical disease.

TYPES OF PRIMARY PSYCHOTIC DISORDERS

- Schizophrenia;
- Schizoaffective disorder;
- Schizophreniform disorder;
- Brief psychotic disorder;
- Delusional disorders; and
- Substance- or medication-induced psychotic disorders.

CLINICAL PRESENTATION (SIGNS AND SYMPTOMS)

- Delusions and hallucinations;
- Disorganized thinking and speech;
- Premorbid features: Mood changes, neurocognitive impairments, functional decline, social isolation;
- Prodromal symptoms: Presence of psychiatric symptoms that do not meet full diagnostic criteria; delusions or hallucinations which are not serious enough to require clinical care (social irritability, poor job function, belief in magic or paranormal experiences);
- Agitation/aggression;
- Catatonia;
- Apathy, flat affect;
- Neurocognitive deficits; and
- Functional impairments.

COMPLICATIONS OF PSYCHOTIC DISORDERS

- Suicidal thoughts or attempts;
- Self-harm/injury;
- Anxiety disorders;
- Depression;
- Attention-deficit/hyperactivity disorder (ADHD);
- Metabolic disorder;
- Substance use;
- Inability to work or attend school;
- Social isolation;
- Homelessness;
- Legal and financial problems; and
- Being victimized or traumatized.

PSYCHOTIC DISORDER MANAGEMENT

- The etiology of the psychosis must first be determined: Rate of onset, age of onset, type of hallucinations, rule out medical or substance causes from primary psychiatric causes. The specific psychiatric diagnosis is determined by the time, course, and quality of symptoms.
- Medication;
  - Antipsychotics (multiple classifications);
  - Combination psychotherapeutic agents;
- CBTs;
- ECT; and
- Confinement for management.

RESOURCES

- American Psychological Association (www.apa.org)
- National Alliance on Mental Illness (www.nami.org)

SUBSTANCE USE DISORDER

SUD is a mental disorder that affects a person's brain and behavior, leading to the inability to control the use of substances such as legal or illegal drugs, alcohol, or medications. Individuals with a SUD may also experience a co-occurring mental disorder and vice versa.

RISK FACTORS

- Genetic predisposition;
- Stress;
- Trauma;
- Anxiety;
- Depression;
- PTSD;
- Being male;
- Having another mental disorder;
- Peer pressure;
- Lack of family involvement or support;
- Anxiety, depression, and loneliness; and
- Taking highly addictive prescription medications.

CLINICAL PRESENTATION (SIGNS AND SYMPTOMS)

- Frequent use of substances like alcohol, tobacco, opioids, or illicit drugs;
- Negative effects as a result of use;
- Dependence on two or more substances;
- Sudden weight loss;
- Pupils are smaller than usual;
- Changes in appetite or sleep patterns;
- Slurred speech;
- Impaired coordination of tremors;
- Deterioration of physical appearance or changes in grooming practices;
- Unusual odors on breath, body, or clothes;
- Paranoia, fearful, anxious;
- Fatigue versus periods of excess energy;
- Behavioral changes: Secretive, relationship problems;
- Changes in spending habits;
- Inability to meet obligations and responsibilities;
- Reckless behavior; and
- Legal trouble.

COMPLICATIONS OF SUD

- Move to multiple types of substances;
- Risk of contracting infectious disease;
- Accidents while under the influence;
- Suicide;

- Relationship problems;
- Work or school issues;
- Legal and financial problems;
- Short-term or long-term physical health problems; and
- Changes in the brain's structure and function.

MANAGEMENT OF SUD

- Detoxification;
  - Supervision usually required;
- Therapies:
  - Behavioral, cognitive, and dialectical
  - Therapeutic communities
  - Assertive community treatment
  - Contingency management
- Medications (opioids, tobacco, and alcohol)
- Self-help groups:
  - Alcoholics Anonymous
  - Narcotics Anonymous

RESOURCES

- National Institute of Mental Health: https://www.nimh.nih.gov/health/topics/substance-use-and-mental-health#:~:text=A%20substance%20use%20disorder%20(SUD,most%20severe%20form%20of%20SUDs
- National Institute on Drug Abuse: https://nida.nih.gov/nidamed-medical-health-professionals/screening-tools-prevention
- Substance Abuse and Mental Health Services Administration: https://findtreatment.samhsa.gov/

ATTENTION-DEFICIT/HYPERACTIVITY DISORDER

Attention-deficit/hyperactivity disorder (ADHD) manifests in childhood with symptoms of hyperactivity, impulsivity, and/or inattention. These symptoms affect cognitive, academic, behavioral, emotional, and social functioning.

CLINICAL PRESENTATION (SIGNS AND SYMPTOMS)

ADHD is a syndrome with two categories of core symptoms: hyperactivity/impulsivity and inattention. Each core symptom has its own pattern and course of development.

- Hyperactivity and impulsivity:
  - Excessive fidgetiness
  - Difficulty remaining seated when required
  - Restlessness
  - Difficulty playing quietly
  - Excessive talking
  - Difficulty in waiting turns

  - Blurting out answers too quickly
  - Interruption or intrusion of others
  - Becoming bored with a task quickly
  - Difficulty focusing attention or completing a single task or activity
- Inattention:
  - Failure to provide close attention to detail
  - Difficulty maintaining attention at school, play, or home activities
  - Seems not to listen even when directly addressed
  - Fails to follow through (homework, chores)
  - Difficulty organizing tasks
  - Avoids tasks that require consistent mental effort
  - Loses objects required for tasks (schoolbooks, sports equipment)
  - Easily distracted by irrelevant stimuli
  - Forgetfulness in routine activities
- Impaired functioning: Children with ADHD experience impairment in academic, occupational, and social skills. These impact the ability to make and maintain relationships and friendships. The behaviors associated with ADHD may result in peer rejection which results in poor self-esteem and an increased risk of anxiety and depression.

TESTING TO DIAGNOSE ADHD

- ADHD occurs in both children and adults but is most often diagnosed in childhood. Evaluation should be initiated no earlier than 4 years of age. Symptoms should be present, and a comprehensive evaluation should include medical, developmental, educational, and psychosocial assessment. See Table 9.5.

COMPLICATIONS OF ADHD

- Children with ADHD often have other conditions that make management difficult, including:
  - Poor self-esteem
  - Accidents and injuries
  - Substance use
  - Delinquent or risky behavior
  - Trouble interacting with peers
  - Excess weight and eating disorders
  - Sleep problems

ADHD MANAGEMENT

- Behavioral therapies, especially for preschool-aged children
- Alternative therapies conducted by schools and employers:
  - Educational support and assistance
  - Self-management programs
- Medications

TABLE 9.5 Differential Diagnosis for Attention-Deficit/Hyperactivity Disorder (ADHD) in Children and Adolescents[a]

	Methods to distinguish from ADHD
Developmental abnormalities or variations	
Intellectual disability	Psychometric testing
Giftedness	Psychometric testing
Normal variation	History
Neurologic or developmental disorders	
Learning disability	Psychometric testing
Language or communication disorder	Psychometric testing
Autism spectrum disorders	History; structured observation
Neurodevelopmental syndromes (e.g., fetal alcohol syndrome, fragile X syndrome, Klinefelter syndrome, childhood cerebral adrenoleukodystrophy)	History; examination; genetic testing
Seizure disorder	History; electroencephalography if clinically indicated
Sequelae of central nervous system trauma or infection	History
Motor coordination disorder	History; examination; occupational therapy evaluation
Emotional/behavioral disorders	
Depression or mood disorder	Broadband behavior scale; mental health evaluation
Anxiety disorder	Broadband behavior scale; mental health evaluation
Oppositional defiant disorder	Broadband behavior scale; mental health evaluation
Conduct disorder	Broadband behavior scale; mental health evaluation
Obsessive compulsive disorder	Broadband behavior scale; mental health evaluation
Posttraumatic stress disorder	Broadband behavior scale; mental health evaluation
Adjustment disorder	Broadband behavior scale; mental health evaluation
Psychosocial or environmental problems	
Child abuse or neglect	Medical history; psychosocial history; examination
Stressful home environment	Psychosocial history

(continued)

TABLE 9.5 Differential Diagnosis for Attention-Deficit/Hyperactivity Disorder (ADHD) in Children and Adolescents[a] (*continued*)

	Methods to distinguish from ADHD
Inadequate or punitive parenting	Psychosocial history
Parental psychopathology or substance abuse	Psychosocial history
Inappropriate educational setting	Symptoms occur at school but not at home
Frequent school absence	Psychosocial history
Selected medical conditions	
Hearing or vision impairment	Hearing and vision screen
Sleep disorder	History; sleep study as indicated by clinical findings
Iron deficiency anemia	Complete blood count and other hematologic studies as indicated
Lead poisoning	Measurement of blood lead level
Endocrine disorders (e.g., thyroid disease, diabetes mellitus)	Laboratory studies as indicated by clinical findings
Cardiac disorders (e.g., heart failure)	Medical history; echocardiograph/pediatric cardiology consultation as indicated
Substance abuse	History; toxicology screening
Food allergy	History; allergy testing as indicated
Undernutrition	Assessment of growth parameters
Medication side effects	History

[a]These conditions may mimic or co-occur with ADHD.

Source: Data from Attention-deficit and disruptive behavior disorders. (2000). In *Diagnostic and Statistical Manual of Mental Disorders* (4th edn text revision., p. 85). American Psychiatric Association; Leslie, L. K., & Guevara, J. P. (2009). Attention-deficit/hyperactivity disorder. In T. K. McInemy (Ed.), *American Academy of Pediatrics Textbook of Pediatric Care* (p. 1201). American Academy of Pediatrics; Subcommittee on attention-deficit/hyperactivity disorder, Steering committee on quality improvement and management, Wolraich, M., Brown, L., Brown, R. T., DuPaul, G., Earls, M., Feldman, H. M., Ganiats, T. G., Kaplanek, B., Meyer, B., Perrin, J., Pierce, K., Reiff, M., Stein, M. T., & Visser, S. (2011). ADHD: Clinical practice guideline for the diagnosis, evaluation, and treatment of attention-deficit/hyperactivity disorder in children and adolescents. *Pediatrics, 128*, 1007; Krull, K. (2022, May 31). Attention deficit hyperactivity disorder in children and adolescents. *UpToDate*. https://www.uptodate.com/contents/attention-deficit-hyperactivity-disorder-in-children-and-adolescents-clinical-features-and-diagnosis?search=ADHD&topicRef=623&source=see_link

RESOURCES

- ADHD Parents' Medication Guide: https://www.aacap.org/App_Themes/AACAP/docs/resource_centers/resources/med_guides/ADHD_Medication_Guide-web.pdf
- Other Concerns and Conditions with ADHD: https://www.cdc.gov/ncbddd/adhd/conditions.html
- National Institutes of Mental Health: https://www.nimh.nih.gov/health/topics/attention-deficit-hyperactivity-disorder-adhd
- American Academy of Pediatrics: https://publications.aap.org/pediatrics/article/144/4/e20192528/81590/Clinical-Practice-Guideline-for-the-Diagnosis?autologincheck=redirected

AUTISM SPECTRUM DISORDER

Autism spectrum disorders (ASD) are caused by genetic or environmental factors or a combination of these. For some, the cause is strictly a genetic mutation. Examples include Rett syndrome or fragile X syndrome. A combination of prenatal plus postnatal environmental factors may also play a role. Nongenetic factors could include parental age, maternal nutrition, metabolic status, infection during pregnancy, prenatal stress, and exposure to certain toxins, heavy metals, or drugs. The prevalence of ASD is still not well defined, but the latest statistics from 2020 suggest Hong Kong, South Korea, the United States, Japan, and Ireland hold the highest prevalence of cases. Statistics from low-income countries are not definitive due to a lack of assessment and diagnostic tools. Researchers are also examining the role of the GI system in ASD. Many individuals with ASD report GI dysfunction. The estimated prevalence of GI disturbances within the autistic population range between 20% and 86%. Abdominal pain, bloating, diarrhea, constipation, or gastroesophageal reflux are the most commonly reported GI problems, leading to a hypothesis of "leaky gut" leading to chronic inflammation. Individuals with ASD present with abnormal microbial composition which might exacerbate GI pathology and inflammatory processes. Changes to the gut microbiota and "leaky gut" directly or indirectly elicit inflammatory processes that impact cerebral function, thereby contributing to the neuropathology of ASD (Sauer, 2021).

TESTING TO DIAGNOSE AUTISM

- Historically, diagnosis of ASD featured a triad of impaired social interactions, verbal and nonverbal communication deficits, and restricted, repetitive behaviors. Despite recent advancements, there are no reliable biomarkers. Clinical diagnosis of ASD involves assessing behaviors and other disorders that may co-occur with ASD.
- There is a lack of universal screening instruments and inconsistent use, but that aside, several standardized screening tools exist. These include:
  - The Screening Tool for Autism in Toddlers and Young Children (STAT™)
  - Autism Diagnostic Observation Schedule (ADOS™)
  - Diagnostic Instrument for Social Communication Disorders (DISCO)
  - Social Communication Questionnaire (SCQ)
  - Childhood Autism Rating Scale (CARS)
  - *DSM-5*
  - M-CHAT (Lordan, 2021)

CLINICAL PRESENTATION (SIGNS AND SYMPTOMS)

- The clinical features of ASD include impairments in speech, social interaction, and repetitive or restrictive behaviors. ASD typically begins to manifest by age 3 years. Early indicators may be lack of response to one's name and discomfort maintaining eye contact. Symptoms related to social functioning and cognitive ability persist into adulthood. Communication skills may improve over time, but intellectual functioning and IQ tend to not change over time.
- The following are key features that guide diagnosis:
  - Delay in speech development
  - Learning impairment
  - Difficult social interactions
  - Impacted executive function and organized thinking
  - Difficulty processing stimuli
  - Difficulty planning steps to complete an activity
  - Behaviors may be rigid and ritualized
  - Difficulties with independent behaviors o initiating tasks
  - Stereotyped actions such as hand flapping, rocking of the body, repetitive words, or phrases
  - Sensory fixations, adherence to a specific routine
  - Aggression, hyperactivity, and impulsivity (Sauer, 2021)

MANAGEMENT/TREATMENT OF AUTISM

- Treatment of ASD is a controversial topic; approaches include attempts to improve the abilities, skills, and quality of life with a variety of behavioral and educational therapies:
  - Applied behavior analysis
  - Discrete trial training
  - Verbal behavioral intervention
  - Treatment and Education of Autistic and related Communication-Handicapped Children (TEACCH)
  - Developmental approaches (SLP, OT)

RESOURCES

- Treatment and Intervention Services for Autism Spectrum Disorder: https://www.cdc.gov/ncbddd/autism/treatment.html
- Autism Speaks: https://www.autismspeaks.org/interventions-autism
- Autism Science Foundation: https://autismsciencefoundation.org/treatment-options/

DEMENTIA

Dementia is an acquired disorder characterized by a decline in cognition: learning, memory, language, executive function, complex attention, perceptual-motor, and social cognition. As the world's population ages, the burden of dementia increases. Over 55 million people live with dementia worldwide with nearly 10 million new cases every year. Dementia results from a variety of diseases and injuries that primarily or secondarily affect the brain.

TYPES OF DEMENTIA

- Alzheimer's disease (the most common type of dementia);
- Vascular dementia;
- Mixed dementia;

- Dementia with Lewy bodies;
- Severe brain injury; and
- Frontotemporal dementia.

RISK FACTORS

- Age;
- Genetics;
- Cardiovascular disease;
- Unhealthy eating habits;
- Excessive alcohol use;
- Depression;
- Smoking; and
- Diabetes.
- Risk factors that may be reduced with proper management:
  - Depression
  - Medication side effects
  - Excessive use of alcohol
  - Thyroid problems
  - Vitamin deficiencies

DIAGNOSTIC TESTS FOR DEMENTIA

There is no one test to diagnose dementia. There is only one definitive way to diagnose Alzheimer's is by postmortem examination. The following can be used in the workup for dementia:

- Cognitive and neurological tests;
- Brain scans (stroke, tumor);
- Psychiatric evaluation; and
- Genetic tests.
- Precivity AD (examines beta amyloid and APO E in the blood; this test will determine if plaques can be seen on a brain PET scan).

DEMENTIA MANAGEMENT

- There is no cure for dementia but, if diagnosed early, some medications may help slow the progression. Medications used in Alzheimer's may be used to slow the progression of dementia.
- Medications:
  - Acetylcholinesterase inhibitors (Cholinesterase inhibitors)
  - Donepezil
  - Rivastigmine (Exelon)
  - Galantamine (Reminyl XL, Aucumor XL, Galsya XL, Gatalin XL)
- Cognitive stimulation and behavioral therapies
- NMDA receptor antagonist
  - Memantine

RESOURCES

- Alzheimer's Association: www.alz.org
- Agesp ace: https://www.agespace.org/dementia/treatments-used-dementia
- National Institute on Aging: https://www.nia.nih.gov/health/what-is-dementia

REFERENCES

Alvernia University. (2022). *Behavioral health vs mental health*. Author. https://online.alvernia.edu/program-resources/behavioral-health-vs-mental-health/

American Psychiatric Association. (2022). *What is a substance use disorder*? Addiction and Substance Use Disorders. https://www.psychiatry.org/patients-families/addiction-substance-use-disorders/what-is-a-substance-use-disorder

American Psychological Association. (2022). *APA dictionary of psychology*. Author. https://dictionary.apa.org/behavior-disorder

Heidenreich, P. E. (2022). *2022 AHA/ACC/HFSA guideline for the management of heart failure*. American College of Cardiology/American Heart Association Joint Commission on Clinical Guidelines. https://doi.org/10.1016/j.jacc.2021.12.012

Krull, K. (2022, May 31). Attention deficit hyperactivity disorder in children and adolescents. *UpToDate*. https://www.uptodate.com/contents/attention-deficit-hyperactivity-disorder-in-children-and-adolescents-clinical-features-and-diagnosis?search=ADHD&topicRef=623&source=see_link

Lordan, R. E. (2021). Autism spectrum disorders: Diagnosis and treatment. In A. Grabrucker (Ed.), *Autism spectrum disorders*. Exon Publishing. https://doi.org/10.36255/exonpublications.autismspectrumdisorders.2021.diagnosis

Malla, A. R. (2015, May). Mental illness is like any other medical illness: A critical examination of the statement and its impact on patient care and society. *Journal of Psychiatry and Neuroscience*, *40*(3), 147–150. https://doi.org/10.1503%2Fjpn.150099

Medicine, N. L. (2020, May 30). Mental disorders. *MedlinePlus*. https://medlineplus.gov/mentaldisorders.html

National Institutes of Mental Health. (2022, August). *Suicide prevention*. Author. https://www.nimh.nih.gov/health/topics/suicide-prevention

PSMJ. (2018, September 18). PSS-3: Three question suicide screener for the ER. *Patient Safety & Quality Healthcare*. https://www.psqh.com/analysis/pss-3-three-question-suicide-screener-for-the-er/

Sauer, A. E. (2021). Autism spectrum disorders: Etiology and pathology. In A. E. Sauer (Ed.), *Autism spectrum disorders*. Exon Publications. https://doi.org/10.36255/exonpublications.autismspectrumdisorders.2021.etiology

Shumway, K. (2021, September 22). Working with suicidal clients: 6 things you should know. *Time2Track*. https://blog.time2track.com/working-with-suicidal-clients-6-things-you-should-know

Tracy, N. (2019, October 23). Brain disorders: Mental disorders vs. Behavioral disorders. *Healthy Place*. https://www.healthyplace.com/other-info/mental-illness-overview/brain-disorders-mental-disorders-vs-behavioral-disorders#:~:text=The%20primary%20difference%20between%20a,also%20have%20physical%20roots%2C%20however

CHAPTER 10

Assessing the Adult Patient Through Application of the Integrated Case Management Complexity Assessment Grid

Rebecca Perez

OBJECTIVES

- Define the Integrated Case Management Complexity Assessment Grid
- Demonstrate the point scoring for each complexity item
- Define the professional case manager's actions with the scores

Introduction

This chapter puts into practice the method of integrated case management. A case study is examined and what was learned from the patient is applied to the Integrated Case Management Complexity Assessment Grid (ICM-CAG). The case is examined in detail looking at the patient's risk and possible actions to consider for a care plan. Examination of each of the risk elements will help case managers to better understand the application of the ICM-CAG as well as how to systematically address all domains of health.

Basics of the Adult Integrated Case Management Complexity Assessment Grid

The Case Management Society of America's (CMSA's) ICM-CAG was adapted in 2006 from the ICM-CAG developed in Europe and published in *The Integrated Case Management Manual: Assisting Complex Patients Regain Medical and Mental Health* (Kathol et al., 2010) and CMSA's *Integrated Case Management: A Manual for Case Managers by Case Managers* (Fraser et al., 2018).

CMSA embraced the methodology developed by the INTERMED Foundation. CMSA's adaptation, the ICM-CAG, that has been evolving since 2006, is a tool used in conjunction with a comprehensive assessment to systematically demonstrate the presence of strengths and risks. The completion of a comprehensive assessment and use of the ICM-CAG exceed assessment guidelines as outlined in *CMSA's Standards of Case Management Practice.*

This chapter also discusses conducting a comprehensive assessment using the ICM-CAG to guide case managers in determining levels of health risk. Understanding risk helps healthcare professionals develop a prioritized plan of care. As scores are applied to the individual risk elements in the ICM-CAG, a final score is created. Scores greater than 30 indicate complexity—the higher the score, the greater the complexity. Periodic reassessment using the ICM-CAG can be done as a means of demonstrating outcomes. As work is completed to reduce risk and improve health, the risk score decreases. When examining the domains and elements, examples are provided to assist in scoring. However, not every patient's situation will be covered by the examples. The case manager will need to use critical thinking to determine risks not listed. What is most important is to evaluate if risk to health and well-being are present, and if so, what level or how severe is the risk. Does mitigation of the risk require immediate action, or can the risk be prioritized lower than other identified challenges?

When working with complex patients, an assessment may take more time than anticipated, and should be conducted as a conversation, not as an interrogation. When assessing a patient who experiences a level of complexity, case managers may need to complete the

TABLE 10.1 Integrated Case Management Complexity Assessment Grid

Date:	**HEALTH RISKS AND HEALTH NEEDS**					
Name:	**HISTORICAL**		**CURRENT STATE**		**FUTURE RISK**	
Total Score =	**Complexity Item**	**Score**	**Complexity Item**	**Score**	**Complexity Item**	**Score**
Biological domain	PSMC		Symptom severity/ impairment		Complications and life threat	
	Diagnostic dilemma		Diagnostic therapeutic challenge			

(continued)

TABLE 10.1 Integrated Case Management Complexity Assessment Grid (*continued*)

Date:	**HEALTH RISKS AND HEALTH NEEDS**					
Name:	**HISTORICAL**		**CURRENT STATE**		**FUTURE RISK**	
Total Score =	**Complexity Item**	**Score**	**Complexity Item**	**Score**	**Complexity Item**	**Score**
Psychological domain	Barriers to coping		Treatment choice		Mental health threat	
	Mental health history		Mental health symptoms			
Social domain	Work and leisure		Environmental stability		Social risk	
	Relationships		Social support			
Health system domain	Reimbursement and provider access		Getting needed services		Health system deterrents	
	Treatment experience		Provider and patient collaboration			
Comments						
(Enter pertinent information about the reason for the score of each complexity item here. For example, poor patient adherence, death in family with stress to patient, nonevidence-based treatment of migraine, etc.)						
Scoring System: **0** = no need to act **1** = mild risk and need for monitoring or prevention **2** = moderate risk and need for action or development of intervention plan **3** = severe risk and need for immediate action or immediate intervention plan PSMC, persistent, sustained medical conditions.						

Biological Domain Items		Psychological Domain Items	
PSMC	In the last 5 years: Chronic conditions, persistent complaints, and history of physical injury/trauma	Barriers to coping	In the last 5 years: Problems handling stress and/or problem-solving (gambling, drinking, chronic complaining, feigning illness, participation in other risky behaviors)
Diagnostic dilemma	In the last 5 years: Historic problems in the diagnosis of physical illness; diagnostic effort	Mental health history	At any time in the patient's life: Diagnosis, treatment of, or admission for mental illness

(*continued*)

TABLE 10.1 Integrated Case Management Complexity Assessment Grid (*continued*)

Date:	**HEALTH RISKS AND HEALTH NEEDS**					
Name:	**HISTORICAL**		**CURRENT STATE**		**FUTURE RISK**	
Total Score =	**Complexity Item**	**Score**	**Complexity Item**	**Score**	**Complexity Item**	**Score**
Symptom severity/ impairment	In the last 30 days: Physical illness symptoms, severity, and presence of impairment		Treatment choice	In the last 30 days: Has the patient refused or resisted treatment; or have they made choices about whether or not to follow prescribed treatment, for various reasons		
Adherence ability	In the last 30 days: What has been interfering with the ability to follow a treatment plan (finances, social determinants, behaviors, etc.)		Mental health symptoms	In the last 30 days: Is the patient experiencing mental health symptoms, such as depressed mood, overexcitability, delusions, hallucinations, suicidal ideation, nervousness, etc.		
Complications and life threat	In the next 3–6 months: What are anticipated or expected difficulties in diagnosis, treatment, or response to treatment without CM intervention		Mental health threat	In the next 3–6 months: Risk of persistent personal barriers or poor mental condition without case management intervention		
Social Domain Items			Health System Domain Items			
Work and leisure	In the last 5 years: Working actively, able to meet financial obligations; actively working but unable to meet financial obligations; retired from employment; full-time student; full-time parent; full-time, stay-at-home partner; caregiver; volunteer. Participation in hobbies, clubs, player on sports teams, regularly scheduled social events, family outings/ events, entertaining, travel, etc.		Reimbursement and provider access	In the last 5 years: the patient has had a means to pay for healthcare (insurance, Medicare, Medicaid, etc.) and has choice in finding trusted providers		

(*continued*)

TABLE 10.1 Integrated Case Management Complexity Assessment Grid (*continued*)

Date:	**HEALTH RISKS AND HEALTH NEEDS**					
Name:	**HISTORICAL**		**CURRENT STATE**		**FUTURE RISK**	
Total Score =	**Complexity Item**	**Score**	**Complexity Item**	**Score**	**Complexity Item**	**Score**
Relationships	In the last 5 years: Able to make and maintain relationships		Treatment experience	In the last 5 years: Experiences with doctors or the health system; using ED or urgent care instead of a primary care physician (PCP)		
Environmental stability	In the last 30 days: The patient is in a safe and healthy environment, able to meet financial obligations, without violence or abuse, has access to healthy food and outdoor activities		Getting needed services	In the last 30 days: Logistical ability to get needed care at service delivery level		
Social support	In the last 30 days: The patient has readily available social support		Provider and patient collaboration	In the last 30 days: Communication and collaboration between providers and between patient and providers		
Social risk	In the next 3–6 months: The patient will not be able to work, support themselves or family, have social supports or a safe place to live without CM intervention		Health system deterrents	In the next 3–6 months: Risk of continued poor access to and/or coordination of services if without case management intervention		

assessment in more than one encounter, especially if the assessment is conducted telephonically. It is often much easier to conduct a comprehensive assessment when meeting the patient face-to-face or with a video visit. The ICM-CAG is scored based on the results of the completed comprehensive assessment to determine risk; specifically, what risks are the major contributors to a patient's complexity. Over time, as the case manager works with the patient, the risk score will reduce, and health and quality of life will improve (Table 10.1).

The ICM-CAG has continued to evolve since the first grid was published in 2010. Each domain examines where a member's risks or strengths may lie. The risk elements have been updated but continue to review history, status, and future risk or vulnerability. The risk elements are scored 0 to 3 with 0 being no risk and 3 being severe risk. The individual elements are totaled providing an overall risk score. The highest possible risk score is 60; a score of greater than or equal to 30 indicates complexity.

The four domains and the updated individual risk elements are explained in the section that follows.

ICM-CAG Domains

Each of the four ICM-CAG domains has five risk elements. The elements review history, current status, and future risk relevant to the specific domain. The detail about each risk element and strategies to decrease risk are outlined. For consistency in the scoring of the risk elements, the criteria used are reviewed:

1. Time frames
   a. History
   b. Current status
   c. Future risk

History encompasses the last 5 years. Collecting a patient's history allows case managers to understand challenges the patient has experienced in the more recent past. Knowing the patient had an appendectomy at age 12 is not relevant to their health today, so the patient's history record is capped at 5 years. However, if the patient has been treated for diabetes and heart disease for at least the last 5 years, these are conditions for that additional assessment and management will affect the case manager's work with the patient, as well as in care planning.

In the case of mental health history, the patient's entire life is examined. Any mental health or behavioral diagnoses, or challenges at any age, impact future risk and vulnerability. For example, a 47-year-old patient may not report any symptoms of depression recently, but at the age of 14 years was very depressed due to bullying at school and was hospitalized for self-mutilation (cutting). This history may impact future risk of recurrence of a depressive condition or disorder. To recap, the historical elements in all four domains, look back at the last 5 years (5 years ago to today), *except for mental health history*, that assesses the patient's lifetime.

For the current status and in all domains, the last 30 days are examined to encompass what the patient has experienced in this short time frame. This includes physical and behavioral symptoms, as well as social and care-related challenges. Based on what a case manager has learned from history and current status, the level of risk the patient may experience over the next 3 to 6 months without case management intervention can be determined.

Health Domains

BIOLOGICAL DOMAIN

The elements in this domain assess a patient's physical condition(s), duration, and severity. This includes existing chronic conditions, persistent physical symptoms, and history of physical trauma or injury. The following questions may be asked: How difficult was it to come to a diagnosis? Were significant resources utilized? How severe are the patient's symptoms? Do they result in disability for the patient? Does the patient have the ability to follow a treatment plan? Do determinants like finances, health literacy, or poor understanding interfere?

Once these elements are examined and scored, the level of risk that the patient will likely face in the next 3 to 6 months without case management intervention can be determined. The goals related to the biological domain should encompass helping the patient/family/caregiver understand their conditions, how other health domains interfere and affect physical health, and what the barriers are in preventing improvement. Examining these risk factors will help with implementation of interventions to support self-management based on ability for health improvement, health stability, and improved quality of life.

To gain a better understanding of the information needed to accurately score the present risk and suggested actions, each risk element in the biological domain is examined in the section that follows.

PERSISTENT, SUSTAINED MEDICAL CONDITIONS

Score	Risk Level	Action
0 = Less than 3 months of physical dysfunction and/or an acute condition	No risk	• No action required
1 = More than 3 months of physical dysfunction or symptoms, or intermittent dysfunction or symptoms for the past 3 months, e.g., pain, weight loss, nausea/vomiting, etc.	Mild risk	• Review with the patient their understanding of why the symptoms or dysfunction have occurred, and any contributing factors • Monitor to determine if the symptoms continue • Ensure that the patient is following up with the primary care or specialty provider
2 = Presence of one chronic disease/illness	Moderate risk	• Determine the patient's understanding of the condition and treatment • Assist the patient in simplifying management if it appears needed • Ensure the patient is keeping medical appointments • Evaluate control of the condition by reviewing any symptoms and what metrics are regularly completed: e.g., for a patient with diabetes, when was the last HgA1c completed and the results? For a patient with hypertension, how often is blood pressure checked and what was the most recent reading?

Score	Risk Level	Action
3 = More than one chronic disease/illness	Severe risk	• Are the conditions well-managed? • Customize any actions related to the results of the assessment: e.g., the patient has not had an HgA1c in over a year—important to schedule as soon as possible; a patient with heart disease who advises of intermittent chest pain—schedule an appointment with the provider as soon as possible, or refer to the emergency department if having acute symptoms • Evaluate the number of providers involved in the patient's care and report findings to the treating providers ensuring all are aware

DIAGNOSTIC DIFFICULTY

Score	Risk Level	Action
0 = No difficulty with the diagnosis of a condition; diagnosis was made easily; e.g., blood pressure has been elevated for 3 months	No risk	• No action needed
1 = A diagnosis was arrived at relatively quickly; e.g., patient exhibiting flu-like symptoms, COVID test performed and was positive for COVID-19	Mild risk	• Observe for any changes in the patient's clinical status
2 = Diagnosis made but only after considerable diagnostic workup; e.g., patient diagnosed with multiple sclerosis (MS) but only after blood work, MRI, and lumbar puncture	Moderate risk	• Review with the patient their understanding of the condition(s), prescribed treatment, what improvements are expected, and over what time frame • Assess how the patient managed the diagnostic period • Discuss what we can do to support the patient to experience a positive outcome • If the patient is having difficulty with the diagnosis, ask if they have discussed this with the physician(s) and would the patient like the case manager to communicate their concerns

Score	Risk Level	Action
3 = After significant diagnostic workup, no firm diagnosis has been made	Severe risk	• Presence of symptoms triggering multiple diagnostics, including invasive testing • Customize any interventions based on what we learn • Ask the patient what concerns them the most about not reaching a diagnosis • Offer to communicate these concerns to all involved providers

SYMPTOM SEVERITY AND IMPAIRMENT

Score	Risk Level	Action
0 = No physical symptoms or symptoms are resolved by treatment; e.g., migraine headaches are controlled by regularly scheduled Botox injections	No risk	• No action required other than to observe efficacy of current treatment
1 = Mild symptoms, but do not interfere with daily function; e.g., arthritic pain in hands but still able to knit and crochet, able to work in the garden	Mild risk	• Observe for worsening symptoms
2 = Moderate symptoms that interfere with daily functions; e.g., chronic back pain that requires rest and analgesics; may miss 1–3 days of work	Moderate risk	• Ensure primary care and other involved providers are aware of symptoms • Ensure patient is following up with providers as required • Be aware of any follow-up testing that may be ordered for worsening symptoms • Make sure patient understands condition, what to report to providers, and when to seek immediate care • If assistive interventions are required (e.g., physical therapy, durable medical equipment [DME]), assist in facilitation and coordination

Score	Risk Level	Action
3 = Severe symptoms that result in an inability to perform most daily functions; e.g., patient with chronic obstructive pulmonary disease (COPD) is unable to climb the stairs to the second floor of their home, vacuum, or walk one block to the market; a patient with multiple sclerosis is chairbound and requires assistance to bathe and use the toilet	Severe risk	• Determine what care is needed to ensure safety. Determine if the impairment is life-threatening • Update the patient's providers with any concerns or risks • Customize other actions based on what was learned from the assessment • Assess what current interventions help the patient most, what is working • Assess what is not working, where challenges lie • Evaluate the presence of social support that can aid with those activities too difficult for the patient to perform or complete • Facilitate and coordinate with collaboration from the treating physician, and provide services that might result in comfort or improvement; e.g., rehabilitation, home care

ADHERENCE ABILITY

Score	Risk Level
0 = Ability to follow a treatment plan; the treatment plan is uncomplicated	No risk
1 = The treatment plan is slightly complicated or there are interferences that make the treatment plan a bit complicated.	Mild risk
2 = The treatment plan is slightly complicated or there are deterrents interfering with the patient's ability to follow the prescribed treatment; i.e., the medication is costly and the patient has difficulty paying for it every month. These challenges may increase risk of worsening health.	Moderate risk
3 = The client is unable to follow the prescribed treatment plan due to physical symptoms, behaviors, or other determinants. These challenges place the patient at high risk of worsening health.	Severe risk

COMPLICATIONS AND LIFE THREAT

Score	Risk Level	Action
0 = Little to no risk of worsening physical symptoms and/or limitations in activities of daily living	No risk	No action required
1 = Mild risk of worsening physical symptoms and/or limitations in activities of daily living without case management intervention. Will require monitoring	Mild risk	• Encourage adherence to treatment and observe for any barriers that may appear • Work with patient to remove barriers
2 = Moderate risk of worsening physical symptoms and/or substantial limitations in activities of daily living without case management intervention	Moderate risk	• Work with the patient to address any causes for nonadherence, especially determinants • If behavioral conditions are a cause, work to coordinate needed behavioral services • Ensure patient and provider are communicating and each understands each other's goals and concerns • Monitor appropriate clinical tests and utilization; e.g., blood sugar, blood pressure, blood chemistries, scans, admissions, emergency department visits, etc. • Case management intervention may be intermittent or long term
3 = Severe risk of physical complications associated with permanent loss of function and/ or risk of death	Severe risk	• Escalate activities outlined for moderate risk • Customize actions based on assessment • Perform frequent reassessment of physical symptoms and response to prescribed treatment • Case management intervention will need to continue until risks are reduced or mitigated • If appropriate, coordinate long-term, palliative, or hospice care

PSYCHOLOGICAL DOMAIN

This domain examines an individual's ability to adapt and cope with their environment; the potential for developing a mental health disorder; follow a physician's treatment plan; and respond to treatment for psychiatric illnesses that lead to dysfunction and suffering. This also includes substance use disorders and behavioral conditions without the presence of mental illness.

BARRIERS TO COPING

Score	Risk Level	Action
0 = The ability to manage stress, life situations, and health concerns by seeking support or participating in activities that result in relaxation and satisfaction, e.g., seeking medical advice, hobbies, social activities, meditation, yoga, etc.	No risk	• No action required
1 = Limited coping skills, such as a need for control, denial of illness, and irritability/impatience	Mild risk	• Help the patient identify stressors and support to reduce stress levels • Encourage counseling to gain insight into positive coping strategies
2 = Impaired coping skills, such as chronic complaining, alienation of support system, substance use (self-medication) but without serious impact on medical conditions, mental health, or social situation	Moderate risk	• Encourage counseling to gain insight into positive coping strategies that may include specific stress-reduction techniques or conflict-resolution training • Recommend Employee Assistance Program (EAP) for any work-related stressors • If living arrangements, work location, or social activities or relationships seem to cause stress, discuss with the patient strategies to change to reduce and eliminate stressors • Screen for alcohol/substance use/abuse if needed • Consider reaching out to the patient's provider if substance/alcohol abuse are of concern or if the patient may benefit from a mental health professional referral'

Score	Risk Level	Action
3 = Poor or absent coping skills manifested by destructive behavior like substance abuse/dependence, gambling, promiscuity, psychiatric illness, self-mutilation, suicide attempts, and failed/failing social relationships	Severe risk	• Engage patient to determine stressors • Customize actions based on what was learned in the assessment • Assist in the development of a crisis intervention plan that may include the patient's support system and providers • Collaborate with providers for a mental health referral for assessment and treatment recommendations • Support and encourage mental health treatment with the patient • Collaborate with the patient's care provider for a referral to substance/alcohol abuse treatment if appropriate • Support and encourage participation in substance/alcohol abuse treatment if appropriate

MENTAL HEALTH HISTORY

Score	Risk Level	Action
0 = No history of mental health problems or conditions	No risk	• No action required
1 = Known mental health problems or conditions, but resolved or without clear effects on daily function; e.g., well-controlled anxiety or depression	Mild risk	• Encourage regular primary care screenings for mental conditions with intervention, if appropriate • Check for access to support from mental health professionals • If medication ordered, assess for adherence and efficacy

Score	Risk Level	Action
2 = Known mental health conditions that have clear effects on daily function, the need for therapy, medication, day treatment, or a partial inpatient program	Moderate risk	• Ensure the patient's understanding of potential for recurrence of mental health conditions by using lay language • Support medication adherence and monitor for efficacy • Understand the potential for medical and physical condition interactions, if indicated • Facilitate and coordinate visits and regular follow-up with a psychiatrist and/or mental health team (psychologists, social workers, nurses, substance use disorder and other counselors); provide support when conditions destabilize • Facilitate, coordinate, and support follow-up with the patient's care provider • Refer to a medical home, if available, to ensure all needed services are provided in onsetting • Monitor patient symptoms over time (e.g., Patient Health Questionnaire-9 [PHQ-9] and generalized anxiety disorder-7 [GAD-7]) • Assist with communication among physical and mental health-treating clinicians
3 = Psychiatric admissions and/or persistent effects on daily function due to mental illness	Severe risk	• Monitor symptoms • Support medication adherence • Include customized actions based on interview • Facilitate communication between the mental health team for mental conditions and with the primary care providerss who care for concurrent physical illness • Collaborate with providers to develop transition plans that will prevent readmissions • Support, encourage, and assist the patient to make and keep appointments with providers, especially mental health providers • Facilitate and coordinate any outpatient services ordered by the treating physician to help stabilize the patient's mental illness(es) • Facilitate and coordinate appropriate social support for the patient to prevent symptom exacerbation and readmission

Treatment Choice

Score	**Risk Level**	**Action**
0 = Interested in receiving treatment and willing to cooperate actively	No risk	• No action required
1 = Some ambivalence or hesitation, though willing to cooperate with prescribed treatment	Mild risk	• Educate patient/family about illnesses • Initiate discussions with patient about willingness to recognize conditions and follow prescribed treatments using motivational-interviewing and problem-solving techniques to facilitate change • Explore other barriers to treatment adherence • Inform providers of adherence problems and work with them to consider alternative interventions, if needed • Monitor adherence and response to any prescribed treatment
2 = Considerable resistance and nonadherence; hostility or indifference toward healthcare professionals, OR patient making choices about treatment based on their circumstances that result in not completely adhering or only partially adhering to prescribed treatment (both medical and mental health treatment)	Moderate risk	• Evaluate prescribed treatment, the patient's ability, and willingness to adhere • Actively explore and attempt to reverse other sources of resistance (e.g., family member's negativism, religious objections, cultural influences, and relationships with treating physician)
3 = Active resistance to important medical care	Severe risk	• Attempt to determine the source of resistance • Ask permission to share expected outcomes of prescribed treatment and consequences of resistance so that patient can make an informed decision • Include customized actions based on interview • Collaborate with treating clinicians in considering and instituting alternative interventions • If needed, work with case management medical director to find second opinion practitioners • If significant resistance exists and is pervasive, consider discontinuation of case management

MENTAL HEALTH SYMPTOMS

Score	Risk Level	Action
0 = No mental health symptoms	No risk	• No action required
1 = Mild mental health symptoms, such as problems with concentration or feeling tense or nervous but do not interfere with current functioning	Mild risk	• Ensure the patient is receiving primary care treatment with access to support from mental health professionals • Facilitate communication among all treating providers
2 = Moderate mental health symptoms, such as anxiety, depression, or mild cognitive impairment, that interfere with current functioning	Moderate risk	• Facilitate mental health evaluation • Ensure that acute maintenance and continuation of treatment is being provided by primary care providerss with mental health support • Facilitate primary maintenance and continuation of treatment provided by primary care providers in a medical home, if possible, with mental health specialist assistance; e.g., a psychiatrist and mental health team (psychologists, social workers, nurses, substance abuse counselors, etc.) when condition destabilizes, becomes complicated, or patient demonstrates treatment resistance • Evaluate and assess symptoms and document using the PHQ-9, GAD-7, and patient report; report concerns to providers • Develop a crisis plan with the patient and with provider input
3 = Severe psychiatric symptoms and/or behavioral disturbances; e.g., violence, self-inflicted harm, delirium, criminal behavior, psychosis, hallucinations,or mania	Severe risk	• Assess the patient's safety for self and others • Include customized actions based on interview • Support active and aggressive treatment for mental conditions by a mental health team working in close collaboration with the patient's primary care provider • When possible, encourage geographically collocated physical and mental health personnel to facilitate ease of coordinating appointments and treatment; e.g., medical home or primary care provider practices in the same vicinity • Evaluate and assess symptoms and document using the PHQ-9, GAD-7, and patient report; report any concerns immediately to providers; always make patient safety a priority

MENTAL HEALTH THREAT

Score	Risk Level	Action
0 = No evidence of new or worsening mental health conditions	No risk	• No action required
1 = Need to observe for worsening mental health/ behavioral symptoms	Mild risk	• Facilitate and coordinate access to appropriate mental health supports and services • Support and encourage follow-up care with providers and perform intermittent mental health assessments, to monitor symptoms, e.g., PHQ-9 and GAD-7 • Encourage and support coping and stress-reduction activities; can be formal or informal
2 = Worsening mental health symptoms	Moderate risk	• Assist the patient in knowing where and from whom to get assistance: primary care provider, psychiatrist, counselor, and the like • Assess symptoms related to depression and anxiety by using tools. such as PHQ-9 and GAD-7 • Facilitate communication among medical and behavioral providers as necessary; facilitate access to an integrated medical home if possible • Promote and encourage adherence to prescribed treatment • Involve caregivers of the patient if agreeable and receive consent in all activities
3 = Severe and persistent worsening of a known mental health disorder	Severe risk	• Assess for patient safety and the safety of family or caregivers. Include interventions that are specific to the patient's prescribed treatment: medication, therapy, or other more aggressive interventions • Work with the patient's clinicians to understand the clinical goals and assist the patient with understanding and with removal of barriers to achieve goals • Patient may need long-term case management involvement • The patient may require inpatient or intensive outpatient psychiatric admission to stabilize condition

SOCIAL DOMAIN

In the social domain, the patient's safety, support, and independence are assessed. The social domain examines the patient's ability to work, to support themselves and others as appropriate, attend school, meet financial obligations, be a caregiver for another, function in social situations, have a safe living environment, access social support when needed, and have quality social relationships. The ability to support oneself and important others, and participate in activities that bring joy, fulfillment, and happiness, reduce the potential for experiencing determinants that contribute to poor health. Addressing health needs becomes significantly more of a challenge if social supports are lacking or absent. Another consideration might be the "work/life" balance that is essential to all health and well-being.

Work and Leisure

Score	Risk Level	Action
0 = Patient works or has retired from gainful employment, is furthering education, is a stay-at-home parent or homemaker, volunteers time, has leisure activities that include clubs, hobbies, travel, and sports	No risk	• No action required
1 = Patient works or is retired (as described in item 0), but without leisure activities	Mild risk	• Discuss with the patient past experiences with leisure activities what have they enjoyed • Is the patient interested in resuming or finding a leisure activity?
2 = Patient has leisure activities but does not work now or for the last 6 months	Moderate risk (excludes retirees)	• Discuss with patient their ability to work, willingness to work, or to go to school • Make referrals to appropriate resources: Social Security for disability, social services for educational and vocational resources, job placement services • If unable to return to work, provide information on how to access public assistance programs or resources to assist with disability applications if health-related • Follow-up in a timely manner to ensure the patient has been able to access any needed resources and assist as necessary • Encourage any interest in leisure activities
3 = No work for more than 6 months and without leisure activities	Severe risk (excludes retirees)	• Explore the impact of not having a job and income; has this impacted the ability to access health services? • Access to public assistance may be more of an urgency; look for community resources that could assist in the interim

Relationships

Score	Risk Level	Action
0 = No social disruptions; no dysfunctional relationships	No risk	• No action required
1 = Mild social disruptions or interpersonal problems; arguing with family or friends but usually resolving differences with time	Mild risk	• If possible, observe the patient's interactions with family or providers • If the patient allows, engage family in conversations with the patient
2 = Moderate social dysfunction, social relationships are tenuous, no strong friendships or family ties, would rather be alone. The patient is victim to overbearing caregivers who control social interactions	Moderate risk	• Encourage the patient to include family or other supporting acquaintances to be involved in care • Assess if social issues have any impact on the patient's health; e.g., has no one to call when sick • Assess if the patient is open to working with a counselor to improve social skills • Explore with the patient if there are social activities in that they might be willing to participate • Engage caregivers to determine cause of social controls; support socialization for the patient as long as safety is not an issue
3 = Severe social dysfunction social isolation unable to "get along" with family, friends, coworkers, and neighbors; argumentative and hostile	Severe risk	• Engage patient in conversation about social support: Do they have any? Do they want support? What do they think needs to happen to secure support? • Facilitate behavioral health assessment due to disruptive and/or destructive behaviors • If no mental health threat, recommend the patient participates in support groups and/or counseling to address behaviors

Environmental Stability

Score	Risk Level	Action
0 = Stable housing, stable living arrangements, able to live independently	No risk	• No action required

Score	**Risk Level**	**Action**
1 = Stable housing with support of others; e.g., family available to assist, receiving home care or home- and community-based services, or living in an institutional setting like assisted living, group home, or long-term care facility. Usually able to meet financial obligations but may require assistance with resources for rent/mortgage, food, utilities, daily essentials; current housing is stable	Mild risk	• Facilitate and coordinate additional support where and when needed; this may require looking for community supports or resources, when services are not reimbursed; e.g., church volunteers, extended family, friends, or coworkers willing to provide support • Locate community resources that can assist with financial obligations, such as rent/mortgage, food, or utilities • Make frequent assessments for potential changes in the patient's needs
2 = Unstable housing; e.g., no support at home or living in a shelter; inability to meet financial obligations related to housing; neighborhood is unstable (patient is afraid to go out at night, fearful of walking in the neighborhood, living far from social support and food sources); there may be need to change the current housing situation	Moderate risk	• Consult with social services or community housing resources to explore housing options if this is what the patient wants • Consult with social services or community resources to assist with meeting financial obligations; explore with the patient their willingness to include family and friends in providing more support • Be timely with follow-up on availability and coordination of needed resources
3 = No current satisfactory or safe housing; e.g., homeless, transient housing (couch surfing), or dangerous environment (abuse, neglect, dwelling is in severe disrepair or compromised by disease vectors); an immediate change is needed	Severe risk	• Immediately connect the patient with safe housing; e.g., emergency shelter or shelter with trusted individual. Safety is the priority. If abuse or neglect is present, contact the appropriate local authority to assist in getting the patient to a safe place. Follow-up with options as soon as the patient is safe and in safe housing; consult with social services and/or community housing resources. • Follow-up on coordination of safe housing is a prioritized action • If appropriate, contact housing authority for needed repairs or mitigation of other unsafe living situations unrelated to violence; e.g., vermin or insect infestations, unsafe structures

SOCIAL SUPPORT

Score	Risk Level	Action
0 = Assistance is readily and always available from family, friends, coworkers, or acquaintances (e.g., church or club members)	No risk	• No action required
1 = Assistance is generally available from family, friends, coworkers, or acquaintances but may be sporadic and not always available when needed	Mild risk	• Assess what assistance is needed • Discuss with patient who are their supports? Ask patient to provide names and availability; suggest to patient development of a "call list" with whom to call first, second, third, etc. • Develop contingency plan for assistance when no one is available; e.g., transportation to appointments, what to do in an emergency
2 = Limited assistance from family, friends, coworkers, or acquaintances; e.g., family does not live close, patient has a limited social circle	Moderate risk	• Discuss with patient and social supports who can assist and when • Develop contingency plan for assistance when no one is available; e.g., transportation to appointments, what to do in an emergency • Assess for in-home support by home health agencies or volunteer organizations if appropriate
3 = No assistance available from family, friends, coworkers, or acquaintances at any time	Severe risk	• Assess for the need and availability of in-home supports; e.g., home and community-based services • Coordinate needed transportation, access to food • Discuss with patient and providers the need for transfer to a setting that will provide more safety and support; e.g., assisted living, retirement community, group home

Social Risk

Score	Risk Level	Action
0 = No risk present that warrants the need to change the living situation; dwelling is safe, social supports are present, and the patient can meet financial obligations	No risk	• No action required
1 = Some assistance might be needed to ensure social supports are available when needed, or there is a need to monitor changes	Mild risk	• Work with the patient to determine if current supports will be available in the future • If in-home supports are needed, determine the length of time needed and availability of the services for that period • Make sure contingency plan is developed for long-term use
2 = Risk exists that would result in the patient having little to no social support, will be unable to meet financial obligations or keep medical appointments	Moderate risk	• Work with the patient and any available support to determine if the current support will continue to be available, regardless of frequency • Explore availability of community and social resources to assist with financial obligations, access to food, etc. • Review benefits/reimbursement to ensure any coordinated services can be extended long term and evaluate if the patient is eligible for any services/reimbursement currently not in play • If unable to extend in-home services, community resources, and social support, explore placement options
3 = Immediate; need for the determination of any support, assistance with meeting financial obligations, emergency planning, and/or placement in a safe environment	Severe risk	• Explore with the patient next steps to improve health status going forward • Expedite placement to a safe environment if home-based options are not feasible • Help the patient understand the need for a safe environment

HEALTH SYSTEM DOMAIN

There is a belief that if an individual gets the right diagnosis and prescribed treatment, there is no reason to believe that their health will not improve. But often no heed has been paid to an individual's challenges in getting needed services. This domain examines where and how a patient accesses care. Do they have resources for reimbursement, and do they have faith and trust in their providers? Trust in the healthcare providers' ability to navigate the system directly impacts health.

REIMBURSEMENT AND PROVIDER ACCESS

Score	Risk Level	Action
0 = The patient has health benefit coverage with little to no financial burden; providers are geographically convenient, and are sensitive and aware of culturally diverse groups.	No risk	• No action required
1 = Some difficulty accessing care; long travel to providers; limited access to specialists like psychiatrists; long waits to get appointments; high deductibles, high pharmacy co-pays; providers who meet preferred cultural practice of language not readily available	Mild risk	• Assist the patient in researching providers who meet their preferences for culture or language • Assist patients in making appointments • Discuss medications with high co-pays with pharmacy staff or medical director to see if peer-to-peer could result in more affordable medication • Facilitate telehealth visits when providers are not geographically convenient or with providers who culturally and linguistically appropriate
2 = Difficulty accessing care due to geography, language, culture, insurance coverage, or premiums; limited provider network. The risk is similar to the description for mild risk, but everything is more complicated. Act on this risk more quickly addressing the interventions outlined in mild risk	Moderate risk	• Speak with provider offices to facilitate expedited appointments or coordinate multiple appointments in 1 day so that travel is reduced • Assist with filling gaps in care; e.g., lack of counselors; facilitate telephone or telecommunication software for access to counseling services • If insurance costs are too high, explore what other options may be available to the patient
3 = No adequate access to care due to geography, language, culture, insurance coverage, high deductible or co-pays, or premiums; benefits for some services are excluded, such as mental health or substance abuse treatment	Severe risk	• Immediately act on the interventions outlined for mild and moderate risk • Contact social services to see if the patient might qualify for access to specialty clinics • Collaborate with the patient's pharmacy for prescription drug assistance • Work with social worker to make sure the patient is receiving any and all healthcare benefits and programs for that they are eligible (i.e., dual eligibility)

TREATMENT EXPERIENCE

Score	Risk Level	Action
0 = No problems with healthcare providers	No risk	• No action required
1 = Less than positive experiences with healthcare systems, organizations, or providers; less than satisfied with providers, have not been able to find a provider that instills trust and caring; feels treated like a number, not a person	Mild risk	• Ask the patient to describe their experiences • Ask the patient if they were able to follow prescribed treatment plans • Ask the patient to describe the attributes of the perfect provider • Help the patient better prepare for provider visits by coaching them on the types of questions to ask; recommend the patient write down the questions to take to appointments
2 = The patient may have changed providers many times due to dissatisfaction; no primary care provider; sees multiple providers; might be using the emergency department or urgent care instead of making appointments with a primary care provider	Moderate risk	• Use questions from the mild risk category • Have the patient describe the conflicts and then assist the patient in resolving conflicts with practitioners if possible by communicating their concerns or coach the patient on how to inform the provider about their dissatisfaction • Review the recommended treatment plan with the patient; ask if this is a plan the partient can follow and if not, why not; facilitate communication of those concerns to the provider • If conflicts do not seem to be resolved, ask the medical director to speak with the provider • If the patient is still not happy with the provider, help the patient find a new provider
3 = Repeated provider conflicts; emergency department use	Severe risk	• Attempt to utilize the strategies outlined in moderate risk • Speak with providers for their perspective to see if a mental health evaluation is warranted • Coach the patient on how to resolve conflicts with their provider(s). If conflicts cannot be resolved, assist the patient in finding a new primary care provider • Educate the patient on when and how to use the emergency department; emphasize how repeated use interferes with condition-changing care and health improvements

GETTING NEEDED SERVICES

This category relates to the logistics of getting care: easy access to needed services, transportation to appointments, care is coordinated and delivered in a timely manner; assistance as needed and warranted is received.

Score	Risk Level	Action
0 = No difficulty getting services	No risk	• No action required
1 = Some difficulties in getting to appointments or needed services like medications, medical supplies, durable medical equipment, etc.	Mild risk	• Explore the barriers preventing access • Coordinate and facilitate the services need to ensure adequate access • Communicate with supplying providers to ensure they can fulfill care in a timely manner • If mental health or substance use services are needed but not reimbursed, assist the patient in locating low-cost or free community services
2 = Routine difficulties in coordinating and/or getting to appointments or receiving needed services	Moderate risk	• Assist the patient in getting appointments when convenient and in booking multiple appointments in one day • Facilitate consistent and reliable transportation • Facilitate referrals to specialists; intervene if the patient is unable to secure a timely appointment for their condition • Help the patient locate and facilitate needed mental health or substance use services when appropriate
3 = Inability to coordinate and/or get to appointments or needed services	Severe risk	• Include interventions from moderate risk • Determine what is interfering with getting needed services • Explore available services and resources in the patient's community or nearby

Provider and Patient Collaboration

Score	Risk Level	Action
0 = Patient able to communicate effectively with all practitioners and practitioners communicate with each other; there are no problems with coordination of care	No risk	• No action required

Score	Risk Level	Action
1 = Primary care practitioner coordinates all care, including mental health services; limited communication if patient has more than one practitioner; patient does not always understand prescribed treatment; the patient does not know how to communicate with a provider; does not know what questions to ask	Mild risk	• Coach the patient on how to communicate with providers. • Communicate with primary care provider that if assistance is needed in the coordination of care, case management can assist • Make the patient aware that integrated practices are available; e.g., patient-centered medical home (PCMH) or health home • Facilitate communication among practitioners and provide medication lists, appointment dates, etc. • Coach the patient to update the primary care provider of any services received outside of the primary care practice
2 = Lack of communication among providers related to a patient's conditions and ordered treatment; the patient does not know how to communicate with the provider; does not keep the primary care provider informed of care sought outside of the primary care practice; does not relay side effects or challenges with prescribed treatment	Moderate risk	• Include interventions from mild risk • Help the patient schedule same-day appointments for different problems. Patient can be instructed to bring summary of each visit to the next session • Communicate with all practitioners so that you can facilitate coordination of needed care and services • Suggest accessing care at an integrated clinic (e.g., PCMH or health home)
3 = No communication among providers and no responsible party for care coordination resulting in delayed or missed care and services or adverse events related to prescribed care that is contraindicated; the patient does not participate in any shared decision-making related to their care	Severe risk	• Include interventions from moderate risk • Attend provider visits with the patient if possible • Speak with treating practitioners on behalf of the patient, with the patient's permission (may need to have written consent) • Provide treating providers a list of medications or other prescribed treatments to prevent adverse events

HEALTH SYSTEM DETERRENTS/VULNERABILITY

Score	**Risk Level**	**Action**
0 = No risk or concern that care between medical and behavioral providers is not coordinated; no issues with insurance or reimbursement	No risk	• No action required
1 = Mild risk of health system challenges, such as insurance coverage restrictions, geographical access to care, inconsistent or limited communication among providers, or inconsistent coordination of care without case management intervention	Mild risk	• Examine with the patient any insurance coverage restrictions or deterrents like high deductible, or coinsurance, exclusions • Investigate community resources for services not covered by insurance; e.g., counseling, other mental health services • Determine with the patient if they have the resources to maintain insurance coverage • If there is a threat to maintaining coverage, strategize how to mitigate that threat • Is it possible for the patient to continue to see providers who are not geographically convenient? • Continue to facilitate communication among providers
2 = Moderate risk of health system challenges related to insurance coverage restrictions, potential loss of insurance coverage, geographical access to care, poor communication among providers, and poor care coordination without case management intervention	Moderate risk	• Include interventions from mild risk • Assist with finding resources to continue affordable health insurance coverage if unable to maintain current coverage • Facilitate care in a medical home to improve communication and care coordination if possible
3 = Severe risk of health system challenges, such as no health insurance, limited coverage, providers resistant to communication, and no obvious coordination of care	Severe risk	• Include all interventions for moderate risk but elevate the priority for implementation

The following case study assessment is an application of the ICM-CAG:

CASE STUDY

Randy is a 45-year-old construction worker admitted to the hospital 2 weeks ago with chest pain and shortness of breath. Randy is single, lives with his elderly, frail mother, and has been laid off work for 3 months. He was diagnosed with hypertension and atrial fibrillation 4 years ago. He is morbidly obese with a BMI of 42. During this recent admission, Randy required cardioversion for uncontrolled atrial fibrillation, was newly diagnosed with type 2 diabetes, congestive heart failure, and central sleep apnea. Randy's blood sugar on admission was 600; he had significant edema in his lower extremities and elevated brain natriuretic peptide (BNP). Two sleep studies were required to diagnose central sleep apnea. Cardiac testing during the admission revealed a low ejection fraction. He was able to ambulate only 50 to 75 feet on admission but is now able to ambulate 100 to 150 feet without getting short of breath. Randy's length of stay was 10 days. He was discharged on insulin, with instructions to test his blood sugar at least twice per day, to follow-up with his primary care provider in 7 days, and to see a cardiologist. Randy receives care from a university clinic staffed by residents and medical students. He rarely sees the same resident twice. A BiPap was ordered for Randy to use during sleep. Randy did not receive insulin or testing supplies for 3 days after discharge due to poor communication between the patient and the hospital. Randy did not understand that he had to take the prescriptions to the pharmacy to be filled; he thought the hospital had already sent the orders. Randy called the university clinic, but they had no record of his discharge orders.

Randy does not have a history of any mental or behavioral conditions. He does, however, seem to be a bit nonchalant about recent health events. Randy shared that his dad had diabetes and "it was no big deal." It is important to note that Randy's father passed away from renal failure as a result of his diabetes. He also shared that he wants to return to work.

Randy's line of work is very physical, carrying heavy loads, shoveling, and transporting rock, working in the elements, and the like. He does not seem to have a good understanding about the seriousness of his conditions.

As stated earlier, Randy has been laid off from work for the last 3 months. He has been a member of a bowling team for the last 10 years with the same teammates. He has a sister in town, but she is a single mother working two part-time jobs. Randy lives with his mother, who owns the home, and he is a caregiver for his mother, helping with cooking, household chores, and transportation. Randy has health coverage through his construction union, but eligibility is maintained by hours worked. Unless he returns to work, his health coverage will lapse in 4 months.

Date:	**HEALTH RISKS AND HEALTH NEEDS**					
Name: Randy	**HISTORICAL**		**CURRENT STATE**		**VULNERABILITY**	
Total Score = 36	**Complexity Item**	**Score**	**Complexity Item**	**Score**	**Complexity Item**	**Score**
Biological domain	Persistent, sustained medical conditions	**3**	Symptom severity/ impairment	**3**	Complications and life threat	**3**
	Diagnostic difficulty	**2**	Adherence ability	**3**		
Psychological domain	Barriers to coping	**1**	Treatment choice	**1**	Mental health threat	**2**
	Mental health history	**0**	Mental health symptoms	**0**		
Social domain	Job and leisure	**1**	Environmental stability	**1**	Social vulnerability	**3**
	Relationships	**0**	Social support	**2**		
Health system domain	Reimbursement and provider access	**1**	Getting needed services	**3**	Health system deterrents	**3**
	Treatment experience	**2**	Provider collaboration	**3**		

Scoring System:
0 = no vulnerability or need to act
1 = mild vulnerability and need for monitoring or prevention
2 = moderate vulnerability and need for action or development of intervention plan
3 = severe vulnerability and need for immediate action or immediate intervention plan

Randy has always accessed care at the university clinic where his mother seeks care; the clinic is 50 miles from his residence. Randy never sees the same physician twice as the clinic is staffed by medical school residents. Randy's mother is a Medicare and Medicaid recipient and has always sought care at the clinic. Even though Randy has health coverage through his union, he has continued to attend the clinic because he was responsible for getting his mother to her appointments. Randy's current health coverage will expire in 4 months due to the time off work. He has the option of paying Consolidated Omnibus Budget Reconciliation Act (COBRA) insurance for a time but will need to eventually find another method of health coverage.

Rationale for Scoring

Review the reasons for that the documented risk scores were applied to the ICM-CAG based on the information learned from Randy's assessment.

Biological Domain

- **Chronic Illness Score = 3**: Randy has a 4-year history of hypertension and atrial fibrillation. Two weeks ago, he was diagnosed with diabetes, heart failure, and central sleep apnea during the recent admission; a high BMI resulted in a diagnosis of morbid obesity.
- **Diagnostic Difficulty Score = 2:** Two sleep studies were conducted to diagnose the central sleep apnea. This condition differs from obstructive sleep apnea but causes the same complications. The diabetes was not diagnosed before this admission that makes us concerned that this may have been missed during any previous clinic visits.
- **Symptom Severity Score = 3:** Randy had shortness of breath and chest pain that resulted in the recent admission. He also is limited in ambulation because of these symptoms, that are considered severe.
- **Adherence Ability Score = 3:** Randy appears to have a poor understanding of the seriousness of his condition which contributes to his inability to adhere to a treatment plan. The seriousness of his conditions will require behavioral changes to improve diet, activity, follow-up visits, and medication.
- **Complications and Life Threat Score = 3:** Without the assistance of case management, Randy's chronic conditions will likely continue to be uncontrolled. The severity of his current conditions could lead to severe disability or death.

Psychological Domain

- **Barriers to Coping Score = 1:** While Randy does not appear to have difficulty coping, his reaction to the seriousness of his medical conditions may indicate a form of denial; there is a need to observe and question a bit deeper regarding his ability to cope.
- **Mental Health History Score = 0:** Randy has no history of mental illness.
- **Treatment Choice Score = 2:** Worsening health indicates Randy has not taken steps to control his conditions. His lack of insight may not be conscious or intentional, but his cavalier attitude is concerning.
- **Mental Health Symptoms Score = 0:** Randy exhibits no symptoms of any mental or behavioral conditions.
- **Mental Health Threat Score = 2:** This score may be surprising, but Randy's lack of concern for his worsening health over the next 3 to 6 months without case management support and interventions, will result in further inability to cope with his serious health conditions. His lack of understanding, or laissez-faire approach to health, will prevent improvement.

Social Domain

- **Work and Leisure Score = 1:** Randy has been off work for 3 months and has participated in leisure activities being a longtime member of a bowling team. Randy has a personal goal of returning to work.
- **Relationships Score = 0:** There is no evidence that Randy has any difficulties with developing or maintaining relationships.
- **Environmental Stability Score = 1:** Randy lives with his mother who owns the home. However, because he is out of work, there is a potential that it may be difficult to pay for living expenses. He also functions as a caregiver.
- **Social Support Score = 2:** Randy is his frail elderly mother's primary caregiver and his sister has limited ability to assist. Randy has his bowling team friends but we do not yet know if any of them are available to assist Randy if needed. There is no plan in place should Randy's health decline.
- **Social Vulnerability Score = 3:** There are serious concerns about what will happen because Randy will likely be unable to return to work any time soon, if ever. Will he have needed financial resources to buy food, pay utilities, and so on? Since he is the primary caregiver for his mother, if his health worsens, who will care for her and be there to assist him?

Health System Domain

- **Reimbursement and Provider Access Score = 1:** Randy has had good health coverage and access to providers nearby but has chosen to seek care from a university clinic 50 miles away. His eligibility for health coverage is based on hours worked. If he does not return to work soon, he will lose coverage in 4 months.
- **Treatment Experience Score = 1:** Randy has seen a different practitioner with nearly every visit to the clinic. This has likely contributed to the poor management of his conditions.
- **Getting Needed Services Score = 3:** Randy has access to care but has chosen to seek care at the university clinic where his mother seeks care. His recent decline in health, specifically the diagnosis of significantly uncontrolled diabetes, is likely due to inconsistent care and communication by the clinic staff. He did not receive diabetes medication and testing supplies after dischargedue to a poor care transition.
- **Provider Collaboration Score = 3:** It is unclear if the discharge orders were received by the university clinic. Randy did not receive needed supplies or instructions; even when he called the clinic, it seemed they were unaware of his discharge needs. He rarely sees the same provider twice at the clinic; communication at the clinic appears to be inconsistent.
- **Health System Deterrents Score = 3:** Randy is at significant risk of worsening health unless the case manager can assist him in maintaining insurance coverage. His health will likely not improve without assistance from providers who better communicate and address his needs. He will need to access a primary care physician and appropriate specialists closer to his home.

REFERENCES

Fraser, K., Perez, R., & Latour, C. (2018). *CMSA's integrated case management: A manual for case managers by case managers* (1st ed.). Springer Publishing Company.

Kathol, R. G., Perez, R., & Cohen, J. S. (2010). *The integrated case management manual: Assisting complex patients regain physical and mental health.* Springer Publishing Company.

CHAPTER 11

Assessing the Pediatric Patient Using the Integrated Case Management Complexity Assessment Grid

Rebecca Perez

OBJECTIVES

- Interpret the Integrated Case Management (ICM) process for children/adolescents with health complexities
- Compare the similarities and differences between the adult and pediatric complexity assessment grids
- Demonstrate the need for assessment of family issues related to pediatric caregiving
- Demonstrate the professional case manager's actions with the scores and patient-centered plan of care

Introduction

Adults are not exclusive in experiencing complexity. Pediatric patients can experience complexity as well, but the case manager's approach to support them is very different from that of the adult. As a result, the Case Management Society of America (CMSA) developed a version of the Integrated Complexity Assessment Grid for use with children and youth. This chapter outlines how best to address the risks that exist for children and adolescents experiencing complex medical and behavioral conditions that may be further complicated by social and health system barriers. Pediatric-integrated management (PIM) follows the same standards of practice for adult case management.

However, there exists unique challenges when assisting children/youth and their families with health complexity in addition to having to consider the contributions of caregivers/parents, teachers, coaches, and peers in their child-specific assessments and care plan development. Children/youth are at as great a risk for multiple factors contributing to health complexity as adults; therefore, an approach to integrated pediatric case management parallels the approach taken with adults. This will allow those case management programs that understand the importance of correcting mental health issues as a means of reversing persistent physical symptoms to include a child/youth component in their case management services, particularly if they have already decided to provide adult-integrated case management (ICM) and have a child/youth population to serve as well.

Basics of the Pediatric Integrated Care Management Complexity Assessment Grid

The pediatric version of the Integrated Case Management Complexity Assessment Grid (PIM-CAG) was originally developed with input from pediatric psychiatrists, pediatricians, child psychologists, and pediatric case managers under the guidance of the developers of the original Integrated Case Management Complexity Assessment Grid (ICM-CAG). There is some overlap between the Adult CAG and the Pediatric CAG, but additional risk elements have been added to the PIM-CAG to be inclusive of the special needs of the child and adolescent. Like the ICM-CAG, the PIM-CAG is specifically developed for use by case managers rather than by treating practitioners. To re-emphasize, the role of case managers is to uncover barriers to improvement, coordinate care and services, and advocate and support the patient so that they can eventually reach a level of self-management. It is not the case manager's role to diagnose or treat, so it is not necessary to know all physical or mental health interventions that may be involved. With assessment and use of the PIM-CAG, case managers can identify the barriers preventing health improvement and work with the patient, family, guardian, or caregiver in obtaining the necessary care and services that will impact the child's health and well-being. As with adults, one item could trigger multiple actions by the case manager involving more than one health domain.

The PIM-CAG goes far beyond assessing risks in physical and mental health. It includes factors that influence the ability of the child or adolescent to maximize their health by assessing cognitive functioning, family relationships, relationships with friends, school experiences, adverse life events, and the health and abilities of the parent/caregiver/guardian. What is most important to understand is that the approach to working with children and adolescents must be different. Children and adolescents are not small adults: Their world view is very different; their needs are very different. So must be the approach to be helpful and effective.

Similarities and Differences Between the Pediatric Integrated Management Complexity Assessment Grid and the Integrated Case Management Complexity Assessment Grid

Like the ICM-CAG, the PIM-CAG is used to conduct an ICM assessment since it provides a method through which illness and life situation complexity can be prioritized by assigning levels of risk and then acted upon on behalf of the child/adolescent. Risk elements are reviewed as they pertain to the child and adolescent. For those readers who may be providing case management intervention to this population but are less familiar with conditions and challenges of the pediatric population, review Chapter 9 to learn more about behavioral challenges in children and then make sure to become familiar with how medical conditions are treated. For example, diabetes in a child will have nuances not found in the treatment of adults. Pediatric cancers and hematological disorders also are treated differently than in adults. For an adult, chemotherapy may be administered in the outpatient setting, but a child may require an acute care admission to receive treatment. Remember, it is the case manager's professional responsibility to understand the conditions that their patients face.

An additional caveat to working with the pediatric population is the need to focus on parents/caregivers/guardians, and health and well-being of the child are not functionally capable of meeting the child's needs, the case manager may have some very difficult interventions to consider. The parent/guardian/caregiver may need the interventions of a case manager for assistance in managing their own challenges so that they can be a support to the child. The case manager may also find parents/guardians/caregivers who are not providing a safe environment for the child: perhaps the child is in danger of injury; if so the case manager will be required to report these concerns to the appropriate authorities. This can be uncomfortable, especially if one has been working with the child's support system for some time. Ultimately, the child is the case manager's patient, and they must always act in the child's best interest (Table 11.1).

TABLE 11.1 Additional Elements for Assessment for the Child Versus the Adult

Pediatric Risk Assessment	**Additional Assessment Elements**
Psychological	
Cognitive development	As children grow and mature, any evidence that cognitive development is not following standard growth and development milestones indicates risk without intervention. Case managers must investigate any deficit, whether existing or potential, and work with the parent/caregiver/guardian to coordinate services that will result in improved cognition

(continued)

TABLE 11.1 Additional Elements for Assessment for the Child Versus the Adult (*continued*)

Pediatric Risk Assessment	**Additional Assessment Elements**
Barrers to coping	Children have very different coping mechanisms from adults. Children rely on emotion to express and share anxieties, fears, anger, sorrow, and grief, and they need the adults in their lives to validate these emotions (National Association of School Psychologists [NASP], 2021). Examples of how these emotions may manifest (NASP, 2021): Preschooler: • Thumb sucking • Bedwetting • Clingy • Fear of the dark • Behavior regression Elementary school children • Irritability • Aggression • Nightmares • School avoidance Adolescents • Sleep and appetite disturbances • Agitation • Increase in conflicts • Delinquent behavior If the parent/guardian/caregiver has an infant with complex needs, xamine their coping mechanisms and not the infant's
Adverse developmental events	Physical or psychological events that can impact the child's expected psychological or physical development are examined in this element. Adults can be impacted by adverse events but not in the same way as a child. Depending on the severity of an event, a child's entire lifetime may be impacted. For example, a child born to a mother who abused alcohol may be diagnosed with fetal alcohol syndrome (FAS). Children with FAS have physical and mental damage that may include dysmorphic facial features, difficulty learning, and exhibit behavioral challenges (Centers for Disease Control and Prevention [CDC], 2022). Children with FAS will need special education and social services. Trauma, whether it be physical or emotional can impact a child's behavior. Evidence of the impact of trauma at a young age may not manifest, but recognizing that trauma occurred is a risk factor that should be included in the assessment and care planning. While there may be no apparent effects in our assessment, a history of trauma will be a constant when examining future risk

(*continued*)

TABLE 11.1 Additional Elements for Assessment for the Child Versus the Adult (*continued*)

Pediatric Risk Assessment	**Additional Assessment Elements**
Social Domain	
Learning ability	If a child is old enough to have been exposed to formal learning, we examine if the child is achieving expected milestones and keeping pace with peers. If the child is not old enough for formal learning, there is no evidence of historical risk. but the case manager will want to monitor or educate the parent/caregiver/guardian on what to watch for and where to find resources
Family and social relationships	The Adult ICM-CAG examines how well the patient has been able to make and maintain relationships. For the pediatric patient, we assess whether the child has friends at school or in their neighborhood and play or socialize with these friends. Do parents/caregivers/guardians have stable family relationships, friends, or relationships in the community? Is there evidence that relationships are not stable or are they isolated from others?
Caregiver/parent health and function	This element examines the health and well-being of the parent/caregiver/guardian. We look for evidence that they have physical, emotional, or psychological challenges that could impact their ability to care for the child
Child and adolescent support system	This element and the next replace the adult social support element. The child hopefully has a stable parent/caregiver/guardian but is there anyone else in the child's life that they can be available for support? This can be another relative, neighbor, or family friend
Caregiver/family support	In addition to other support for the child, we examine whether the parent/family/caregiver has any support from friends, family, or other social services. Just like with the adult patient, who can the parent/caregiver/guardian call when they need help?
School and community participation	For the adult, we examine their history related to work and leisure, but for the child, we look at their current participation in school and the community. School can be viewed as the child's "work" and their leisure activities may include playing sports, being a girl or boy scout, participating in clubs, or other activities outside of school and home. If the child is not yet old enough, this may be an area to monitor

The Child/Adolescent and Caregiver/Parents Interview and Assessment

ICM is based on the relationship developed between the case manager and the patient to support health improvement and reduce impairment. The PIM-CAG is scored similarly to the ICM-CAG based on the assessment discussion with the parent/guardian/caregiver. Depending on the child, the child's age, and parental consent, the child may participate in the assessment and care-planning processes. Adolescents should be part of the assessment discussion insofar as they can understand the issues and parents are accepting of the inclusion.

As part of the usual process, the case manager should review any data related to risk, clinical notes, and/or claims information available about the child/youth. One most important tasks to complete before working with any child or adolescent is to determine the identities of the legal guardians. Once those individuals are identified, the case manager should define any issues related to confidentiality. Determine how they will be honored, and then determine the expectations of the parent/guardian and child or adolescent. For example, are there any issues with parental relationships like separation or divorce, custody, or disagreements about how to address the child's needs? Are there custody limitations, such as one parent is the primary contact and decision-maker? Does one parent have limited visitation or access to the child? If the patient is an adolescent, how will the case manager work with the parent/guardian when the adolescent wishes to participate in their own care? Parents/caregivers/guardians may want to shield the child/adolescent from worry, while the adolescent may want to know the details. Negotiation with all concerned needs to occur to ensure participation and engagement in case management intervention. Very young children will not likely be involved in the assessment and care-planning process. Older children and adolescents may wish to participate and the negotiation that must take place includes what the parent/guardian is comfortable with the child knowing, and how much autonomy will be afforded to the child/adolescent. It is natural for parents and caregivers to want to protect their children or those in their care, but case managers can also help them understand that taking responsibility for one's health cannot start too soon. Allowing the child/adolescent to be actively involved in their health will result in improved self-management as they grow and mature. Case managers must be sensitive to an adolescent's developing independence. Some adolescents may welcome complete transparency with the parent/guardian while others may want to keep some information confidential. At the beginning of the relationship development, the parent/caregiver/guardian and patient need to understand that information that may be harmful or helpful will be disclosed only as appropriate. States may have very specific laws and regulations related to the age of consent or how information should be shared between parent/caregiver/guardian and patient. The case manager must become aware of and familiar with the laws in the jurisdiction in which they practice.

Pediatric Integrated Case Management Assessment Grid Scoring Sheet

Children and adolescents experiencing health complexity will likely need long-term case management intervention. The assessment process may take more time than would be typically seen with the complex adult patient,—more time to understand the relationships between the patient, parent/caregiver/guardian, other family members; providers; school; and friends. While more effort is required by the case manager, relationship development will likely be more successful and necessary to assist the child/adolescent in moving toward improved health (Table 11.2).

The PIM-CAG contains 25 items in four domains, whereas the IM-CAG contains 20 items in four domains. The scoring range for the PIM-CAG, therefore, is from 0 to 75 while the scoring range for the IM-CAG is from 0 to 60. You will notice that risk elements in the social domain are expanded to address the special needs of the child/adolescent. Risk scoring for history examines the child's entire life. Current risk elements examine the last 30 days. Future risk examine the next 3 to 6 months just as the Adult CAG.

The new items that have been added to the PIM-CAG include: cognitive development, adverse developmental events, learning ability, parent/caregiver/guardian health and function, child/adolescent support, parent/caregiver/gaurdian support, and school and community participation. These items recognize and capture the complexity that may be experienced by children and adolescents.

While cognitive deficits can occur in adults (e.g., various dementias), these differ in the child or adolescent. This risk element encompasses the presence of intellectual disabilities, as well as the spectrum of developmental disorders like autism or pervasive developmental disorder. Children and adolescents with deficits in cognitive development may need specialized educational settings, support personnel in the home, and assistance with socialization since development delay is not understood and is often handled ineffectively due to lack of understanding by nonprofessionals.

Adverse developmental events has been added to the psychological domain to bring awareness of both physical and behavioral exposures that have historically impacted, or may impact in the future, cognitive abilities, emotions, or behaviors. These include, but are not limited to, toxic exposures like lead, traumatic brain injuries, trauma such as physical or psychological abuse and neglect, or other central nervous system illnesses that may occur because of birth trauma, like cerebral palsy. While some of the adverse events are the result of a physical or biological event, typically a greater risk is seen in behavioral or mental illness symptoms. If there are coexisting physical symptoms or conditions, these can be captured in the biological domain.

Children and adolescents do not work in the traditional sense—their "work" is attending school and participating in school and community activities like school clubs, sports, boy, and girl scouts, 4H clubs, and so on. The two risk elements added to the assessment are historical learning ability and current school and community participation. School performance is examined that includes their ability to be successful in school, attendance, and behavior at school and with peers. If risk is assessed, the case manager may need to assist in facilitating more involvement by parents/caregivers/guardians,

TABLE 11.2 Pediatric Integrated Management Complexity Assessment Grid

Date:	**HEALTH RISKS AND HEALTH NEEDS**					
Name:	**HISTORICAL**		**CURRENT STATE**		**VULNERABILITY**	
Total Score =	**Complexity Item**	**Score**	**Complexity Item**	**Score**	**Complexity Item**	**Score**
Biological domain	PSMC		Symptom severity/ impairment		Complications and life threat	
	Diagnostic difficulty		Adherence ability			
Psychological domain	Barriers to coping		Treatment choice		Learning and/or mental health threat	
	Mental health history		Mental health symptoms			
	Cognitive development					
	Adverse developmental events					
Social domain	Learning ability		Residential stability		Family/school/ social system risk	
	Family and social relationships		Child/adolescent support system			
	Parent/ caregiver/ guardian health and function		Parent/caregiver/ guardian support			
			School and community participation			
Health system domain	Reimbursement and provider access		Getting needed services		Health system deterrents	
	Treatment experience		Provider collaboration			

Scoring System:
0 = no vulnerability or need to act
1 = mild vulnerability and need for monitoring or prevention
2 = moderate vulnerability and need for action or development of intervention plan
3 = severe vulnerability and need for immediate action or immediate intervention plan

school administrators, and health providers. Know that past performance in school will be an indicator of future performance.

Parent/caregiver/guardian health and function has been added to provide a general assessment of the person(s) responsible for the child's or adolescent's health, well-being, and safety in order to better understand the ability of the parent/guardian to meet the needs of a child or adolescent with complex health needs. If the parent/caregiver/guardian is incapable of meeting the child's needs, case managers must facilitate actions and interventions to compensate for any lack of ability on the part of the parent/caregiver/guardian. This element demonstrates the strengths of the parent/caregiver/guardian or may indicate the need for more significant intervention to keep a child safe.

Child/adolescent support is essentially the same as the ICM-CAG social support element. Evaluated is who else in the child or adolescent's life can support, mentor, and contribute to the growth and development of the child such as a grandparent or other family member, coach, or teacher who is actively involved in the child's life. Also assessed is parent/caregiver/guardian support for the presence of assistance in case of emergency or crisis: Who is available to assist the parent/caregiver/guardian if they are unable to care for the child/adolescent such as in the case of illness or when other urgent/emergent situations arise?

Please refer to the Adult ICM-CAG grid to guide the scoring of the risk elements that mirror the ICM-CAG. Following is an examination of the risk elements that are unique to the pediatric population and examples of actions to mitigate risk.

Scoring for the Psychological Domain

Cognitive Development

0 = No cognitive impairment

- No action required

1 = Possible developmental delay or immaturity; low IQ (mild risk)

POSSIBLE ACTIONS

- Assist in establishing level of impairment, including the capacity of child to communicate physical needs and symptoms by coordinating referrals for appropriate testing.
- Discuss level of impairment and needs with caregivers, educator, and the pediatrician to ensure appropriate placement in school system.
- Assess need for remedial educational assistance and home support; facilitate completion of an individual educational plan (IEP) to meet the child's/youth's educational needs.

- Maintain communication with the school system and medical providers regarding the child's/youth's progress with learning.

2 = Delayed development; mild or moderate cognitive impairment (moderate risk)

POSSIBLE ACTIONS

Determine the level of cognitive delay and how it was evaluated.

- Assess and assist with home support for the child/youth based on functional capabilities and respite for parent/caregiver/guardian related to assimilation of social skills; provide relief for parent/caregiver/guardian from day-to-day caregiving.
- Assess and share child's/youth's ability to communicate.
- Ensure the child/youth has access to all available services.
- Consult with the available education resources and make necessary referrals so that the child/youth has every opportunity to thrive and grow.

3 = Severe and pervasive developmental delays or profound cognitive impairment (severe risk)

- Determine the level of dysfunction and needed supports.
- Ensure parents/caregivers/guardians have access to needed resources and supports to deal with severe developmental delays.
- In extreme circumstances, placement may be required; work with providers and parents/caregivers/guardians to facilitate a transition as difficult as this.

ADVERSE DEVELOPMENTAL EVENTS

0 = No identified developmental traumas or injuries (e.g., physical or sexual abuse, meningitis, lead exposure, drug abuse, exposure to infection, or other untoward prenatal exposures)

- No action required

1 = Traumatic prior experiences or injuries with no apparent or stated impact on child/youth (mild risk)

- While at the time of assessment there may appear to be no untoward effects of early trauma or exposure; observation is warranted as the child/youth grows and develops.

2 = Prior traumatic experiences or injuries with potential relationship to impairment in child/youth (moderate risk)

- Facilitate needed testing and evaluation for the extent that the trauma or exposure has affected the child/youth.

- Facilitate appropriate interventions to reduce the resulting effects of the trauma or exposure.

3 = Traumatic prior experiences with apparent and significant direct relationship to impairment in child/youth (severe risk)

- Determine the extent of trauma and impact to the child/youth.
- Ensure the immediate safety of the child/youth.
- Urgently coordinate needed services to address the impairments experienced due to trauma and exposures.

Social Domain

LEARNING ABILITY

0 = Performing well in school with good achievement, attendance, and behavior; not yet attending school

- No action required

1 = Performing adequately in school although there are some achievement, attendance, and behavioral problems (e.g., missed classes, pranks; mild risk)

- Encourage parent/caregiver/guardian to become more closely involved with the child's teachers and administrators. Encourage parent/caregiver/guardian to create a plan for improvement with the teacher and other school support staff.
- Assist parent/caregiver/guardian to find needed resources to improve school achievement.

2 = Experiencing moderate problems with school achievement, attendance, and/or behavior (e.g., school disciplinary action, few school-related peer relationships, academic probation; moderate risk)

- Recommend parent/caregiver/guardian closely work with teachers and counselors to determine strategies to improve achievement, attendance, and reduce disruptive behavior.
- May need to refer to additional counseling or tutoring resources outside of school.

3 = Experiencing severe problems with school achievement, attendance, and/or behavior (e.g., homebound education, school suspension, violence, illegal activities at school, academic failure, school dropout, disruptive peer group activity while at school; severe risk)

- Urgently assist with facilitation of additional resources and referrals for counseling, tutoring.

- Facilitate pediatrician visit for evaluation and possible referrals to other providers.
- Work with parent/caregiver/guardian, providers, and school to create safe environments for the child/youth, siblings, classmates, family members.

FAMILY AND SOCIAL RELATIONSHIPS

0 = Stable nurturing home, good social and peer relationships

- No action is required

1 = Mild family problems, minor problems with social and peer relationships (e.g., parent/caregiver/guardian–child/youth conflict, frequent fights, marital discord, lacking close friends; mild risk)

- Offer to facilitate counseling to address family problems or the child's/youth's challenges with making friends

2 = Moderate level of family problems, inability to initiate and maintain social and peer relationships (e.g., parent/caregiver/guardian neglect, difficult separation/divorce, alcohol abuse, hostile parent/caregiver/guardian, difficulties in maintaining same-age peer relationships; moderate risk)

- Collaborate with providers and school to encourage family counseling or counseling for the child's/youth's inability to maintain relationships or to cope with family discord.
- Involve social services to assess family dysfunction and risk to child's/youth's safety.

3 = Severe family problems with disruptive social and peer relationships (e.g., significant abuse, hostile child custody battles, addiction issues, parental criminality; for the child: complete social isolation, little or no association with peers; severe risk)

- Immediately notify social services or appropriate authorities if there is a risk of danger to the welfare of the child/youth or other family member.
- Notify the child's/youth's providers, teachers, and social services of concerns with social isolation; facilitate referral to appropriate mental health providers.

PARENT/CAREGIVER/GUARDIAN HEALTH AND FUNCTION

0 = All parent/caregiver/guardians physically and mentally healthy (no risk)

- No action required

1 = Physical and/or mental health issues, including poor coping skills, and/or permanent disability, present in one or more parent/caregiver/guardian, but do not impact parenting (Mild Risk)

- Discuss with parent/caregiver/guardian the challenges and contributors to difficulty in coping and facilitate any and all available resources to assist with coping.
- Assess any needed assistance related to existing disabilities and make any appropriate referrals.
- Provide resources to the parent/caregiver/guardian to obtain defined assistance.

2 = Physical and/or mental health conditions, including disrupted coping mechanisms, and/or permanent disability, present in one or more parents/caregivers/guardians, that interfere with parenting (moderate risk)

- Facilitate referrals to resources to assist with coping and disability assistance.
- Assist parent/caregiver/guardian in making needed appointments for counseling and other mental health services.
- Provide information on resources that may assist the parent/caregiver/guardian with compensation for any physical disability.

3 = Physical and/or mental health conditions, including disrupted coping mechanisms, and/or permanent disability, present in one or more parent/caregiver/guardian, which prevent effective parenting and/or create a dangerous situation for the child/youth (severe risk)

- Immediately contact the patient's providers to advise of a dangerous situation.
- Work with social services to ensure the parent/caregiver/guardian and child have a safe environment, even if just temporary.
- Reassure the parent/caregiver/guardian that you will assist in making sure there are no interruptions in the care and services received by the child/youth.

CHILD/YOUTH SUPPORT

0 = Supervision and/or assistance readily available from other family/caregivers, friends/peers, teachers, and/or community social networks (e.g., spiritual/religious groups) at all times (no risk)

- No action required

1 = Supervision and/or assistance generally available from another family member/caregiver, friends/peers, teachers, and/or community social networks; but possible delays (mild risk)

- Ascertain who besides parent/caregiver/guardian are able to provide support, caring, and supervision such as friends or teachers.
- Determine how readily available this support is—if needed, how quickly can the support respond to the child's needs?
- Create a plan with the parent/caregiver/guardian and other family/friend/teacher/community assistance so that these supports are available when needed.

2 = Limited supervision and/or assistance available from family/caregiver, friends/peers, teachers, and/or community social networks (moderate risk)

- Determine who can be identified as support other than the parent/caregiver/guardian, and how quickly they could respond to the needs of the child/youth.
- If the identified support cannot be available when needed, look for alternative supports that can be included, like after-school care or community activities.
- Create a plan of who to call first, second, and so on.

3 = No effective supervision and/or assistance available from family/caregiver, friends/peers, teachers, and/or community social networks at any time (high risk)

- Look to the community to establish supports other than parent/caregiver/guardian.
- Get permission to speak with extended family members to ascertain their ability to support the child/youth.
- Work with school and social services to see what programs might be available to address the child's/youth's need for additional emotional support.

SCHOOL AND COMMUNITY PARTICIPATION

0 = Attending school regularly, achieving and participating well, and actively engaged in extracurricular school or community activities (e.g., sports, clubs, hobbies, religious groups; no risk)

- No action required

1 = Average of 1 to 2 days of school missed/per month or minor disruptions in achievement and behavior with few extracurricular activities (mild risk)

- Discover the reason for missed school days.

- Strategize with parent/caregiver/guardian on how to prevent missed school days.
- Work with parent/caregiver/guardian and patient to learn what the child/youth is interested in; for example, hobbies, sports, games.
- Encourage parent/caregiver/guardian to connect patient to activities.

2 = Average of 2 to 4 days or more of school missed/month and/or moderate disruption in achievement or behavior with resistance to extracurricular activities (moderate risk)

- Discuss with parent/caregiver/guardian the cause of the child/youth missing school so frequently.
- Discuss with parent/caregiver/guardian and child/youth their interests: sports, clubs, art, music, and so on.
- Contact patient's school to help facilitate parent/caregiver/guardian communication with teachers and school counselors to develop a plan to improve attendance, performance, and participation.

3 = Truant or school nonattendance with no extracurricular activities and no community connections (severe risk)

- All of the interventions included in the moderate risk category; however, these need to implement urgently, immediately.

Following is an example of an integrated assessment for a complex pediatric patient.

CASE STUDY

Danny is an 8-year-old boy currently residing with his second foster family. Danny was placed in the foster care system at age 5 after his mother was sentenced to federal prison on drug-trafficking charges. Danny was diagnosed with attentiondeficit/hyperactivity disorder (ADHD) at age 3 while attending a Head Start program. At age 6, he was diagnosed with von Willebrand's disease after an injury at school. After this incident, his first foster parent asked that Danny be placed elsewhere because she found his behavior and the new diagnosis of a hematological disorder far too stressful and beyond her capabilities.

Danny has struggled in school due to his ADHD. He is often separated from his class due to disruptive behavior and is extremely active, finding it difficult to sit or be inactive for any length of time. There is also concern that he may have a learning disability as his reading level does not equate to the expected grade level. To date, he has not had any testing. He loves to play outdoors and play sports, especially football and baseball, but gets very frustrated and angry when he is not allowed to play. He has been to the emergency department three times in the last 6 months due to injuries, with one resulting in an admission due to excessive bleeding from a fall at school; these visits addressed large hematomas that occurred while playing football and jumping off a swing. He has required infusion of factors to address hematomas and the bleeding. Danny has a pediatrician and pediatric oncologist, and his new foster family ensures he keeps all appointments. Danny has health coverage through his state's Medicaid program for Children with Special Healthcare Needs. There are no concerns with access to needed care and services.

Danny has been with his new foster family for 2 years. Sharon and Bill are committed to Danny and want to provide him with a safe and loving home. They admit his behaviors are challenging and sometimes they are overwhelmed because he is so active, and they fear that he will continue to injure himself. But their priority is to make sure Danny feels secure and loved and to better address his ADHD so that he can feel successful in school and learn to better control his impulses preventing significant injuries. Sharon and Bill would like to find resources that would give them the right information and approach to help Danny understand the need to avoid injury and would like to find some additional support outside of school to address his ADHD. At present, Danny is not taking any medication to address ADHD symptoms, but Bill and Sharon wonder if medication might help Danny do better in school.

Pediatric Integrated Complexity Assessment Grid Scoring Sheet

Date:	**HEALTH RISKS AND HEALTH NEEDS**					
Name: Danny	**HISTORICAL**		**CURRENT STATE**		**VULNERABILITY**	
Total Score = 44	**Complexity Item**	**Score**	**Complexity Item**	**Score**	**Complexity Item**	**Score**
Biological domain	Persistent, sustained medical conditions	**2**	Symptom severity/ impairment	**2**	Complications and life threat	**3**
	Diagnostic difficulty	**1**	Adherence ability	**2**		
Psychological domain	Barriers to coping	**2**	Treatment choice	**0**	Learning and/or mental health threat	**3**
	Mental health history	**2**	Mental health symptoms	**1**		
	Cognitive development	**2**				
	Adverse developmental events	**2**				

Date:	**HEALTH RISKS AND HEALTH NEEDS**					
Name: Danny	**HISTORICAL**		**CURRENT STATE**		**VULNERABILITY**	
Total Score = 44	**Complexity Item**	**Score**	**Complexity Item**	**Score**	**Complexity Item**	**Score**
Social domain	Learning ability	**2**	Environmental stability	**0**	Family/school/social system vulnerability	**2**
	Family and social relationships	**3**	Child/adolescent support system	**1**		
	Caregiver/parent health and function	**2**	Caregiver/family support	**1**		
			School and community participation	**2**		
Health system domain	Reimbursement and provider access	**0**	Getting needed services	**2**	Health system deterrents	**2**
	Treatment experience	**0**	Provider and patient collaboration	1		

Scoring System:
0 = no vulnerability or need to act
1 = mild vulnerability and need for monitoring or prevention
2 = moderate vulnerability and need for action or development of intervention plan
3 = severe vulnerability and need for immediate action or immediate intervention plan

Biological Domain

- **PSMC = 2:** There is presence of a serious medical illness for which there is no cure, and which requires immediate intervention (von Willebrand's)
- **Diagnostic Difficulty = 1:** Condition was easily diagnosed after traumatic injury
- **Symptom Severity = 2:** Condition requires urgent intervention when a bleeding event occurs; requires implementation of safety measures to prevent bleeding events
- **Adherence Ability = 2:** Danny's foster parents are able to and do adhere to Danny's treatment plan, but Danny's behaviors make it challenging to prevent injury
- **Complications and Life Threat = 3:** Danny requires urgent interventions to prevent life threat. Without case management intervention to assist with needed care coordination, Danny is at risk of death from hemorrhaging

Psychological Domain

- **Barriers to Coping = 2:** Danny has exhibited anger and frustration because he is not allowed to play sports. He does not understand why and acts out as a result.
- **Mental Health History = 2:** Danny has been diagnosed with ADHD without any known treatment.
- **Cognitive Development = 2:** Danny's reading level does not equal his school grade level. It appears no testing has been done to assess a learning disability.
- **Adverse Developmental Events = 2:** Danny was removed from his mother's care and custody at age 5 and was placed in the foster care system. It is unknown if Danny's mother used substances during her pregnancy; if so, it could be a contributor to a possible learning disability.
- **Treatment Choice = 0:** Danny's foster parents are actively involved in Danny's care and want to be more proactive in addressing his challenges.
- **Mental Health Symptoms = 1:** While not true mental health symptoms, Danny's inability to sit quietly and his temper indicate a need to observe for any deterioration in behavior.
- **Mental Health Threat = 3:** Unless Danny's behaviors are better managed, he is at risk of continued delayed development as well as physical risk.

Social Domain

- **Learning Ability = 2:** Danny's reading level does not equate to the expected school grade level. There is no known learning disability, but no testing has occurred.
- **Family and Social Relationships = 3:** The effects of removal from his mother's care at a young age is unknown. He has been in the care of two foster care families in 3 years. His first foster care guardian could not manage his behaviors or medical condition. Any other family connections are unknown.
- **Caregiver/Parent Health and Function = 2:** Danny's mother was convicted of felony (drug trafficking) and sent to prison; as a result, Danny was placed in the foster care system. His first foster parent could not manage his behavior or medical condition. His current foster parents seem better equipped and prepared to care for him, but this history is essential for any possible future vulnerability.
- **Environmental Stability = 0:** Danny's current foster parents are able to meet all his needs for a safe environment.

- **Caregiver/Family Support = 1:** Danny's current foster family appears very supportive and caring, but other available supports to Danny are unknown.
- **School and Community Participation = 2:** Danny regularly attends school except for physical health events. He loves to play sports, but these are risky activities in his circumstance. Danny has no other known interests or hobbies.
- **Family/School/Social System Vulnerability = 2:** There is need to assist the foster care family to find support for them so that they can continue to care for Danny. In order to improve his school successes, additional resources need to be implemented and there is a need to find social activities that Danny enjoys but do not put him at risk of injury.

Health System Domain

- **Reimbursement and Provider Access = 0:** Danny has health coverage through his state's program for children.
- **Treatment Experience = 2:** Danny has been in the emergency department for injury and emergent administration of desmopressin (DDAVP).
- **Getting Needed Services = 2:** Danny receives the care he needs but his foster parents would like assistance in helping Danny understand why some sports are unsafe for him. Danny has not received any treatment for his ADHD and his foster parents are also interested in exploring treatment options.
- **Provider and patient Collaboration = 1:** There is no evidence that Danny's providers are not in good communication with one another or with Danny's Foster parents, however they would like to discuss treatment for ADHD.
- **Health System Deterrents = 2:** Without case management assistance, there may be delays in discussing and electing ADHD treatment.

Summary

Danny is a child who will need support and intervention throughout his formative years, and perhaps beyond. Most importantly, the case manager will be providing his foster family with the tools they need to manage his physical safety and to prevent medical complications, and also support his emotional and academic development. He remains in foster care and there is likely some insecurity for Danny; the case manager will need to ensure that every possible resource is provided to the foster family for success.

REFERENCES

Centers for Disease Control and Prevention. (2022, November 4). *Fetal alcohol syndrome disorders*. Author. https://www.cdc.gov/ncbddd/fasd/facts.html#:~:text=Fetal%20alcohol%20spectrum%20disorders%20(FASDs)%20are%20a%20group%20of%20conditions,a%20mix%20of%20these%20problems

National Association of School Psychologists. (2021). *How children cope with ongoing threat and trauma: The basic pH model*. Author. https://www.nasponline.org/resources-and-publications/resources-and-podcasts/school-safety-and-crisis/mental-health-resources/trauma/how-children-cope-with-ongoing-threat-and-trauma#:~:text=A%20child%20who%20utilizes%20his,adults%20in%20his%2Fher%20life

CHAPTER 12

Targeted Care Planning and Care Transitions

Rebecca Perez

OBJECTIVES

- Demonstrate targeted care planning based on assessed risk
- Define the critical elements for improving transitions of care for patients
- Demonstrate a safe and effective care transition

Introduction

Care planning is one of the fundamental actions of every case manager collaborating with a patient to improve health outcomes. Care planning with the patient should also include providers as they play an integral role in helping a patient achieve the identified goals that result in health improvement and stabilization. This chapter focuses on the aspects of targeted care planning and transitions of care, including examining risk assessment in care planning, defining the critical elements of improving transitions of care, and demonstrating safe and effective care transition methods.

Targeted Care Planning

Case managers base their care plans on the results of a comprehensive assessment of physical psychological, social, and health system domains, and what is important to a patient. Family and caregivers should be included in the assessment and the development of a care plan. Care plans are like road maps, providing information on the current state of the patient and where the care of the patient is heading. This "road map" illustrates how to get from point A to point B.

For example, a case manager is working with Sam, whose uncontrolled diabetes has resulted in a nonhealing ulcer on the bottom of his foot. He has already has had two hospital admissions for infections and debridement of the ulcer. What are the concerns? A major concern is that the ulcer will worsen and ultimately result in amputation of the foot. So, what is the goal? The goal is a healed diabetic foot ulcer that will avoid amputation. And how will a healed foot ulcer be achieved? The case manager will consider many variables and options when developing this care plan. Developing a care plan for Sam may seem amazingly simple if one is only wearing their clinician's hat. But take that hat off for a moment and become a detective; think Sherlock Holmes with his deerstalker hat and magnifying glass. Before the care plan can be developed, the case manager must understand and discover what has or has not occurred to result in poorly controlled diabetes, and why has the nonhealing ulcer persisted. .

The case manager's comprehensive case management assessment reports on Sam's medical history and treatment, but not necessarily how his condition advanced or what occurred causing a nonhealing foot ulcer. Using the Integrated Case Management Complexity Assessment Grid (ICM-CAG) to examine and prioritize risk will help in this discovery. The case manager discovers that Sam lives alone, has a history of depression, has no close family or social ties, does not have a good relationship with his primary care provider, cannot always afford to buy healthy foods, and is unable to drive because the ulcer is on the bottom of his right foot. He has not been attending medical appointments and is ordering fast food delivery because he cannot get to the grocery store. He has not been regularly checking his blood sugar; his last A1c was over 6 months ago, and, at that time, it was 9.2. He also has neuropathy in his feet and had been prescribed orthotic diabetic shoes, but he has not been wearing them.

Sam has multiple risks and now the case manager must prioritize them to create a care plan that will result in the goal of a healed foot ulcer and no amputation. Before putting that clinician hat back on, the case manager should be sure to spend some time talking to Sam about what is important to him. What does Sam see as the barriers to better diabetes management? He tells you that while he does not have any close family ties as most of his family is deceased, he does enjoy attending religious services and the socials that follow on Sundays at the church near his apartment. He does have a few former work acquaintances that he talks to every couple of months, but he does not engage further because he does not believe they want a "guy with bad diabetes hanging around." He is a retired copyright editor from the local newspaper and only has a modest pension in addition to his Social Security benefits. His health coverage is with a Medicare Advantage plan.

The case manager would begin Sam's targeted care plan by examining the patient's challenges:

- Nonhealing foot ulcer
- Uncontrolled diabetes
- Unable to drive

- History of depression
- Nonadherence to a diabetic diet
- Not keeping medical appointments
- Lack of social support
- A desire to participate in social activities

Once the challenges are identified, they are prioritized. Based on the priority, the goals for the care plan are established.

Case Management Goals

A customary practice of some case management organizations is to construct goals as actions. Goals are not actions. Action verbs should be avoided when constructing goals. Actions are interventions, and interventions are needed to achieve a goal. This may take thinking differently, but this process is simpler, more efficient, and effective. SMART goals require a "time" for goal achievement, but it makes more sense to time the completion of interventions. SMART goals are defined as specific, measurable, achievable, relevant, and time bound. Unfortunately, many in the case management profession allocate a specific time to a goal, when in actuality, the time-bound or time-based requirement of a SMART goal is more about an end date for the prioritized tasks, rather than a specific period of time.

With a clinician's hat now firmly on, consider all the things that need to happen to improve diabetes management and heal Sam's ulcer. When collaborating with complex patients, there will be many issues that need to be addressed, but with an integrated approach, the patient's needs and issues are prioritized based on risk. Where does the greatest risk lie? If the foot ulcer does not heal, another infection is likely, the neuropathy will worsen with continued poor diabetes management, and his already compromised peripheral circulation will only worsen. He is depressed, which contributes to his lack of motivation for diabetes management. His lack of social contacts is contributing to the depression. All of these issues need to be addressed but the priority, the greatest risk, lies with the nonhealing ulcer.

A mistake would be to try and address everything at once. This would not only result in delays in addressing the greatest risk but would also overwhelm the patient. Individuals with complexity need to solve problems in increments. Allow the patient, and the case manager, to experience some successes, however small, as the success will encourage and instill confidence to achieve more.

For Sam, the number one goal is a healed foot ulcer. This goal, when achieved, will reduce the danger of amputation and a return to activity. Subsequent goals are to address social needs like food insecurity, a return to the social activities he enjoys, and depression. For now, let's place the focus on the priority goal.

Goal 1: Healed Foot Ulcer*

*If SMART goals are a focus of your organization, you will want to put a time frame on this goal, but it would be difficult to judge the length of time it will take to heal the ulcer.

Interventions

1. Establish an appointment with Sam's primary care physician (PCP).
2. Coordinate nonemergent transportation to the appointment.
3. Review diabetic medications, Sam's ability to obtain them and his understanding of adherence.
4. If acquiring medication is burdensome, work with a pharmacist to find reduced-cost medications.
5. Discuss a wound consult with PCP; make appointment and arrange transportation.
6. Coordinate wound care supplies, home health, follow-up appointments, and transportation.
7. Work with the patient on adherence to diabetes management: regular glucose testing, wearing diabetic shoes for off-loading of the wound, taking medications as prescribed, keeping all appointments.
8. Arrange Meals on Wheels for healthy meals until Sam can drive again.
9. Investigate if Sam is taking advantage of all benefits available with his Medicare Advantage plan.

As these interventions are implemented and response is monitored, the goal identified by Sam—a return to social interactions—can start.

Goal 2: Social Connections (In 60 to 90 Days)

1. Ask Sam if he is comfortable reaching out to his church to see if volunteers are available to take him to Sunday services.
2. If Sam is not comfortable, offer to make the call.
3. If no volunteers are available, investigate other forms of transportation to church activities.
4. Talk with Sam about his former work friends and ask if he is interested in establishing a closer relationship with them.

After 90 days of working with Sam, rescore his ICM-CAG. By this time, Sam's risk score should decrease, and the lower score is evidence of improvement as a result of case management intervention. Rescoring the ICM-CAG every 90 days is recommended until the patient graduates from case management service.

Transitions of Care

Transitions of care are the movement of patients from one healthcare practitioner, level of care, and/or one setting to another, as their condition and care needschange. For successful transitions of care, case managers should use their critical thinking skills, taking a holistic approach and knowing that their research makes the arguable inarguable. The case manager should focus on communicating any changes to the healthcare team, which improves patient outcomes, especially those with complex injuries or diagnoses.

Integrated Case Manager Skills Required for Successful Transitions of Care

- The ability to coordinate medical and behavioral interventions
- Professional, yet empathic demeanor
- Focus on patient-centered autonomy and assisting the patient in defining goals
- The ability to bring patients into a collaborative partnership with meaningful communication between , family, and the care team.
- The ability to not only engage stakeholders but turn that engagement into activation.

Activation is an integral part of the transition process (Will et al., 2019). This involves the talent of the case manager to instill the knowledge, skills, confidence, and resources to patients to manage their disease state in an active and informed manner. A patient-centered approach meets patients at their personal level of readiness to learn and accomplish their health-related goals. Focus is on patient/provider shared decision-making in all phases of their treatment. Patients with the highest levels of activation display interest and involvement, and actively decide the best course of involvement for themselves. In addition, high activation levels are associated with decreased healthcare costs. The case manager coordinates cost-effective plans, providing high-quality continuous care that eliminates duplication of services and wasted benefit dollars. These are often dollars which can be hard to track but occur when there is one case manager from beginning to case closure. Fragmented care can be avoided by fewer case manager handoffs. The role of the case manager is to communicate with clients and providers to reassess, educate, and develop a care or treatment plan. Most importantly, the case manager must promote self-efficacy and engage patients in their treatment protocol.

The case manager is responsible for facilitation and coordination of care for the patient while communicating with the interprofessional care team, involving the patient in the decision-making process to minimize fragmentation in the services provided, and preventing risk for unsafe care and suboptimal outcomes (Will et al., 2019). To facilitate effective and competent performance, the professional case manager should demonstrate knowledge of health insurance and funding sources, healthcare services, human behavior dynamics, healthcare delivery and financing systems, community resources, ethical and evidence-based practice, applicable laws and regulations, clinical standards and outcomes, and health information technology and digital media relevant to case management practice. The skills and knowledge base of a case manager may be applied to individual patients such as in the hospital setting, or to groups of patients such as in disease, chronic care, or population health management models. Often case managers execute their responsibilities across settings, providers, over time, and beyond the boundaries of a single episode of care. They also employ the use of health and information technology and tools. Successful interdisciplinary teams are able to improve the patient care experience and outcomes by increasing the coordination of services, integrating healthcare for the patient's wide range of health needs, empowering patients as active partners in care, and helping them to problem-solve by exploring options of care, when available, and alternative plans, when necessary, to achieve desired outcomes (Perez, 2022).

Care Transition Models

The culture of healthcare in the United States has been primarily reactive instead of proactive. Science and technology continually present new and more effective ways to treat illness, but prevention still seems to be a secondary concern. The focus on patient-centered care must also focus on prevention and this movement is slowly becoming more of a priority. Most illnesses can be professionally managed in the outpatient setting. Emergency department visits and admissions need to be viewed as treatment failures. While some admissions are unavoidable, they should not be seen as the standard of care. Helping the patient to learn to self-manage as much as possible in the outpatient setting should be the priority of every healthcare professional. Admissions are an event on the care continuum and should be avoided as much as possible. To promote outpatient or ambulatory care, transitions back to outpatient management need to be safe and effective (Perez, 2022).

There are many transition models that can be implemented in several practice settings: acute care to home, acute care to a clinic, and acute care to rehab or skilled nursing. Using a transition model can ensure a standard process that creates accountability for both the discharging entity and the receiving entity. Accountability and communication are the two areas that will make a transition successful and effective. Each entity must be accountable for the transition, not just the tasks they are required to complete. Until all parties take responsibility for a transition, mistakes or missteps will continue to occur.

Case managers play an integral role in care transitions. Whether you are the hospital case manager initiating the discharge plan with the patient and family or caregiver, or the health plan or post acute case manager taking the passed baton and supporting the patient, family, or caregiver continue on their care continuum.

See Table 12.1 for examples of care transition models.

TABLE 12.1 Examples of Care Transition Models

Mode	Setting	Tools/Components	Key Findings
TCM: https://consultgeri.org/geriatric-topics/transitional-care	Hospital to home	• In-hospital evidence-based nursing care plan • Home visits and phone follow-up with TCM • Holistic focus • Patient and caregiver education and support • Early identification and response • Patient and caregiver on team • Physician nurse collaboration • Open cross-communication • TCM hospital discharge screening tool for high-risk older adults	• Reduced hospital readmissions • Decreased ED visits • Decreased healthcare costs

CTI: http://www.caretransitions.org	Hospital to home	Four pillars of CTI:
		• Medication
		• PHR
		• Follow-up
		• Transition Coach
		  ▪ Hospital visit
		  ▪ Home visit
		• Telephone call in 2 to 3 days
			• Self-sustaining
			• Rehospitalization rates 50%
			• Cost-effective

BOOST: http://www.hospitalmedicine.org/Web/Quality_Innovation/ Implementation_Toolkits/Project_BOOST/Web/Quality_Innovation/Implementation_Toolkit/Boost/Overview.aspx http://caretransitions.org/tools-and-resources/	Hospital to home	• The target • Patient preparation to address situations (after discharge) successfully (patient PASS) • Teach-back process • Risk specific interventions • Written discharge instructions • Technical assistance	• Reduced 30-day readmission rates • Tools well-received by healthcare team and patients • Hospital and primary care provider communication and collaboration

(continued)

TABLE 12.1 Examples of Care Transition Models (*continued*)

Mode	Setting	Tools/Components	Key Findings
Project RED: http://www.bu.edu/fammed/projectred/	Hospital to home	• Diagnosis-related education • Postdischarge appointments, tests, etc. • Medications, diet, exercise-related education • Discharge plan reconciliation with national guidelines/clinical pathways • Emergency plan • Discharge summary transmission • Written discharge plan • Telephone call in 2 to 3 days	• Decreased 30-day re-hospital utilization and emergency department use • Reduced costs per subject enrolled • Increased revenue per discharge
CCM: http://www.improvingchroniccare.org/index.php?p=	Clinic to home	• Community • Healthcare system • Self-management support • Delivery system design • Decision support • Clinical information systems • Organization ACIC • PACIC	• Improved well-being in patients with asthma, diabetes, bipolar disorder, comorbid depression, and cancer
INTERACT: http://www.maseniorcarefoundation.org/Initiatives/Care_Transitions.aspx	Nursing home to hospital	• Resource binder for champions • Case examples • Communication tools • Care path and change in condition cards • Advance care planning tools • Quality improvement	• 17% hospital admission reduction • Medicare savings • Further randomized studies to determine avoidable hospitalizations, morbidity, and cost savings

ACIC, assessment of chronic illness care; BOOST, Better Outcomes for Older Adults Through Safe Transitions; CCM, chronic care model; CTI, care transitions intervention; INTERACT, Interventions to Reduce Acute Care Transfers; PACIC, patient assessment of care for chronic conditions; PASS, preparation to address situations successfully; PHR, Personal health record; RED, Re-engineered Discharge; TCM, transitional care mode.

The case manager should continue to support the complex patient as long as it takes to achieve health stabilization. Whenever possible, the case manager facilitates self-determination and self-care through the tenets of advocacy, shared decision-making, and education. Turn the passenger into a driver while assisting the patient in the safe transitioning of care to the next most appropriate level, setting, and/or provider.

Seven Tips for Clinicians When Communicating Transition Instructions

1. Use plain language.
2. Limit information (3–5 key points).
3. Be specific and concrete, not general.
4. Demonstrate, draw pictures, use models.
5. Repeat/summarize.
6. Teach-back (confirm understanding).
7. Be positive, hopeful, empowering.

CASE STUDY

The following case study highlights how select integrated case management tools are used for safe transitions of care by the case manager and the interdisciplinary team for an individual in an acute care facility following an exacerbation of emphysema and history of atrial fibrillation and depression. The case illustrates how the team can determine educational needs and develop and support the plan of care. Each aspect of the treatment plan requires an assessment of the patient's knowledge and motivation.

A 63-year-old White male presents to the emergency department with complaints of shortness of breath (SOB) upon exertion and at rest. He shows signs and symptoms of a lung infection: productive cough, greenish-yellow sputum, increased dyspnea, tachycardia, fever, and weight loss. He was diagnosed with emphysema at age 53 qualifying for social security disability.

Diagnoses

- Atrial fibrillation,
- Depression, and
- Emphysema.

Past Surgical History

- None

Current Medications

- Escitalopram 10 mg once daily for depression,
- Diltiazem ER 240 mg once daily for atrial fibrillation,
- Long-acting beta agonist, and
- Long-acting anticholinergic.

Economic/Income Status

- Monthly social security income and Veterans pension. Income is limited even with these two sources.

Health Coverage

- Medicare Advantage Plan, and
- Veterans Affairs (VA) benefits.

Social History

- Smoker for 35 years; ceased upon emphysema diagnosis at age 53;
- Averages two to three alcohol drinks per week;
- Divorced for 24 years, one adult daughter; and
- Retired teacher.

Based on presenting symptoms, the emergency physician admitted him to the hospital wih a primary diagnosis of emphysema with exacerbation. The acute care stay was 10 days due to diagnosis of methicillin-resistant *Staphylococcus aureus* in the sputum. The patient became weak during the admission and required a transfer to a skilled nursing facility to finish antibiotics and to receive physical and occupational therapies.

The acute care case manager collaborated with the patient's daughter to settle on a facility that was near where she lived. The discharge orders of antibiotics, continuation of home medications, oxygen at 2 liters/min, and 2 hours of physical and occupational therapy per day were reviewed with the patient and his daughter before sending them to the receiving facility. The expected length of stay in the skilled facility was 2 weeks. The acute care case manager arranged for an ambulance transfer to the nursing facility. The acute care case manager followed up with the facility to ensure the discharge orders were received and that all services would be in place prior to his arrival. The acute care case manager also notified the assigned case manager from the Medicare Advantage plan of the date of transfer and the discharge orders.

The Medicare Advantage plan case manager communicated with the skilled facility during the patient's stay to monitor progress and prepare for discharge to home. The patient will be discharged to his daughter's home as it is no longer safe for him to live alone.

Working closely with the skilled facility created the atmosphere for a safe an effective discharge to the daughter's home. Home oxygen, a walker, and bedside commode were delivered the day before discharge. The patient's daughter will function as his caregiver, taking him to appointments and outpatient physical therapy.

When communication, collaboration, and accountability are employed, transitions can be safe and readmissions avoided.

REFERENCES

Perez, R. (2022). *Case management adherence Guide 2020*. Cognella Academic Publishing.

Will, K. K., Johnson, M. L., & Lamb, G. (2019). Team-based care and patient satisfaction in the hospital setting: A systematic review. *Journal of Patient-Centered Research and Reviews*, *6*(2), 158–171. https://doi.org/10.17294/2330-0698.1695

SECTION IV

Specialty Populations

CHAPTER 13

Trauma Survivors: Trauma-Informed Care

Melanie A. Prince

OBJECTIVES

- Discuss the effects of trauma on the human experience
- Describe trauma-informed approach to care management
- Apply six principles of a trauma-informed approach to integrated case management

Introduction

Survivors of trauma are one of four patient/client groups considered as a specialty population. The goal of this chapter is to provide evidence-based support to the tenets of care for trauma survivors. But why is it important to consider trauma survivors a specialty population? In 1999, the United States Congress enacted Public Law 106-129, Healthcare Research and Quality Act of 1999 and established the Agency for Healthcare Research and Quality (AHRQ). Part of the agency's mission is to enhance the quality, appropriateness, and effectiveness of health services for priority populations (online source: https://www.govinfo.gov/content/pkg/PLAW-106publ129/html/PLAW-106publ129.htm).

Case management can actualize AHRQ's mission intent because the promotion of *quality care and cost-effective outcomes* is a central part of the case management definition (Case Management Society of America, 2022). Trauma survivors are inherently a specialty population because the cohorts identified by law as priority groups may also be deemed at risk for trauma exposure, that is, low-income groups, minority groups, women, children, the elderly, and individuals with special healthcare needs (online source: https://www.govinfo.gov/content/pkg/PLAW-106publ129/html/PLAW-106publ129.htm). However, the Substance Abuse and Mental Health Services Administration (SAMHSA) describes trauma as a "common experience for adults and children in American communities" (online source: retrieved Aug 2022, https://www.samhsa.gov/trauma-violence).

Given that AHRQ identifies priority groups and SAMHSA asserts virtually no boundaries to potential trauma exposure in the United States, the *why* of this specialty population is more significant than the *who* as a rationale for integrated case management (ICM). Research has shown that traumatic experiences are associated with both behavioral health and chronic physical health conditions (online source: retrieved August, 2022, https://www.samhsa.gov/trauma-violence). As case managers develop strategies to assess and care for multi-diagnoses patients, a history of trauma adds another layer of complexity. Because of this added layer of complexity, case managers must broaden their perspective on how to care for patients comprehensively and holistically. Thirkle et al. (2021) conducted studies to determine the most appropriate methodologies, but the bottom line is that Trauma Informed Care (TIC) should become embedded into ICM culture and an understanding of what this means is necessary to begin to understand trauma-informed care and its implementation. A trauma-informed lens is critical to the success of quality care and appropriate, cost-effective outcomes.

What Is Trauma-Informed Care?

There has been considerable research on TIC over the past two decades especially in mental and psychological health disciplines. The National Library of Medicine conducted a literature review and identified several themes and definitions. In the context of this manual, and as the authors advocate for an integrated model of care management, the following Hopper et al. (2010) definition by is relevant:

> *"Trauma-Informed Care is a strengths-based framework that is grounded in an understanding of and responsiveness to the impact of trauma, that emphasizes physical, psychological, and emotional safety for both providers and survivors, and that creates opportunities for survivors to rebuild a sense of control and empowerment" (National Library of Medicine, retrieved August 8, 2022).*

The Hopper definition provides the context for this chapter as TIC is considered from both the providers as well as trauma survivors' perspectives.

What Is Trauma?

What is trauma? Individual trauma results from an event, series of events, or set of circumstances that is experienced by an individual as physically or emotionally harmful or threatening and that can have lasting adverse effects on the individual's functioning and physical, social, emotional well-being. The Missouri Early Connections website provides an excellent description of the types of traumas. There are three main types of traumas: acute, chronic, or complex.

1. Acute trauma results from a single incident.
2. Chronic trauma is repeated and prolonged such as domestic violence or abuse.
3. Complex trauma is exposure to varied and multiple traumatic events, often of an invasive, interpersonal nature. The following are a few examples.

Natural disasters	Sexual abuse
Physical abuse	Domestic violence
Medical injury, illness, or procedures	Community violence
Neglect, deprivation	Traumatic grief
Victim of crime	Kidnapping
Accidents	School violence
Loss	

(Online website, retrieved August 2022, https://earlyconnections.mo.gov/professionals/trauma-informed-care#)

From the providers' perspective, one must be educated and aware of a person's *response* to trauma and how this response influences the mind, body, and spirit. Therefore, the care must be delivered in a way that empathetically considers what people have experienced while also facilitating safety, connection, and healing. (Tolann et al., 2022). Awareness is key. SAMHSA (2021) posits TIC should start from a universal expectation that trauma has occurred, and the patient may be a trauma survivor. SAMHSA's comprehensive research and training content provides a wealth of information on trauma-informed practice, especially its 4-R framework.

4-R Framework

The 4-R framework is a practical guide to delivering TIC: **realize** the impact of trauma, **recognize** the signs and symptoms of trauma, **respond** with awareness and knowledge of trauma-related policies and procedures, and **resist** re-traumatization. WAVE Trust (Worldwide Alternatives to ViolencE) is an international educational charity that works with child survivors of trauma and succinctly depicts the 4-R framework and TIC in Figure 13.1.

FIGURE 13.1 Trauma-informed care and the 4 R's.

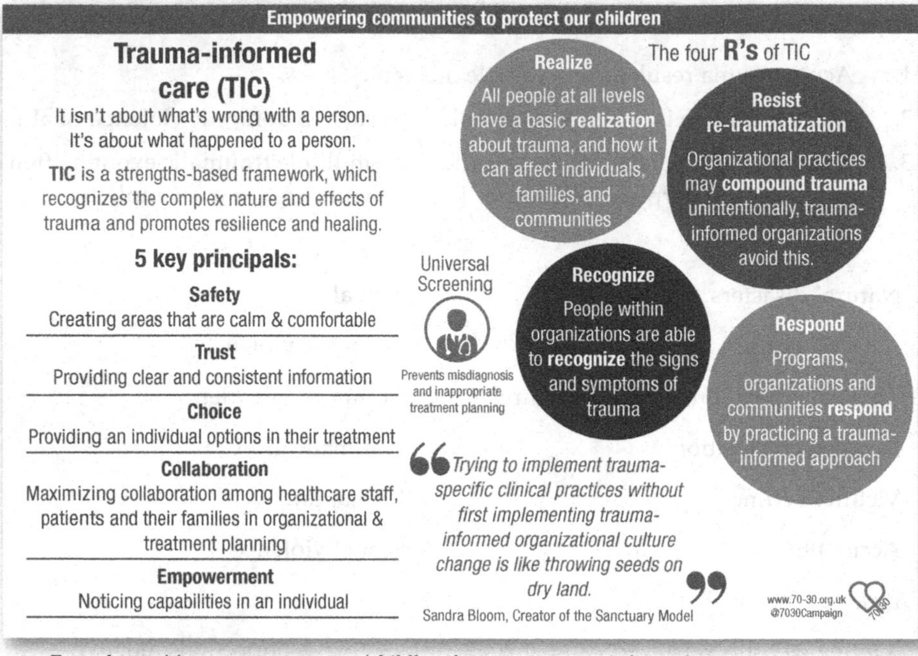

Source: From https://www.wavetrust.org/childhood-trauma-trauma-informed-care

Neurobiology of Trauma

In order to realize, recognize, respond, and resist trauma, case managers must understand how trauma is manifested in patients/clients and what the response looks like. The most practical approach to assessing the influence of trauma exposure is understanding the brain–stress relationship. Shonkoff et al. (2000) states that the brain's development is shaped by genetics and experiences; thus, the brain's functioning is a reflection of our experiences. Trauma causes stress and the human response to stress is a function of the brain's fight or flight instinctual reaction to preservation. The brain reacts to stress and defensive behaviors are initiated. The brain's "defensive response" affects multiple body systems, including the heart, muscles, stomach, lungs, eyes, blood vessels, and gastrointestinal organs. Kozlowska et al. (2015) illustrates the brain–stress relationship in their research analysis of the brain–body defense cascade: arousal, freezing, flight or fight, tonic immobility, collapsed immobility, and quiescent immobility. See Figure 13.2 for an illustration of the neuropathways directly affecting parts of the body such as the heart, gut, muscles, and others (Kozslowska, 2015, p. 265). One can extrapolate how physical ailments may manifest.

FIGURE 13.2 The defense cascade.

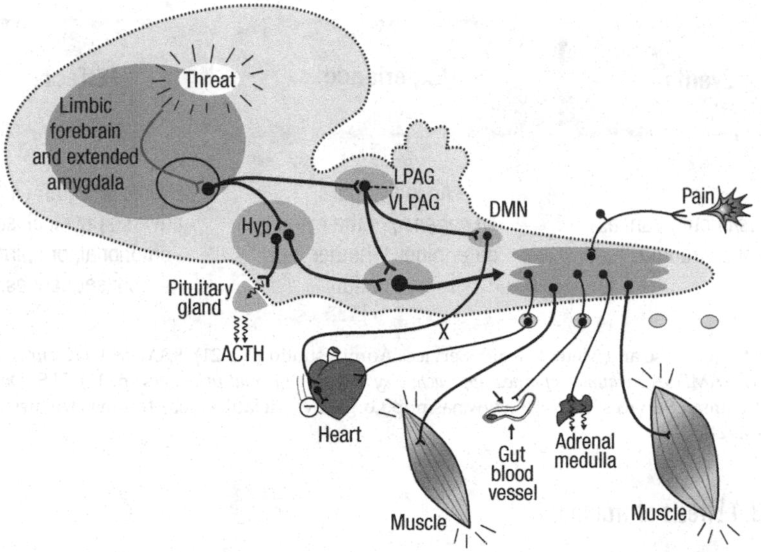

Source: Kozlowska, K., Walker, P., McLean, L., & Carrive, P. (2015). Fear and the defense cascade: Clinical implications and management. *Harvard Review of Psychiatry, 23*(4), 263–287. https://doi.org/10.1097/HRP.0000000000000006

A basic understanding of the neurobiology of trauma can enhance the case manager's assessment of the physical, mental, and sociobiological responses trauma exposure adds to complex care management. To tie this together, a person's genetic expression in the brain combined with experiences of trauma can manifest as bodily, psychological, or behavioral impairments along the care continuum. One way to remember this brain-stress connection in TIC is to assess a patient/client's potential trauma exposure using the three E's: Event, Experience, and Effects (SAMSHA, 2021) of potential trauma exposure (Figure 13.3).

As the case manager develops an ICM plan for patients/clients, the neurobiology of the brain provides the evidence to support a holistic approach to needs stratification and comprehensive, collaborative interventions. With a holistic lens, what do the effects of trauma look like? There is a plethora of literature to answer this question. There are general response effects and human responses to specific types of traumas such as traumatic brain injury, interpersonal violence, chronic exposure to gun violence, repeat disaster experiences, chronic extreme stress, and so on. Dr. Noel Hunter uses three spheres to illustrate what trauma looks like in survivors (Hunter, retrieved August 2022, https://mindclearpsychotherapy.com/trauma-stress-body/). Note the inclusion of coping responses in Figure 13.4 (Hunter, 2022, p. 1, online source). This illustration suggests that social determinants of health (SDoH) are important considerations for TIC of trauma survivors.

FIGURE 13.3 The three E's in trauma: Event, Experience, and Effects.

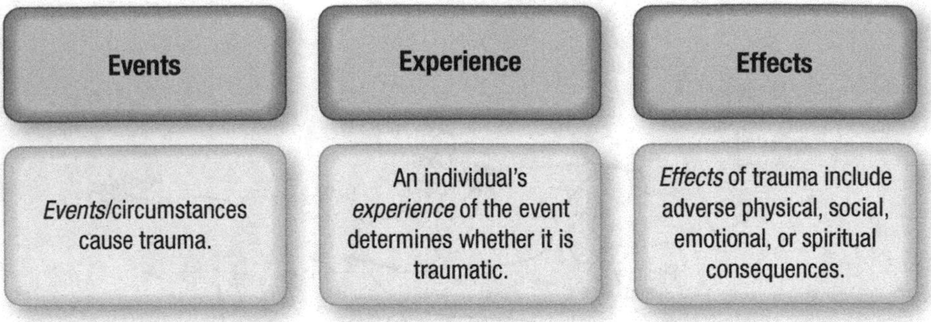
Events
Experience
Effects
Events/circumstances cause trauma.
An individual's *experience* of the event determines whether it is traumatic.
Effects of trauma include adverse physical, social, emotional, or spiritual consequences.

Source: Substance Abuse and Mental Health Services Administration. (2021). *SAMHSA/TIC curriculum instructor's guidance SAMHSA's trauma-informed approach: Key assumptions and principles* (p. 11). U.S. Department of Health and Human Services. https://www.nasmhpd.org/sites/default/files/TraumaTIACurriculumTrainersManual_6-2-21.pdf

FIGURE 13.4 Effects of trauma.

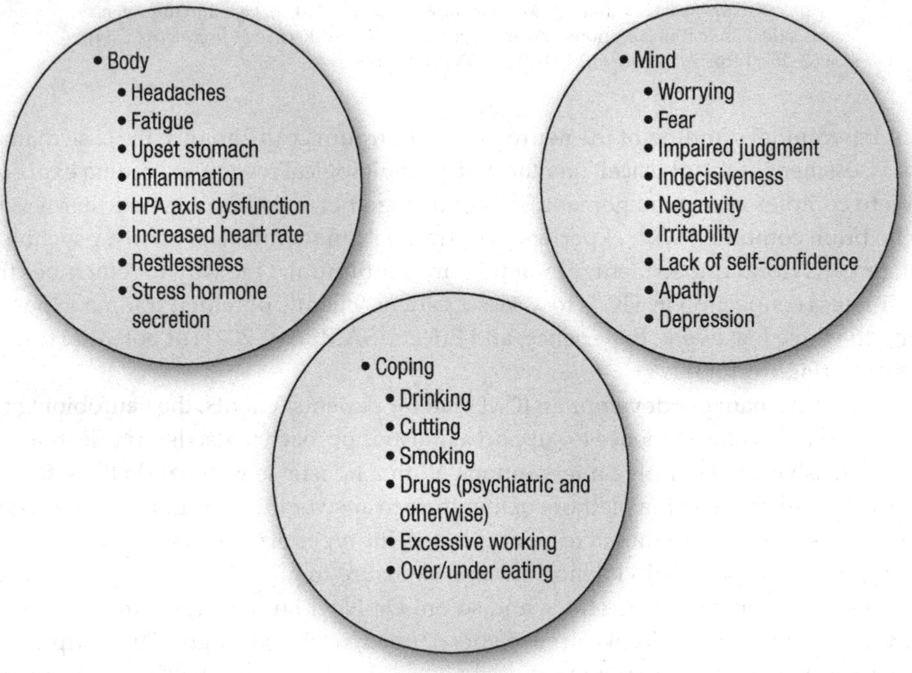
• Body
• Headaches
• Fatigue
• Upset stomach
• Inflammation
• HPA axis dysfunction
• Increased heart rate
• Restlessness
• Stress hormone secretion
• Mind
• Worrying
• Fear
• Impaired judgment
• Indecisiveness
• Negativity
• Irritability
• Lack of self-confidence
• Apathy
• Depression
• Coping
• Drinking
• Cutting
• Smoking
• Drugs (psychiatric and otherwise)
• Excessive working
• Over/under eating

Source: Hunter, N. (2022). Mind clear psychotherapy website. Online source retrieved August 2022. Complex Trauma, Stress and the Body: It's All Connected (mindclearpsychotherapy.com). https://mindclearpsychotherapy.com/trauma-stress-body/

Trauma Informed Care and Social Determinants of Health

Healthy People 2030 defines SDoH as "the conditions in the environments where people are born, live, learn, work, play, worship, and age that affect a wide range of health, functioning, and quality-of-life outcomes and risks" (U.S. Department of Health and Human Services, www.health.gov, retrieved September 2022). The five domains are: Economic Stability, Education Access and Quality, Healthcare Access and Quality, Neighborhood and Built Environment, Social and Community Context. All of these domains can be assessed for traumatic influences, but especially the domains of Neighborhood / Built Environment and Social/Community Context. For example, refer back to Figure 13.3 where the case managers can use the Three E's of a trauma-informed approach to assessment of the Neighborhood and Built Environment. A sample assessment dialogue may be as follows:

- *What types of* ***events*** *occur in the area where you live or within your home that make you feel stressed or distraught? What keeps you from a restful sleep?*
- *How do these* ***experiences*** *make you feel, whether it is neglect, chronic hunger, physical abuse, community violence?*
- *When you experience these types of traumas, what* ***effect*** *does it have on your mind and body? (Or mentally and physically?)*

The Three E's can guide the assessment questions, but it is the **Four R's** that should inform the case manager's overall approach to the ICM of survivors of trauma. Again, the 4 R's are: **realize** the impact of trauma, **recognize** the signs and symptoms of trauma, **respond** with awareness and knowledge of trauma-related policies and procedures, **resist** re-traumatization. SDoH offer a good starting point for TIC assessment.

Tools and Tips for Trauma Informed Care in Integrated Case Management

Zatzick et al. (2011) conducted a study on collaborative care intervention is specialty populations, specific cohorts of patients with posttraumatic stress. The research supports the tenets around ICM. Their Trauma Survivors Outcomes and Support Study used an interdisciplinary team of clinicians in a collaborative care model of integrated care management, including concern elicitation, motivational interviewing, and behavioral elicitation. This study aligns with components of ICM in the context of trauma survivors. The concern elicitation aligns with the earlier points about caring for patients with a universal expectation that trauma may have occurred. Motivational interviewing is a key competency in ICM. Behavioral elicitation represents the *change outcomes* in the lives of trauma survivors and the Zatzick et al. (2011) study utilized nurses and social workers for care interventions.

As case managers develop the care interventions for trauma survivors, SAMHSA (online source retrieved August 2022) offers six guiding principles for TIC. These principles are important resources for both the individual care plan and the systems in which the case manager is driving an ICM approach. Figure 13.5 (CDC, 2022) provides an illustration and explanation of these six principles.

FIGURE 13.5 Substance Abuse and Mental Health Services Administration Trauma Informed Care guiding principles.

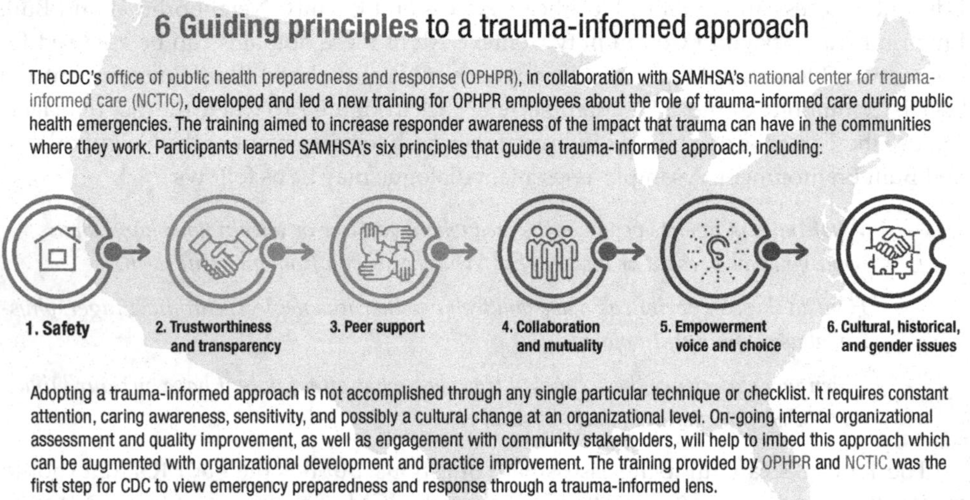
6 Guiding principles to a trauma-informed approach
The CDC's office of public health preparedness and response (OPHPR), in collaboration with SAMHSA's national center for trauma-informed care (NCTIC), developed and led a new training for OPHPR employees about the role of trauma-informed care during public health emergencies. The training aimed to increase responder awareness of the impact that trauma can have in the communities where they work. Participants learned SAMHSA's six principles that guide a trauma-informed approach, including:
1. Safety
2. Trustworthiness and transparency
3. Peer support
4. Collaboration and mutuality
5. Empowerment voice and choice
6. Cultural, historical, and gender issues
Adopting a trauma-informed approach is not accomplished through any single particular technique or checklist. It requires constant attention, caring awareness, sensitivity, and possibly a cultural change at an organizational level. On-going internal organizational assessment and quality improvement, as well as engagement with community stakeholders, will help to imbed this approach which can be augmented with organizational development and practice improvement. The training provided by OPHPR and NCTIC was the first step for CDC to view emergency preparedness and response through a trauma-informed lens.

Source: Center for Disease Control. (2022, December). *Infographic: 6 guiding principles to a trauma-informed approach.*. https://www.cdc.gov/cpr/infographics/6_principles_trauma_info.htm

TABLE 13.1 Sample Trauma Informed Care Checklist for Integrated Case Management

Principle	**Case Manager Checklist**
Safety	Ensure physically and psychologically safe environment during assessment
Trustworthiness and Transparency	The organization and collaborative teams are transparent in the type of resources utilized for TIC (policies, team meetings, patient rights)
Peer Support	Multidisciplinary teams advocate for professional self-care and prevention of vicarious trauma (see glossary for definition of vicarious trauma)
Collaboration and Mutuality	ICM plan includes shared decision-making and promotion of healing relationships internally and externally to the care delivery system
Empowerment Voice and Choice	The organization recognizes the uniqueness of each patient experience and incorporates the positive attributes of patients into the care plan
Cultural, Historical, and Gender Issues	The care plan reflects the organization's policies of cultural humility and connects cultural traditions to the healing process of trauma survivors

ICM, integrated case management; TIC, trauma informed care.
Source: Center for Disease Control. (2022, December). *Infographic: 6 guiding principles to a trauma-informed approach*. https://www.cdc.gov/cpr/infographics/6_principles_trauma_info.htm, SAMSHA, 2022

The SAMHSA principles offer an evidence-based approach to develop tools and tips for case managers. Table 13.1 provides an example of an ICM checklist aligned to TIC principles (not all inclusive).

Tolan et al. (2022) studied TIC in their work with children who experienced trauma. They incorporated the principles of safety and "voice" by way of connecting with children to facilitate therapeutics and treatments. The tips shared by Tolan et al. (2022) are applicable to TIC with adults, beginning with the "expectation" of a traumatic history as noted earlier. To incorporate Tolan et al. (2022) suggestions, case managers should

- Approach the care of complex patients in the same way clinicians assume universal precautions for infection control . . . assume there is a history of trauma.
- Clearly explain why sensitive screening questions or physical contact may be required during the assessment phase and apply cultural considerations.
- Create psychological safety by inquiring about anything in their past might be difficult to answer or experience; empower the patient by asking how to make assessment easier to cope.
- Be astute to physical and nonverbal signs of emotional stress, anxiety, "shutdown."
- Demonstrate an attitude of patience, empathy, kindness, compassion . . . noting this is often challenging due to workload and pace of patient care.

Shame Sensitive Care

Another tip when delivering TIC is to be aware of the lived experience of the trauma survivor. The patient/client may appear to not be forthcoming or nonparticipating. Post-trauma experiences elicit a variety of emotions, such as embarrassment or shame, especially in the case of sexual trauma. Dolezal and Gibson (2022) advocates for shame-sensitive practice as essential to a TIC approach. They noted that "shame is a key emotional after-effect of experiences of trauma, and clinicians may not recognize the subtleness of how shame influences the post-trauma survivor's response. Case managers must be patient and employ all modes of communication skills to assess and support the healing process.

Vicarious Trauma

Merriam-Webster defines the word vicarious as "experienced or realized through imaginative or sympathetic participation in the experience of another" (Merriam-Webster online dictionary, retrieved September 2022). Case management practice standards require case managers to treat patient/clients with empathy. However, one must be cognizant of assuming the lived experiences of trauma survivors and to not become negatively affected. If one is a supervisor or case management leader, SAMHSA (2014a,b) describes the importance of supporting staff with trauma histories and/or staff who spend significant time with survivors of trauma. The goal is to not prompt secondary trauma in staff as they work with individuals experiencing complex trauma. Working with survivors of trauma can produce significant stress in staff. And, as noted earlier, stress can have real effects on the mind and body. Fredericksen (2018) illustrates the effect of stress on the body and when coupled with vicarious trauma, case managers must seek to protect oneself. See Figure 13.6 for a depiction of Fredericksen's stress chart (online source, paceconnection.com, retrieved September 2022).

As case managers, the care management of others also necessitates selfcare of oneself. Figure 13.6 can be used as a reference if one is experiencing personal symptoms in any of the mind and body systems. While vicarious trauma is not a concern for everyone, it should be a consideration if the clinician is feeling triggered or having unexplained stress ailments. If experiencing such issues, always seek the advice of a medical professional.

FIGURE 13.6 How stress affects the body.

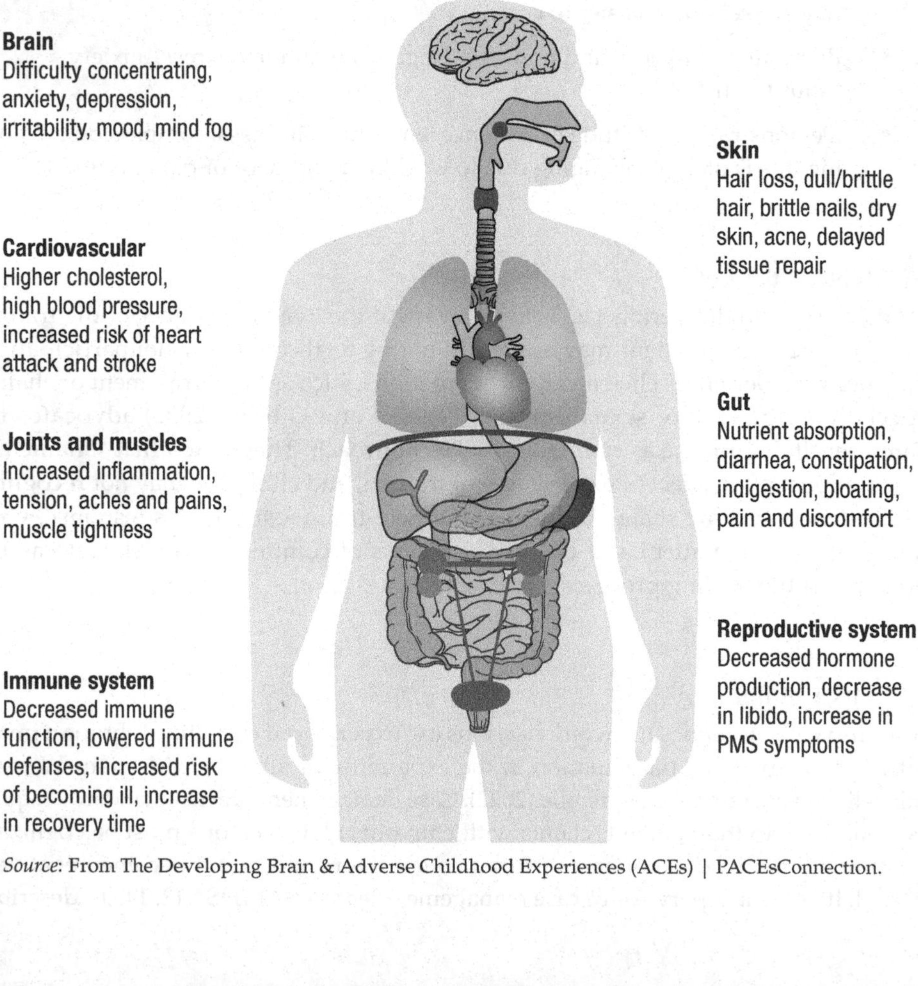

Source: From The Developing Brain & Adverse Childhood Experiences (ACEs) | PACEsConnection.

Trauma Survivor Case Studies

CASE STUDY 1

Homeless Veteran (Sample Dialogue)

"Sandy is placed in a housing and rehabilitation program for homeless veterans. She has been working as a case manager with Tim, a 45-year-old Army veteran who has been homeless for more than 2 years. Tim also has an addiction to opiates and alcohol. Tim has been in the program for 1 month and is likely to remain a resident for another 3 to 4 months. She meets with him weekly to see how he is progressing on the goals that he and the clinical team have established. During these meetings, Tim has begun to disclose his memories of combat in the Mideast, which included seeing friends blown-up from improvised explosive devices and women and children killed by allied forces. When Sandy meets with her field instructor, Matthew, she tells him she does not know how to help Tim: "I'm not a therapist just a case manager." Sandy also becomes teary-eyed as she relates to Matthew some of the experiences that Tim shared with her. Matthew assures Sandy that she does have the skills needed to help Tim with what he has disclosed, and he also validates how difficult it is to hear stories such as Tim's:

Matthew: A lot of our clients have seen and done terrible things. That's why a lot of them end up homeless and addicted. And it's really hard to hear their stories. Over the years, I've learned ways to deal with my feelings. I'm thinking we could take some time to help you do the same. No matter where you work or who you work with, your feelings can get the best of you. But, how about we first talk about how you can be- really how you are—being helpful to Tim.

Sandy: Great, because I feel like I'm not qualified to help him!

Matthew: You're not giving yourself enough credit! First off, you listened to his recollections and expressed your concern for him and sadness for what he experienced, right? That means you validated his experience and what it meant for him. By letting him talk about this, you are helping him manage his feelings.

Sandy: But he needs so much more than I can provide.

Matthew: Well, I agree, that your role doesn't allow you to provide him with in-depth counseling, but as his case manager, you do have the ability to validate his concerns, identify resources that can help him deal with his war experiences, and support the positive changes he has been making. Those are all incredibly important for Tim.

Matthew had not been trained in trauma-informed practice or supervision. However, his work with Sandy is consistent with TI principles. Trauma-informed supervision simultaneously addresses supervisees' potential for indirect trauma and assists them in responding appropriately and in non-traumatizing ways to clients with histories of trauma. The content of field instruction exists within a climate that reflects safety, trust, empowerment, choice, and collaboration.

Safety and trust seemed to already exist in this field instruction relationship, as evidenced by Sandy's willingness to disclose her feelings about her work. Matthew uses his own experiences with indirect trauma to normalize Sandy's reactions and suggests they spend time identifying ways to manage them, which is empowering and reinforces safety and trust. He does not intend to tell her what to do to manage her feelings; he will help her decide this for herself, consistent with collaboration, empowerment, and choice. Finally, Matthew helps Sandy see how she can practice within her role as a case manager and still address in a meaningful way Tim's underlying experience with trauma (Knight, 2019, p. 83).

CASE STUDY 2

School Shooting Survivor (Self-Study)

Janice is a 22-year-old victim of a major vehicular accident. She has a moderate brain injury, two broken ribs and a fractured femur. She is also undergoing tests to determine the extent of injury to her spine. Janice has no significant medical or surgical history. Janice communicates very little with the staff, is not engaged in her care and exhibiting signs of anxiety and depression. The discharge planning nurse contacted the case management department for assistance with Janice's inpatient and post-hospitalization care. Janice recently moves to the area, lives alone in an apartment and has no family or significant others in the local vicinity. She has been referred to you for case management and your first encounter with Janice began with her shouting "I might as well die now because I won't be able to run from the active shooter!" The self-study of this case should include TIC concepts such as the Three E's, Four R's and Motivational Interviewing. Role play or write a sample dialogue of the case manager-patient interaction.

REFERENCES

Case Management Society of America. (2022). *Standards of practice for case management*. Author.

Center for Disease Control. (2022, December). *Infographic: 6 guiding principles to a trauma-informed approach*. https://www.cdc.gov/cpr/infographics/6_principles_trauma_info.htm

Dolezal, L., & Gibson, M. (2022). Beyond a trauma-informed approach and towards shame-sensitive practice. *Humanities & Social Sciences Communications*, *9*(1). https://doi-org.proxymu.wrlc.org/10.1057/s41599-022-01227-z

Frederiksen, L. (2018). The developing brain & adverse childhood experiences. *Online source*. PACEconnection.com https://www.pacesconnection.com/blog/the-developing-brain-and-adverse-childhood-experiences-aces

Hopper, E. K., Bassuk, E. L., & Olivet, J. (2010). Shelter from the storm: Trauma-informed care in homelessness services settings. *The Open Health Services and Policy Journal*, *3*, 80–100.

Hunter, N. (2022). Mind clear psychotherapy website. Online source retrieved August 2022. Complex Trauma, Stress and the Body: It's All Connected (mindclearpsychotherapy.com)

Knight, C. (2019). Trauma informed practice and care: Implications for field instruction. *Clinical Social Work Journal*, *47*, 79–89. https://doi.org/10.1007/s10615-018-0661-x

Kozlowska, K., Walker, P., McLean, L., & Carrive, P. (2015). Fear and the defense cascade: Clinical implications and management. *Harvard Review of Psychiatry*, *23*(4), 263–287. https://doi.org/10.1097/HRP.0000 00000000006

Shonkoff, J. P., & Phillips, D. A (Eds.). (2000). *The developing brain, chapter 8. From neurons to neighborhoods: The science of early childhood development*. National Academies Press. https://www.ncbi.nlm.nih.gov /books/NBK225562/

Substance Abuse and Mental Health Services Administration. (2014a). *SAMHSA's concept of trauma and guidance for a trauma-informed approach*. SAMHSA's Trauma and Justice Strategic Initiative. U.S. Department of Health and Human Services. https://ncsacw.acf.hhs.gov/userfiles/files/SAMHSA_Trauma.pdf

Substance Abuse and Mental Health Services Administration (SAMHSA). (2014b). *Trauma-informed care in behavioral health services. Treatment Improvement Protocol (TIP) Series No. 57*. Section 1, A, Review of the Literature https://www.ncbi.nlm.nih.gov/books/NBK207192/

Substance Abuse and Mental Health Services Administration. (2021). *SAMHSA/ TIC curriculum instructor's guidance SAMHSA's trauma-informed approach: Key assumptions and principles*. U.S. Department of Health and Human Services. https://www.nasmhpd.org/sites/default/files/TraumaTIACurricu lumTrainersManual_6-2-21.pdf

Thirkle, S. A., Kennedy, A., & Sice, P. (2021). Instruments for exploring trauma-informed care. *Journal of Health and Human Services Administration*, *44*(1), 30–44. https://doi.org/10.37808/jhhsa.44.1.2

Tolan, R., Blake, A., & Buisman-Pijlman, F. (2022). Connecting the head to the body – trauma-informed care in practice. *Australian Nursing and Midwifery Journal*, *27*(8), 47. http://proxymu.wrlc.org/login

U.S. Department of Health and Human Services. (2022). *Office of disease prevention and health promotion*. Online Source retrieved September 2022 https://health.gov/healthypeople/priority-areas/social-determ inants-health

Zatzick, D., Rivara, F., Jurkovich, G., Russo, J., Trusz, S. G., Wang, J., Wagner, A., Stephens, K., Dunn, C., Uehara, E., Petrie, M., Engel, C., Davydow, D., & Katon, W. (2011). Enhancing the population impact of collaborative care interventions: Mixed method development and implementation of stepped care targeting posttraumatic stress disorder and related comorbidities after acute trauma. *General Hospital Psychiatry*, *33*(2), 123–134. https://doi.org/10.1016/j.genhosppsych.2011.01.001

CHAPTER 14

Children With Special Healthcare Needs

Kathleen M. Moriarty

OBJECTIVES

- Discover how a child's developmental status impacts how care is delivered
- Summarize how parent/caregiver needs impact the child's needs
- Demonstrate the impact of case management on admissions and lengths of stays for the pediatric patient

Pediatric Population

Providing care to children requires a special approach, especially the hospitalized pediatric patient. After all, children are not just miniature adults. They function differently. They are born into external conditions beyond their control such as poverty and healthcare inequities. They feed and grow differently from adults, their bodies absorb medication differently, and as a result, hospitalized children need an advocate within the family and the care team. Each year, more than 3 million children are hospitalized in the United States. Whether that is a planned event for a procedure or test, or for treatment of a chronic disease, children need a voice. Each hospitalization can have a major impact on the child and the family. If that child is one with multiple diseases or conditions, which often began at birth, hospitalizations can last up to a year or more depending on the complexities and resources available to care for the child. According to the Centers for Disease Control and Prevention (CDC), children with special healthcare needs account for one out of every five children in the United States (McPherson et al., 1998). Physical conditions common to children with special healthcare needs include but are not limited to extreme prematurity, chronic lung disease, bronchopulmonary dysplasia (BPD), multiple congenital and genetic anomalies, gastrointestinal anomalies, and cardiac anomalies.

Pediatric Mortality

Substantial global progress has been made since 1990 in reducing childhood mortality. The total number of deaths in children under 5 years old worldwide has declined from 12.6 million in 1990 to 5 million in 2020 (World Health Organization [WHO], 2020). Since 1990, the global mortality rate for children under 5 years old has dropped by 60%, from 93 deaths per 1,000 live births in 1990 to 37 in 2020 (WHO, 2020). This is equivalent to 1 in 11 children dying before reaching age 5 in 1990, compared to 1 in 27 in 2020 (McPherson et al., 1998). Caring for a critically ill child with multiple organ systems impacted at birth and later is a difficult situation. Critically ill and medically complex children lay heavy emotional, physical, and financial burdens on the family of the child. Health systems are also challenged with rising costs, decreased reimbursement, and greater out- of- pocket expenses passed on to families and caregivers. Even with insurance or Medicaid, family expenses can be significant. Insurance deductibles can run into tens of thousands of dollars per year, while the cost of transportation and parking at the hospital location are substantial. For the primary caregiver, job losses and lost wages are real and can accumulate when caring for complex children.

In addition to physical conditions, one must consider the psychological and behavioral conditions that exist while caring for a pediatric patient. Across the nation, children were in the midst of a growing behavioral health crisis even prior to the COVID-19 pandemic. A decade ago, the CDC reported that one in five children in the United States were diagnosed with a mental health disorder (Bartlett & Stratford, 2021). In 2015, suicide was the second most common cause of death among young people ages 15 to 24 (National Academies Sciences Engineering Medicine [NASEM], 2019). Further concerns for this high-risk population are that every state in the United States has reported experiencing either a high or severe shortage of practicing child and adolescent psychiatrists (Martinelli et al., 2020). Other behavioral health workers including psychologists, social workers, and other therapists suffer from high turnover rates, increased demands, and overwhelming caseloads, resulting in higher rates of burnout and stress (Haseltine, 2021).

For children, the COVID-19 pandemic took a toll on their lives when schools, social routines, and even their home life were completely upended by the pandemic. An estimated 37,300 to 43,000 children lost a parent to COVID-19. The disparities recognized during the COVID-19 pandemic included higher rates of parental loss for Black children (Kidman et al, 2021). These types of disruptions and tragedies experienced by children and adolescents can have lifelong effects. Many children suffered the loss of a family member, especially in communities that were already distressed and economically disadvantaged.

Case managers have learned—and continue to learn—that because of the pandemic, COVID-19 has exacerbated long-standing gaps in the care available for children, especially mental health services. An emphasis on discharge planning and addressing barriers to care and supports needed to stabilize a child in behavioral health crisis is a must. Case managers, particularly social workers trained in behavioral health, are best suited to address the growing behavioral conditions and social determinants of health (SDH). The SDH affecting the pediatric population include poor housing or homelessness, food insecurities, experiencing discrimination, racism, and violence. Gun violence is a community concern and one that cannot be ignored when evaluating health disparities and evaluating health systems. SDHs, such as poverty levels and gun violence, can be tracked within communities by zip code. For hospitals to respond and support the nation's youth, crisis intervention programs are recommended to address public safety and security. The National Institute of Health has released targeted grants to support areas with reported high rates of violent crime. Community violence intervention programs are beginning to support these efforts, such as via the hospital-based violence intervention program, also known as trauma-informed care (TIC) , for individuals who have experienced violence. Several states now incorporate hospital-based intervention reimbursement into Medicaid plans. Getting pediatric patients safely back into their social communities, including schools, allows them to interact with friends and perform social activities that allow them to lead healthy lives both personally and socially.

Health System Challenges

How is case management different in pediatric hospitals? Bower and Reid (2008) offer these five dimensions:

1. Every patient has a payer, each with unique and increasingly stringent requirements.
2. Community resources are scarce, especially for technology-dependent, complex, and chronically ill children.
3. Children, especially those with catastrophic issues, may leave acute care having used much or all of their lifetime allocation of insurance payments.
4. Identification and confirmation of the legal parent and/or guardian is often a challenge.
5. The patient and family are one entity and generally inseparable.

The coordination needed to navigate different healthcare systems, different electronic medical records (EMR) with limited communication, ineffective collaboration, and insurance barriers, is complex. In pediatrics, the case manager must be creative and develop relationships with payer case managers, community resources, and most importantly the patient and their family.

Role of Case Management

Hospital providers and health insurance companies that support case management and care coordination roles often benefit from these roles to help reduce these complex challenges. Introducing case management and care coordination services to support the child and their caregivers has allowed the pediatric population to thrive and reach optimal healthcare outcomes. Case managers continuously strive to give the children in their care the best life possible, understanding that circumstances will be limited to a certain degree because of their chronic health problems. A review of literature published by the American Academy of Pediatrics revealed families were increasingly more satisfied with the overall healthcare experience when working with case managers. With comprehensive case management and care coordination, medically complex children can reach their full potential with better outcomes listed, some of which are listed in the following (Ehlenbach & Coller, 2020; McCarthy et al., 2021):

- Shorter initial hospital stays;
- Fewer readmissions;
- Fewer emergency department visits;
- Early intervention enrollment with the introduction of therapies, accelerating their development;
- Improved coordination with fewer missed appointments; and
- Safe transitions to the home setting.

Benefits of Case Management

General studies of medically complex children and their related medical expenses have found that an effective care coordination program could save 10% to 20% of the overall care expense for this type of child (Berry et al., 2014). The case manager functions as a primary source of support, advocacy, education, and way-finder for a family throughout their child's hospitalization. Figure 14.1 depicts an example of how the case manager interacts with a multidisciplinary care team for a patient born prematurely. In the example, multiple team members are involved in the care for a medically complex neonate ICU patient. The case manager role intersects with numerous team members, gathering information to present to the family in a coordinated way. Case managers fill the gaps in communication and care between the family and care team members. Figure 14.1 illustrates the multiple specialties needed to care for a complex neonate:

- Necrotizing enterocolitis (NEC)—requiring pediatric surgery
- Intraventricular hemorrhage (IVH)/hydrocephalus/seizures—requiring neurology and neurosurgery
- Tracheostomy placement—requiring ear, nose, and throat specialist long-term mechanical ventilation—requiring pulmonary habilitation program (PHP)
- Retinopathy of prematurity (ROP)—Requiring Ophthalmology Specialists
- Adrenal insufficiency—requiring endocrinology
- Family support services (FSS): Licensed clinical social workers (LCSW), certified child life specialists, board certified chaplain
- Discharge planning: Clinical case management and utilization management RNs

FIGURE 14.1 Multidisciplinary care coordination.

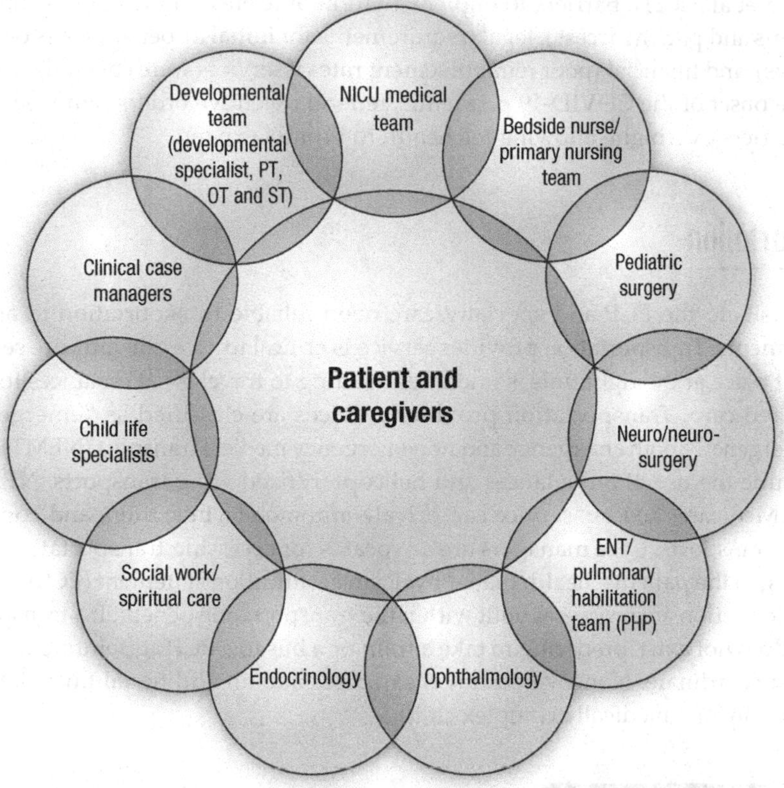

Source: Developed at the Ann and Robert H. Lurie Children's Hospital, Care Coordination, 2021.

Case Manager Role in Family Communication

Immediate access to healthcare is vital for this population. Having families activate a more direct communication tool to their provider, such as EMR two-way communication, allows for a single source of truth for the medical history of that child. In the case manager role, one of the most important tasks to achieve prior to discharge is the activation of the EMR and how to navigate a message to the provider in their native language that is best understood. Beyond electronic communication, in-person assessment and treatments are inevitable such as office visits with the primary care physician (PCP) and specialists involved in the child's care.

Telehealth

Telehealth has made its way to pediatric care because of the COVID-19 pandemic, however not without challenges. While telehealth can have an immense impact on removing some barriers to care (e.g., time and travel constraints, infection prevention in office settings), other barriers may persist. Limited data from 2020 show that many barriers to care caused by racial and social disparities were mirrored with telehealth implementation (Chunara et al., 2021). Barriers to implementation of telehealth included technological (platforms and patient access), legal (requirements for initial in-person visits or variable state laws), and financial (poor reimbursement rates if services were covered) challenges. With the onset of the COVID-19 pandemic, federal executive orders removed many of these barriers overnight, allowing telehealth to rapidly expand.

Transportation

Office visits to the PCP and specialty care need reliable transportation to and from appointments. Transportation provider service is critical to access healthcare services at the right place at the right time, sometimes needing to travel great distances for highly specialized care. Transportation provider services are classified as "emergency" or "nonemergency." Both emergency and nonemergency medical transport (NEMT) services can include the use of ambulances and helicopter/fixed wing transports. NEMT also include Medicare, taxicab, service car, private automobile, bus, train, and commercial airplane transports. Case managers are advocates for accessing transportation benefits according to the patients' health plan. Physician certification statement (PCS) forms and pre-authorization are processes built within the transportation benefit. If a transportation benefit does not exist, preparing to take a train or a bus to a PCP appointment can takes weeks to coordinate. Noncovered travel expenses add an additional financial burden on the family of a medically complex child.

CASE STUDY 1

Jose was born extremely premature with multiple defects. With a genetic workup, Jose was diagnosed with CHARGE syndrome, where C stands for Coloboma, an irregularly shaped pupil, often described as a shape of a keyhole; H for *H*eart anomaly, usually tetralogy of Fallot with pulmonary stenosis, ventricular septal defect, right ventricle hypertrophy, and an overriding aorta; blockage of the airway is usually identified as choanal *A*tresia; R is for growth *R*etardation; G for *G*enital abnormalities, seen often with males more than females; and lastly, E is for *E*ar anomalies often with deafness. Distintctive facial features may also be present including 'square-shaped' head or facial asymmetry. CHARGE syndrome is an autosomal dominant or sporadic condition that affects structures derived from rostral neural crest cells. A gene associated with CHARGE syndrome has been identified on chromosome 8 and involves mutations. It also includes abnormalities in the development of the eyes and midbrain. An early eye exam identified the typical "keyhole" shaped pupil. Other ear, nose, and throat abnormalities included a blockage of his nasal passage and ear abnormalities. Treatment requires medical and surgical treatment for the defect such as cardiac surgery; physical, occupational, and speech therapy are usually indicated. Medically complex babies need multiple surgeries due to the multiple systems involved. In this case study, Jose's anticipated problems involve feeding, growing, developing, and doing the things that normal developing children do. Jose has eight providers that round daily. Coordinating and helping Jose's family navigate through that can be a challenge. While hospitalized, Jose's invasive treatments requiring anesthesia and sedation were clustered, allowing him to receive care that is streamlined. Jose's family does not own a car, English is their second language, and they live 25 miles from the hospital. In preparation for discharge, managing follow up appointments, medications, and day-to-day care needs a case manager is needed to help navigate through the process. Jose's case manager is the key point person—the same face and the keeper of the knowledge throughout the admission and one less unknown for the family preparing for the transition of care. Communication is key and filling in gaps in communication with the coordination of interpreter services is often the role of the case manager. For successful follow-up care, the case manager confirms and accesses transportation services through the state, allowing Jose's family to adhere to follow-up appointments.

CASE STUDY 2

Sophia is a child born prematurely with multiple cardiac and respiratory anomalies. Her condition is too complex to be cared for at the local hospital so shortly after birth, she was transferred to a pediatric medical center. She underwent several tests and procedures immediately after delivery due to acute respiratory failure. Sophia was diagnosed with bronchopulmonary dysplasia (BPD) requiring mechanical ventilation. In addition to prematurity, BPD can be caused by malformation of the lungs, pneumonia, and other infections of the newborn. BPD patients spend many months in the hospital to develop their lungs and adjust ventilation settings to provide more oxygen with lower breaths. This chronic lung disease often causes poor growth and development. Treatment includes mechanical ventilation, medication to support lung function, and antibiotics to fight infection. There is no cure for BPD but it can be treated and most infants go on to live a long and healthy life. Caring for a medically complex child is a full-time job. Scheduling appointments, caring for home medical equipment, coordinating home nursing (often a medically necessary and covered benefit), and follow-up with the payer for approval comes with complexities. Getting Sophia home to reach growth milestones that are difficult to achieve in the hospital is the goal of the case manager. A child life specialist is another member of the pediatric interdisciplinary team who works with the patient and family to help cope with the challenges of prolonged hospitalizations, disabilities, and illness. Children in the hospital do not do the same things they do at home. At home, supported by the family, surrounded with love and comfort, Sophia can develop and grow in a more natural and optimal way. Getting Sophia home and keeping her at home is the goal of the team. With multiple systems involved, Sophia was prescribed up to 25 medications at discharge. Hospital case managers coordinating care provided instructions for medication administration, allowing the caregivers to gain confidence in caring for their child. Pictograms are used by case managers to provide a helpful guide that pairs active medical problems with their respective specialty service, with relevant medication, and when follow-up appointments are necessary. Utilizing tools to promote medication adherence results in reduced complications and adverse events.

CASE STUDY 3

Julia is a 12-year-old child with cerebral palsy that was caused by lack of oxygen to her brain during birth. Cerebral palsy is Julia's underlying chronic condition. She has multiple organ systems impacted by the cerebral palsy that include respiratory, neurologic, and musculoskeletal complications such as, pneumonia, seizures requiring multiple medications for control, and muscle spasticity that results in spinal malformation, chronic pain, and poor alignment. Julia and her family rely heavily on durable medical equipment (DME) to maintain an active lifestyle. The family has housing challenges due to living in a third-floor walkup. As a result, the case manager worked closely with family services to investigate other housing options. Knowing what resources are available and tapping into resources is a skill set every case manager needs. Coordinating weekly care conferences allows for regular cadence to track progress or change direction if needed.

Executing the Case Management Process

Communication is key to case manage a complex child such as Julia during hospitalization. Recurrent communication with the family, providers, and members of the care team is a case manager function. Achieving ongoing understanding of the needs of the child and family is often discussed during family care conferences coordinated by the case manager responsible for care coordination activities. Healthcare findings, treatment plans, and the trajectory of care are discussed. Documentation of care conferences in the EMR allows for a single source of proactive care planning and follow- up action items. The case manager is often the individual who manages the roles and responsibilities of the healthcare team members and shares the goals of care to support the child's quality of life. The importance of empowering the child's primary caregiver, often the parent, cannot be stressed enough. The case manager assesses the family preferences, teaches caregiving skills, assists with home caregiving activities, supports physical and emotional health, addresses financial and social issues, and encourages shared decision-making (Berry et al., 2014).

The case manager meets with caregivers regularly to foster a trusting relationship and partnership. They develop an individualized plan to support each patient and caregiver's unique needs. The case manager provides caregivers with guidance and resources to successfully navigate the hospital system, health coverage options from state and commercial health plans, and identify barriers to caregivers participating in patient's care and implements appropriate interventions. For example, Sophia's case manager coordinates tests and procedures with members of the care team so Sophia does not have to undergo anesthesia multiple times. Partnering with bedside nursing colleagues helps to gain insights into a family's coping, comprehension of the child's condition, and training. The case manager should partner with nursing teams to establish caregiver learning goals and support nursing by providing appropriate educational resources to caregivers.

The case manager checks in regularly with the primary medical team (PMT) to assess a patient's status and plan for next steps. The PMT appreciates regular information sharing to keep them up to date with the family's concerns or questions. The case manager needs to anticipate the potential barriers a family may face related to discharge, that include:

- Collaboration with PMT to coordinate family care conferences,
- Documentation in the EMR or other appropriate documentation systems the results of care conferences followed by plan of care updates,
- Advocate for consistency in care through partnership with PMT and other providers, and
- Partner with all providers to develop an outpatient follow up plan and develop a provider contact list for the caregiver.

The case manager is a member of the pediatric interdisciplinary team with a primary focus on care coordination. In a 60-bed neonatal ICU unit, the case manager focuses on the high-risk patients and anticipates challenges or barriers related to discharge information. The case manager coordinates discharge planning meetings and works with the interdisciplinary team to facilitate key events such as caregiver training via a 24-hour stay in the hospital with the child. Most pediatric hospitals require this 24-hour stay be performed by two individuals that will be the primary caregivers in the home. Each caregiver must complete a separate 24-hour stay providing total patient care. Care includes preparing and administering medications (preferably from home supplies), taking and recording vital signs, completing activities of daily living for the child (washing, toileting, diapering, feeding), and, if applicable, monitoring any wound site for infection and monitoring the child for signs and symptoms of infection and/or rejection.

Licensed social workers are members of the interdisciplinary team and may also function as a case manager. They will typically report to the case management department or a Family Self-Sufficiency (FSS) department consisting of other licensed professionals that are often unique to pediatric case management. These may include child life, housing, spiritual care, and interpreter services. The case manager also collaborates with FSS to assess and support the coping needs of the family unit. These professionals attend family care conferences to help support caregivers through decision-making. They are great partners to ensure caregivers are connected to community resources prior to discharge. Developmental team members facilitate services such as physical, occupational, and speech therapies and developmental specialties. For certain populations in pediatric care, developmental rounds are used to remain informed of the patient's developmental progress and allow caregivers to participate in their child's therapy sessions. The complex process of discharging patients from acute care hospitals requires effective collaboration between multidisciplinary teams and patients. Miscommunication about patient instructions and follow-up appointments can lead to posthospital adverse events, patient dissatisfaction, and delays in discharge (Patel et al., 2019). Figure 14.2 is a helpful guide that allows caregivers to learn the active problems and their associated resources specific to the needs of the child.

Executing a safe transition plan for the complex pediatric patient can take weeks to months. Once an expected discharge date is identified by the team, the case manager and care coordinator are responsible for completion of many tasks. This can include arranging CPR training of the caregivers, obtaining authorization for medication, durable

FIGURE 14.2 Caregiver's guide to active problems and associated resources for their child.

Icon	Service	Health problem	Provider	Daytime contact information	After-hours contact information	Medication	Appointment
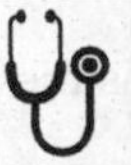	Pediatrician	Healthcare maintenance					
Additional information: - Feeding schedule as of ***:							
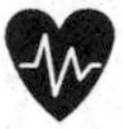	Cardiac electro-physiology						
Additional information:							
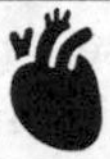	Cardiology						

Source: Developed at the Ann and Robert H. Lurie Children's Hospital, Care Coordination, 2021.

medical equipment and other specialty services such as home nursing that are unique to this population. One challenge a hospital case manager encounters is the need for authorization for medically necessary medication or supplies that are specific to the patient's needs. Developing a collaborative relationship with the patient's insurance company and their case manager helps prevent delays. A discharge checklist including each provider's contact information supports adherence to the follow-up care needed. Simple, nontechnical, and illustrated engagement tools with optimized readability begin to formulate outpatient follow-up care. For those families with underdeveloped literacy skills, these tools are written in layperson language at the fourth- to sixth-grade reading level for greater understanding. These tools facilitate teach-back and reinforce learning about topics that include the condition itself, when to get help, self-management techniques, how to prepare for doctor appointments, and other related subjects.

Many care management programs have outpatient case managers that manage the transition from inpatient to outpatient. These individuals can be a registered nurse and licensed social worker. Outpatient care coordination fosters a trusting relationship that begins in the hospital while planning for the transition home. An individualized care plan needs to be established to confirm appointments, arrange transportation, connect families with community resources, coordinate with home health/early intervention services, provide condition and parenting education, interface with payers, and address psychosocial needs. To provide continuity of care, these outpatient case managers may perform home visits, and attend initial PCP appointments and specialist appointments as needed. As patient advocates, they support the caregivers when questions arise. The outpatient case manager consults with interdisciplinary team members to ascertain the child and caregiver's needs. It is not unusual to have an outpatient case manager follow the medically complex child and family for 2 to 3 years postdischarge. With care coordination, adherence to follow-up care patient outcomes are improved. Getting the family engaged in their child's healthcare is a key component of self-management, such as Julia with cerebral palsy. Adherence to the care plan is more likely to happen if the patient or caregiver is engaged in their child's healthcare (Perez, 2022). Although future hospitalizations for ongoing treatment are expected, unplanned readmissions are reduced with effective care coordination programs. Parents often express multiple challenges associated with the chronicity of medical management and transitions of care for the medically complex child. Future interventions aiming to improve continuity and communication between admissions, ensure that home services are provided when applicable and prescriptions are filled, and provide comprehensive support for families in both the short- and long-term may help improve patient and family experiences while potentially decreasing readmissions (Leary et al., 2020).

The goal of a pediatric hospital case manager is to provide safe transitions of care. The complexities that exist can be a challenge to the health system but more so to the patient and their families. Measurements of success include reductions in length of stay, unplanned readmissions, and emergency department visits. Increases in completed outpatient appointments, caregiver access, and engagement with the EMR facilitates timely communication; as well as, early intervention for challenges shape successful transitions. Having a care coordination program that can remove barriers and empower the family and caregivers to care for the child is considered a successful discharge and one that every case manager should celebrate. Case management must continue past the acute care episode to support outpatient management and prevent, as much as possible, admissions, readmissions, and complications. The hospital admission is but one event along the continuum; supporting the child and caregiver throughout the continuum is key to continued health stabilization and improvement.

REFERENCES

Bartlett, J. D., & Stratford, B. (2021, January 28). *A national agenda for child's mental health. Child Trends*. https://www.childtrends.org/publications/a-national-agenda-for-childrens-mental-health

Berry, J. G., Hall, M., Neff, J., Goodman, D., Cohen, E., Agrawal, R., Kuo, D., & Feudtner, C. (2014). Children with medical complexity and Medicaid: spending and cost savings. *Health Affairs, 33*(12), 2199–2206. https://doi.org/10.1377/hlthaff.2014.0828

Bower, K., & Reid, M. (2008). *The Center for Case Management, Inc.*

Chunara, R., Zhao, Y., Chen, J., Lawrence, K., Testa, P.A., Nov, O., & Mann, D. M. (2021). Telemedicine and healthcare disparities: a cohort study in a large healthcare system in New York City during COVID-19. *Journal of the American Medical Informatics Association, 28*(1), 33–41. https://doi.org/10.1093/jamia/ocaa217

Ehlenbach, M. L., & Coller, R. J. (2020). Growing evidence for successful care management in children with medical complexity. *Pediatrics, 145*(4), e20193982. https://doi.org/10.1542/peds.2019-3982

Haseltine, W. A. (2021, March 9). *The COVID syndemic: The mental health crisis of mental health workers*. Forbes.com. http://www.forbes.com/sites/williamhaseltine/2021/03/09/the-covid-syndemic-the-mental-health-crisis-of-mental-health-workers/?sh=1c1299d451c2

Kidman, R., Margolis, R., Smith-Greenaway, E., & Verdery, A. M. (2021, April 5). Estimates and projections of COVID-19 and parental death in the US. *JAMA Pediatrics, 175*(7), 745–746. https://jamanetwork.com/journals/jamapediatrics/fullarticle/2778229

Leary, J. C., Krcmar, R., Yoon, G. H., Freund, K. M., & LeClair, A. M. (2020). Parent perspectives during hospital readmissions for children with medical complexity: A qualitative study. *Hospital Pediatrics, 10*(3), 222–229. https://doi.org/10.1542/hpeds.2019-0185

Martinelli, K., Cohen, Y., Kimball, H., & Sheldon-Dean, H. (2020). *Children's mental health report: Telehealth in an increasing virtual world*. Child Mind Institute. https://childmind.org/our-impact/childrens-mental-health-report/

McCarthy, S., Currier, D., Copp, K., & Donovan, K. (2021). Partnering with families of medically complex children transitioning from the hospital to home. *Pediatrics, 148*(1), e2020031617. https://doi.org/10.1542/peds.2020-031617

McPherson, M., Arango, P., Fox, H., Lauver, C., McManus, M., Newacheck, P. W., Perrin, J. M., Shonkoff, J. P., & Strickland, B. (1998, July 1). A new definition of children with special health care needs. *Pediatrics, 102*(1), 137–139. https://www.who.int/data/gho/data/themes/topics/sdg-target-3_2-newborn-and-child-mortality

National Academies Sciences Engineering Medicine. (2019). *U.S. should create national agenda to improve child and youth mental, emotional, and behavioral health, says report*. Author. https://www.nationalacademies.org/news/2019/09/us-should-create-national-agenda-to-improve-child-and-youth-mental-emotional-and-behavioral-health-says-report

Patel, H., Yirdaw, E., Yu, A., Slater, L., Perica, K., Pierce, R. G., Amaro, C., & Jones, C. (2019). Improving early discharge using a team-based structure for discharge multidisciplinary rounds. *Professional Case Management, 24*(2), 83–89. https://doi.org/10.1097/NCM.0000000000000318

Perez, R, & R. S. (2022). Case management adherence Guide 2020. *Case Management Society of Americ a*, 19–42.

World Health Organization. (2020, January 28). *Newborn mortality*. Author. https://www.who.int/news-room/fact-sheets/detail/levels-and-trends-in-child-mortality-report-2021

CHAPTER 15

Integrated Case Management for Veterans

Melanie A. Prince

OBJECTIVES

- Compare the differences between healthcare delivery systems in the Department of Defense (DOD) versus the Department of Veterans Affairs (VA)
- Describe some of the challenges veterans experience with complex illnesses or injuries
- Apply the tenets of integrated case management to the care of the veteran

Introduction

A veteran is "a person who served in the active military, naval, air, or space service, and who was discharged or released therefrom under conditions other than dishonorable" (Office of the Law Revision Council U.S. Code, 2022). The Department of Veterans Affairs (VA) provides a range of benefits to men and women who served on active duty, including health and medical care. The VA offers the full continuum of healthcare services from wellness and primary care to intensive and specialty care programs. Some veterans experience complex illnesses and/or injuries, often complicated by significant physical and behavioral concerns. Care of the veteran involves a whole person approach and the social determinants of health (SDH) are important considerations for a holistic case management approach. The VA case management programs advocate and support the care of the veteran and integrated case management is an effective model for meeting the needs of veteran care. However, it is important to understand the terminology when providing case management services within the VA.

Essential Definitions

The Department of Defense (DOD) and VA are federal healthcare programs with a unique lexicon and organizational structure. An effective clinical case manager will possess knowledge of the lexicon and organizational systems to facilitate transitions of care and integrated case management. Several of the essential definitions are presented in the following.

The Department of Defense and Military Healthcare System

The DOD and VA are not the same healthcare system. The DOD is the governing body for the Military Healthcare System (MHS). The MHS administers healthcare for men and women who are serving on active duty in one of the United States Armed Forces. In other words, it is the medical system for servicemembers currently serving in the military. This population includes the immediate family members of military servicemembers, referred to as dependents, and also includes civilian individuals who are considered active duty when serving in their Armed Services Reserve roles. One easy way to remember the difference is the MHS is healthcare for those who wear a military uniform and their immediate family members.

The Veterans Affairs and Veterans Health Administration

The VA is the governing body for the Veterans Health Administration. The Veterans Health Administration nomenclature is used interchangeably with "VA." For the purpose of this chapter, VA means Veterans Health Administration. The VA is the medical system for those who have once served in the military but are no longer on active duty status. While there may be an occasion where an active-duty military person may receive care in the VA, the system is established for those who are no longer in uniform. This intersection of active duty-to-veteran care is especially highlighted in the Post-9/11 M2VA Case Management Program design to assist with the transition from servicemember to veteran. The veteran population includes service members who separated from the military in accordance with certain criteria and servicemembers who retired from one of the Armed Forces. Under these conditions, the member is considered a veteran. This population also includes the immediate family members (or dependents) of the veteran.

The Military Health System

The MHS is a system that provides both direct care and indirect care to military members and their dependents. Direct care is provided in military treatment facilities (MTFs) such as military hospitals, clinics, diagnostic centers, Centers of Excellence (COEs), or joint MHS-VA medical centers. Examples of direct care facilities are Walter Reed National Military Medical Center in Bethesda, Maryland; Brooke Army Medical Center in San Antonio, Texas; Naval Hospital Jacksonville, Florida; and Joint-Base Elmendorf-Richardson Medical Center in Alaska. As of 2021, the MHS consisted of 706 MTFs, with 144 located overseas, usually on military installations (Health.mil, 2023). This direct care is also called military medicine.

Indirect care refers to healthcare provided by the civilian sector administered by the TRICARE program. TRICARE is a network of hospitals, clinics, ancillary and diagnostic centers, rehabilitative institutions, behavioral health entities, skilled nursing, and other specialty care organizations that have agreed to participate in the program. TRICARE provides services that are unavailable within the direct care (military) institutions. In other words, TRICARE complements the MTFs. Together, TRICARE (indirect) and MTFs (direct) comprise the MHS.

Characteristics of the Veteran Client/Patient

The veteran client/patient is someone who has served on active duty in the past and was either honorably discharged from the military, medically retired due to service-connected injuries or conditions, or retired from active service after a 20-year commitment. In general, these individuals are eligible for care at a VA facility, but they must enroll for care. Veterans are representative of all demographics. It is a myth that VA clients/patients are older and male.

Typical characteristics of veteran clients/patients eligible for or receive case management services are dual or multidiagnoses, serious illnesses, multitrauma, chronic conditions, or wounded-warrior care. The veteran may also have behavioral health conditions or a combination of behavioral and physical health comorbidities. The veteran clients/patients may be the recipients of inpatient, outpatient, or both types of care. What is unique about a veteran client/patient is the comprehensive, holistic nature of concerns that are addressed by case management, such as homelessness, occupational rehabilitation, or housing adaptations.

Veterans Affairs Case Management Structure and Programs

Any of the primary or specialty care services available in traditional civilian sector care are also available within the VA system. As noted earlier, VA program and case management services not only address behavioral and physical health concerns, but also issues informed by the impact of SDH on clinical outcomes. The VA organizational structure allows for case managers to practice in the community as a way to advance the goals of inpatient or outpatient treatment plans. Most notably, the VA restructured its case/care management program to ensure that "traditional case management" is complemented with a rigorous integrated care management approach. The 2019 VHA DIRECTIVE 1110.04 codified Integrated Standards of Practice ensures professionals who provide case management services receive standardized training and that they approach case management from the lens of basic, moderate, or complex levels of care coordination. See Appendix M for more information on the VA Integrated Standards of Practice.

Application of an Integrated Case Management Approach

Oftentimes, veterans are challenged with both physical and mental health conditions. For example, Vietnam War veterans may be suffering with the ill effects of Agent Orange and long undertreated post traumatic stress disorder (PTSD), not to mention the effects of being treated negatively by members of the general population for their service. Those who served in the Middle East theaters beginning in the 1980s have experienced increased incidence of concussive blast injuries as well as PTSD. The components of brain injury involve both physical and behavioral symptoms.

Catastrophic injuries are always a complication of war but advances in the treatment of traumatic injury and battlefield medicine have resulted in increased survival. Survivability of high force injuries (explosions and gunshot) is now upward of 90% compared to 84% in the Vietnam era, and 80% during World War II (Clough & Khan, 2019). The treatment of the associated emotional trauma is more often the challenge. An integrated case management approach is ideal for addressing the needs of veterans facing physical and mental health conditions. The Case Management Society of America's (CMSA) Integrated Case Management Trainingexplores in depth strategies to reduce risk and disease burden for the veteran challenged with complexity. Case managers will require instruction and training not only in navigation of the VA healthcare system, but to gain additional knowledge of the impact of catastrophic, chronic, and co-occurring mental and behavioral conditions.

REFERENCES

Clough, R. A. J., & Khan, M. (2019). Initial CABC: Advances that have lead to increased survival in military casualties. *Trauma, 21*(4), 247–251. https://doi.org/10.1177/1460408619838438

Department of Veterans Affairs. (2019). VHA DIRECTIVE 1110.04(1.). *Veterans Health Administration Transmittal Sheet.* 20420

Health.mil. (2023). *Military health system and Defense Health Agency.* https://www.health.mil/Military-Health-Topics/Access-Cost-Quality-and-Safety/Military-Hospitals-and-Clinics

Office of the Law Revision Council United States Code. (2022). *Title 38 United States Code 101, definitions.* Veterans Benefits. https://uscode.house.gov/view.xhtml?req=granuleid:USC-prelim-title38-section101&num=0&edition=prelim

Post 9-11 M2VA Case Management Program. (2023). *U.S. Department of Veterans Affairs.* https://www.va.gov/POST911VETERANS/Post_9_11_Transition_and_Case_Management_TCM.asp

CHAPTER 16

Maternal and Child Health

Rebecca Perez

OBJECTIVES

- Define maternal and child health
- Explore the causes of maternal and child morbidity and mortality
- Discover the role case management and care coordination play in reducing disparities related to maternal child health

Introduction

This chapter serves as an introduction to the importance of the role case managers play in maternal child health. The content in this chapter will be further developed as part of Case Management Society of America's (CMSA) Integrated Case Management Training.

Maternal and Child Health

The health of mothers and children are interrelated and impacted by many factors. Maternal health is defined as the health of a mother during pregnancy, childbirth, and the postpartum period (Kaiser Family Foundation [KFF], 2022). Child health is defined as the health of a child from birth through the adolescent years, primarily focusing on birth through 5 years of age (KFF, 2022). Newborn health focuses on the health of an infant from birth through the first 28 days of life.

An estimated 5 million children under the age of 5 years of age die primarily from preventable and treatable causes (KFF, 2022). Approximately 295,000 women die during pregnancy and childbirth each year with millions more suffering severe adverse consequences (KFF, 2022).

Maternal and Child Mortality

The causes of maternal mortality can be attributed to inadequate care during pregnancy and lack of access to contraceptives and family/reproductive health services (KFF, 2022) (Figure 16.1).

FIGURE 16.1 Maternal mortality.

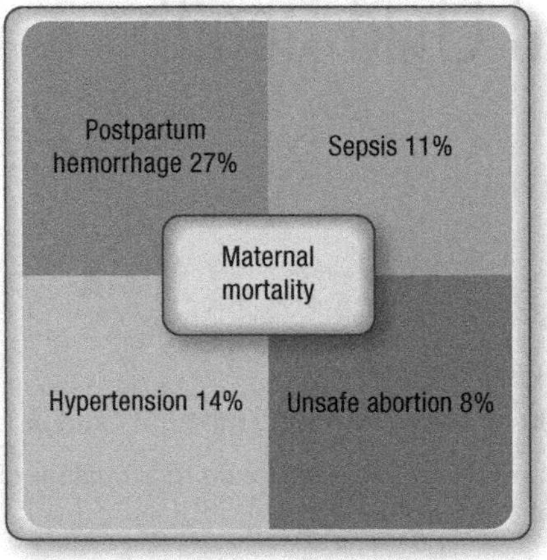

Source: Kaiser Family Foundation. (2022). *The U.S. government and global maternal and child health efforts.* Author. https://www.kff.org/global-health-policy/fact-sheet/the-u-s-government-and-global-maternal-and-child-health-efforts/

Newborn deaths account for most child deaths (47%). Undernutrition is considered one of the primary contributors to these deaths (KFF, 2022) (Figure 16.2).

Healthcare Professionals

To improve the health and well-being of mothers and infants requires effort from healthcare professionals, states, tribes, local communities, and women and families (Office of the Surgeon General, 2020). States, tribes, and local communities help ensure infrastructure and program support for maternal health, and healthcare professionals must provide education, support, and care for women before, during, and after pregnancy. Understanding the factors that contribute to a woman's overall health can mitigate potential pregnancy risks. Healthcare professionals are caring for women from diverse geographical, economic, cultural, and ethnic communities and evidence-based and culturally appropriate care will ensure each woman's needs are met.

Healthcare professionals must increase awareness and utilization of recommended clinical practice tools such as (Office of the Surgeon General, 2020):

FIGURE 16.2 Causes of newborn deaths.

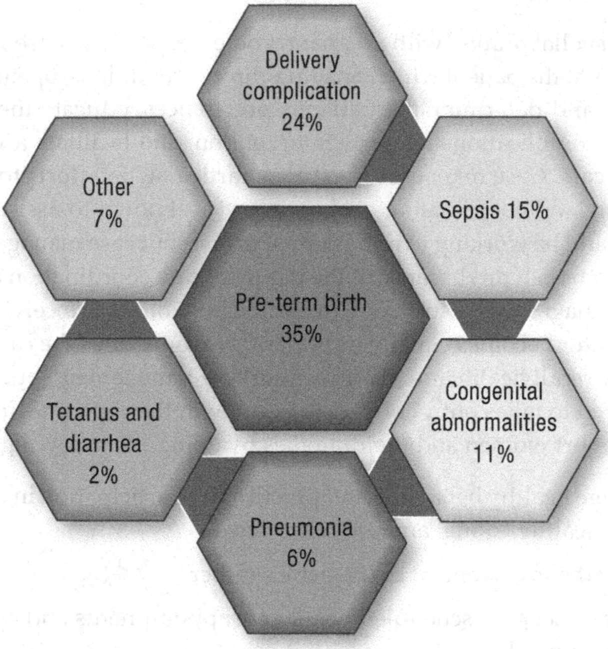

Source: Kaiser Family Foundation. (2022). *The U.S. government and global maternal and child health efforts.* Author. https://www.kff.org/global-health-policy/fact-sheet/the-u-s-government-and-global-maternal-and-child-health-efforts/

- **The Women's Preventive Services Guidelines:** https://www.hrsa.gov/womens-guidelines
- **Bright Futures Guidelines for Health Supervision of Infants, Children, and Adolescents:** https://publications.aap.org/aapbooks/monograph/478/Bright-Futures-Guidelines-for-Health-Supervision?autologincheck=redirected
- **Centers for Disease Control and Prevention:** https://www.cdc.gov/reproductivehealth/maternalinfanthealth/index.html

Racial, socioeconomic, geographic, and cultural disparities contribute to poor outcomes. Healthcare professionals, including case managers, need to increase self- and situational awareness to decrease disparities. All healthcare professionals have a responsibility to identify disparities and then work to create processes and protocols that are culturally and linguistically sensitive, and locate and implement resources that address socioeconomic challenges. This can range from helping the individual access health coverage through an employer or Medicaid and community resources to assist with food and housing.

Case Manager's Role in Maternal and Child Health

The case manager collaborating with pregnant women, especially those with known risk factors, need to assist the patient with managing chronic conditions, openly communicate about pregnancy and determine the patient's preferences, educate the patient on the warning signs of complications for early intervention, and facilitate access to prenatal and postpartum care. Case managers must also participate in efforts to reduce disparities by facilitating and coordinating care and services known to assist. All healthcare professionals should be working to mitigate disparities, but case managers are uniquely positioned to accomplish this because of the nature of care coordination and facilitation.

As the case manager works to ensure the pregnant woman is receiving needed care, their role of educator becomes equally important. Not only does the case manager promote a focus on overall health and chronic condition management, but the mother can also be empowered to take control of her situation with the right information. The case manager can support women and their families by doing the following:

1. Encourage healthy behaviors and practices by participation in regular physical activity, healthy eating, and adequate sleep.
2. Promote the involvement of the baby's father.
3. Encourage keeping scheduled healthcare appointments and assist with transportation if needed.
4. Identify early signs and symptoms of physical or mental illness during and after pregnancy.
5. Continue to support healthy behaviors after delivery.

REFERENCES

Kaiser Family Foundation. (2022). *The U.S. government and global maternal and child health efforts*. Author. https://www.kff.org/global-health-policy/fact-sheet/the-u-s-government-and-global-maternal-and-child-health-efforts/

Office of the Surgeon General. (2020). *The Surgeon General's Call to action to improve maternal health*. US Department of Health and Human Services. https://www.ncbi.nlm.nih.gov/books/NBK568218/#_NBK568218_pubdet_

SECTION V

Interdisciplinary Teams and Using Integrated Case Management to Improve Outcomes

CHAPTER 17

Composition, Roles, and Functions in Value-Based Care and Reimbursement

Rebecca Perez

OBJECTIVES

- Interpret the definitions of value-based care and value-based reimbursement
- Describe some of the quality measures as outlined by the Centers for Medicare & Medicaid Services (CMS)
- Apply the case management documentation process to demonstrate improvement

Introduction

Healthcare delivery and reimbursement models in the United States have been based on fee-for-service (FFS) for decades. FFS reimbursement means that for every service provided, a provider receives reimbursement. Until managed care, this was quite lucrative for some providers—the more services ordered the more the provider was reimbursed. Managed care put some controls into place but reimbursing based on quantity has resulted in overwhelmingly increased healthcare spending. This chapter examines issues surrounding value-based care and reimbursement, quality measures, and application of the case management documentation process.

History

In 2009, the growth of healthcare spending was determined to be "unsustainable" by the Social Security Advisory Board (Health Affairs, 2022). U.S. healthcare spending grew to be 10.8% of the Gross National Product (GDP) between 1970 and 2019. During the COVID-19 pandemic, healthcare spending accounted for 19.7% of the GDP—this level of spending was not predicted to be reached until 2028 (Health Affairs, 2022).

The Affordable Care Act was passed in 2010 and as many pieces of that legislation come to fruition, the United States continues to struggle with healthcare spending. Accountable care or value-based care (VBC) are part of that legislation. Demonstration projects for VBC began not long after the legislation was passed and have produced data to guide the full transition. Smaller healthcare organizations and provider practices as well as rural hospitals will experience more challenges with the shift from FFS to value-based reimbursement (VBR) because of technology and reporting requirements.

Value-Based Care

VBC indicates that providers are reimbursed based on the quality of care provided versus the volume of services provided as in the FFS model. Reactionary healthcare, or care that is delivered once someone gets sick, will be replaced with a focus on wellness. Providers contract with payers (Medicare, Medicaid, and other insurers) to care for a defined set of patients known as attributed patients. Physicians earn financial rewards or avoid negative payment adjustments by meeting specific quality and performance measures that are tied to better long-term outcomes. Measures include vaccine distribution, certain cancer screenings, and specific disease management clinical measures like hemoglobin A1c. (The full list of measures can be accessed at https://www.cms.gov/Medicare/Quality-Initiatives-Patient-Assessment-Instruments/Value-Based-Programs/Value-Based-Programs.)

A sampling of some of the measures includes:

- End-Stage Renal Disease Quality Incentive Program (ESRD-QIP):
  - Transfusion rates
  - Fistula placement
  - Fistula infection rates
- Hospital Readmission Reduction Program (HRRP):
  - Improved care coordination
  - Improved patient/caregiver engagement in the discharge process
  - Readmissions prevention
- Hospital-Acquired Conditions (HAC) Reduction Program:
  - Improved patient safety
  - Implementaton of best practices to reduce hospital-acquired infections
  - Prevention of pressure sores
  - Prevention of hip fracture after surgery

VBC requires a focus on population health, which is the improvement in the health outcomes of a group of individuals. The goal is to optimize outcomes for the entire group by delivering standardized holistic services. Access to preventive care is the foundation of population health whether patients are chronically ill or healthy.

VBC and payments (VBD and VBP) have the potential to reduce excess spending in administrative waste, clinical waste, and other contributors to costs. Delivery systems, health plans, and individual states can decide which spending drivers need to be addressed. The terminology used to describe VBP can be confusing: Value-based payments are also known as alternative payment models (APMs). These are a variety of payment arrangements that have one thing in common: They are not traditional FFS arrangements. These arrangements can be a hybrid of FFS with bonuses for advanced quality models like bundled payments or global capitation. The Healthcare Learning and Action Network developed a framework for APMs (Figure 17.1). The payment models fall into one of four categories but only categories three and four are considered APMs (Health Affairs, 2022).

FIGURE 17.1 Framework for alternative payment models.

CATEGORY 1	CATEGORY 2	CATEGORY 3	CATEGORY 4
Fee-for-service: no link to quality and value	**Fee-for-service: link to quality and value**	**APMs built on fee-for-service architecture**	**Population-based payment**
	2A	3A	4A
	Foundational payments for infrastructure and operations For example, care coordination fees and payments for health information technology investments	**APMs with shared savings** For example, shared savings with upside risk only	**Condition-specific population-based payment** For example, per member per month payments or payments for specialty services, such as oncology or mental health
	2B	3B	4B
	Pay-for-reporting For example, bonuses for reporting data or penalties for not reporting data	**APMs with shared savings and downside risk** For example, episode-based payments for procedures and comprehensive payments with upside and downside risk	**Comprehensive population-based payment** For example, global budgets or the full or a percent of premium payments
	2C		4C
	Pay-for-performance For example, bonuses for quality performance		**Integrated finance and delivery systems** For example, global budgets or the full or a percent of premium payments in integrated systems
		3N	4N
		Risk-based payments not linked to quality	Capitated payments not linked to quality

Source: From Health Affairs. (2022). *Value-based payment as a tool to address excess U.S. health spending*. Author. http://doi.org/10.1377/hpb20221014.526546

The Case Manager's Role in Value-Based Care

The information provided here is a very high-level overview of VBC. How and when these models are implemented will be determined by the organization by which case managers are employed. Successful VBC requires better control of clinical and financial risks that are associated with complex or high-risk patients. Population health requires proven interventions implemented to support the individual and customized to their specific needs. The Centers for Medicare & Medicaid Services (CMS) recognizes case management as a means to improve care, improve patient and provider experiences, and reduce cost (Health Affairs, 2022).

Case managers working one-on-one with high-risk and complex patients can, with the skills and tools suggested in this textbook, (e.g., motivational interviewing, risk prioritization, and targeted care planning), can not only assist in risk reduction and stabilization of conditions, but can encourage and support preventive measures like lifestyle changes and annual screenings, coordinate services that impact psychological and social challenges, and coach patients to participate in shared decision-making for eventual self-management.

Data collected on care coordination and information exchange are requirements for the delivery of VBC. Documentation should include the following: (eHealth Initiative):

- A longitudinal record of the care received which includes any provider or organization.
- Regular medication reconciliation to monitor adherence and prevent any adverse events.
- Regular reassessment of the patient's needs, monitoring and documentation of the patient's progress, response to prescribed treatment, and engagement in care. All this information is to be made available to all providers (preferably with an interoperable electronic health record [EHR]).
- Identification of social supports and tracking of the effect of the services coordinated. Did the services meet the patient's needs? Did the services result in clinical improvements?

In addition, case managers should follow these general guidelines:

- Make the information available to all treating providers which requires better EHR interoperability. In the absence of this, case managers need to be accountable for communication between and among the patient's providers.
- Share the results of interventions.

The practice of case management inherently supports a value-based philosophy by following Case Management Society of America's (CMSA) Standards of Practice for Case Management, which include personalized care plans that target risk and the establishment of trusted relationships that increase the likelihood of a patient engaging in their care. Of greatest importance is that with these efforts, the patient will experience improved health, satisfaction with the care received, and improved quality of life.

Interdisciplinary Team Concepts

Interdisciplinary teams are increasingly prevalent and are central to healthcare reform. Blinders, silos, and territories impede the case manager's view of the full healthcare system. What can case managers do to create change for their patients and become true integrated case managers? The foundation of integrated care is a holistic view of the individual and personal health as complex, integrated systems, rather than a simple sum of independent body systems. It follows that integrated care begins with an assessment of patients for conditions and or the risk of developing conditions in addition to the ones they present. To do so effectively, the case manager must assemble a healthcare team. Teams should focus on a defined goal with parameters, such as a specific unaddressed care need, improvement on a quality measure, a setting, or a patient population. Remember, a case manager's team members come from diverse training and backgrounds within the same specialty. Teams must develop respect, competence, accountability, and trust for each other to define and treat not only patient problems but those affecting process and workflow. Together, team members will determine the team's mission and common goals. The outcomes of the team's work must be deemed superior to individually based outcomes.

In 2013, the Institutes of Medicine published "The Patient-Centered Primary Care Collaborative" that outlined best practices for health professionals working together to advance value- and science-driven healthcare before the advent of VBC. These best practices focused on achieving the Triple Aim by providing safe, high-quality, accessible, and patient-centered care (Institute of Medicine of the National Academies, 2013). Principles for effective team performance include shared goals between health professionals, patient, and family/caregiver; mutual respect for roles and responsibilities; mutual trust, especially combining personal values with the organization's values; communication that is effective and complete; and measurable processes and outcomes (Institute of Medicine of the National Academies, 2013).

Research shows that solving problems collectively leads to improved outcomes (Middleton, 2022). Individuals are more likely to employ innovation if they have the support of a team (Middleton, 2022). Working as part of a team not only leads to improved outcomes for the patient, but personal growth, job satisfaction, and reduced stress for each team member.

Collaborative Partnership Approach to Care

Research suggests that high-functioning interdisciplinary teams share a set of characteristics, including, but not limited to, positive leadership, a supportive team climate, clarity of vision, appropriate skill mix, and respect and understanding of all roles. A team should have a shared mission using improved clinical systems to deliver improved care to a patient population supported by operational and financial systems. Such care is continuously evaluated through improvement processes and effectiveness measurement. Examples include the transition management frameworks employed by organizations.

The Transitional Care Model (TCM) is an example of one such framework. TCM was developed to address preventable hospital admissions. The CMS incentivized providers with additional reimbursement by improving care and outcomes for patients with chronic conditions (Avicenna Medical Systems, n.d.). TCM was designed to counteract the negative outcomes of hospitalization especially for the geriatric population. Improving transitions between the hospital and the community requires a focus on supporting outpatient care by preparing the patient and family/caregiver for self-management (Morkisch et al., 2019). Interventions such as medication management via multidisciplinary communication have been shown to reduce adverse events (Morkisch et al., 2019).

Creating the collaborative team among physicians, pharmacists, nurses, case managers, social workers, allied health, and supporting staff, such as claims adjuster or patient's employer, if applicable, is critical to achieving the goals of the team, the organization, and changing the way we deliver healthcare today. Case managers should collaborate and advocate with all stakeholders to develop a care plan across the care continuum. As the healthcare environment focuses on becoming more cost-effective and efficient, it is important for all disciplines to work as a team in order to:

- Understand the role of each discipline.
- Encourage effective communication.
- Prevent duplication of services.
- Ensure continuity of care.

It is key to develop a communication process that defines how the team will solve differences and build collaboration. Case managers should position themselves as the eyes and ears of physicians, as collaborators in providing good care, and assisting with providing information and education. Case managers should seek to shift from reliance on abstract principles to using past concrete experiences to guide actions. It is also advisable to experience a shift in perception of situations from separate pieces to whole parts with the ability to recognize what is most relevant. For example, the case manager should take information and observations from working with patients to better communicate what has worked and what has not. A group of patients with uncontrolled diabetes will not manifest with the same symptoms or challenges. When the reason for the lack of control is known, the approach to assisting the patient to better control diabetes may differ. Focusing on just diet management and instructing the patient what or how to eat are short-sighted. Perhaps other factors, like the inability to access or pay for healthy food, are the concern.

Case managers should pass from being a detached observer to an involved performer—actively engaged and fully participating. Finally, the integrated case manager should spend less time giving advice, and more time asking questions of the team.

There is no question that industry movement toward integrated health systems, population health management, and VBR requires an interprofessional approach to care coordination using collaborative care teams. Professional integrated case managers are key members of this new team culture in which trust, respect, and multidisciplinary interdependence are required to achieve effective patient outcomes.

Each member of the collaborative care team—whether licensed or unlicensed, clinical or nonclinical—has an important role in care coordination. The key is to verify that all members of the team are crystal clear on their roles, accountabilities, and scopes of practice. The interdisciplinary team members should be complexity- and relationship-focused and serve as resources to each other. This includes making sure that the roles and functions of the professional case manager are not inappropriately delegated to unqualified team members.

Professional case managers are licensed healthcare professionals or those that have advanced degrees in health and human services (CMSA, 2022). And according to these and other professional standards of practice and practice acts, only these individuals can conduct an assessment or coordinate medical care. The assessment and coordination of care cannot be delegated to an individual without these qualifications. Nonlicensed staff can assist with many other activities that support care coordination allowing the case manager to work more closely with the patient and family/caregiver.

CASE STUDY

Virginia is a 65-year-old female who is status-post a below-the-knee amputation. She experienced a postoperative wound infection which delayed her transfer to acute rehabilitation. Virginia was transferred to acute rehabilitation and began gait training with a temporary prosthesis and is ready to discharge home with continued outpatient therapy and fitting of a permanent prosthesis. Virginia is a widow with no surviving children. She lives alone but does have several close friends and a niece that live nearby. Her niece works full-time, and her friends are available intermittently. She is on multiple medications including insulin for type 2 diabetes. As the discharge plan is developed, Virginia will have multiple needs that include safety in the home environment, medication management, outpatient physical therapy, transportation to physical therapy and physician appointments, and assistance with independent activities of daily living (cooking, shopping, cleaning, laundry, etc.) To coordinate and facilitate all of these needs, the team will need to come together with resources and recommendations. As the team lead, the case manager gathers the team to meet and discuss the best options for coordinating the many facets of care for Virginia:

1. Pharmacy: Coordinate home delivery of medications and diabetes testing supplies.
2. Physical and occupational therapies: Home evaluation for safety and scheduling of outpatient therapy visits, and appropriate durable medical equipment for the home.
3. Dietician: Assist with coordinating Meals on Wheels for diabetic diet.
4. Nonclinical support staff: Secure transportation for outpatient therapy, schedule follow-up visits with primary care provider and surgeon, and secure transportation for those visits.
5. Meet with Virginia's niece and friends to see if and when they could assist with shopping, cleaning, laundry, and some meal preparations.

The case manager brings all of the disciplines together to address the patient's needs with each lending their expertise to ensure Virginia's transition home is safe and effective.

Nonlicensed Patient Navigator, Extender, or Health Coach

The professional case manager makes a profound difference in their patient's life. For many years, the patient's outcomes, although positive, were not always recognized as a direct result of the case manager's plan and intervention. Ironically, as the value of case managers becomes visible, the scarcity of professional case managers is notable. The shortage of case managers is directly related to the 2021 U.S. Bureau of Labor Statistics report that we can expect 175,000 registered nurse openings for a 10-year period between 2019 and 2029 and social work positions are expected to only increase by 26,700 over the same time period (White, 2021). Contributing to this shortage is a 9% vacancy rate for nursing faculty (White, 2021). The case manager is needed for chronic illness management, high-risk case management, and integrated case management (ICM). Because of the demand for this service, many organizations are assembling a partnership with a nonlicensed patient navigator, health coach, patient extender, or other organizational titles, to assist in the care coordination of patients. The professional case manager directs a patient-centered model and may utilize patient navigators to reduce barriers to care. The navigators support individual patients through the healthcare continuum as it pertains to their specific disease, ensuring that barriers to care are resolved and that each stage of care is as easy for the patient as possible.

The concept of patient navigation is about providing education and emotional support to patients and guiding them through the healthcare maze under the direction of the professional case manager. The patient navigator benefits not only patients, but also hospital systems and insurance companies. The navigator supports the patient-centered care plan created by the professional case manager, in collaboration with the case manager, patient, and other appropriate partners. Healthcare systems and payers expect positive patient-centered outcomes. The common metrics used to measure outcomes are improved patient and caregiver satisfaction, improved quality, reduced costs, and optimized resources and revenue. Patient navigators work in a variety of settings including communities, hospitals, homes, primary care offices, and tertiary care. The navigators do not require formal clinical training, license, or certification; however, these would be beneficial. It is essential that navigators collaborate with licensed and certified professional case managers to supplement, complement, and assist patients/clients through the healthcare system. They should never be used as a substitute for the professional case manager. Navigators are trained by the professional case manager to recognize potential roadblocks to services.

Examples of a Navigator Role

Navigators are most often seen assisting cancer patients. While some cancer patients experience complexity indicating the need for case management intervention, cancer patients generally are prescribed a treatment protocol that is, for the most part, standardized. Navigators can assist the cancer patient with provider communication, scheduling appointments, and assistance with reimbursement issues. These functions do not necessarily require intervention by a licensed healthcare professional, but certainly someone familiar with how the healthcare system functions.

Another example might be assistance with access to social supports, such as an individual who is unhoused. Navigators can build bridges between communities and resources and service providers to meet specific socioeconomic needs for an individual or group.

REFERENCES

Avicenna Medical Systems. (n.d.). *A guide to understanding Medicare transition of care and chronic care management*. Author. https://cdn2.hubspot.net/hubfs/88260/docs/Avicenna_Care_Management_Whitepaper.pdf?__hstc=184295289.cbcf56e8ea95ce83fb546f94a2874241.1675796492327.1675796492327.1675796492327.1&__hssc=184295289.1.1675796492327&hsCtaTracking=2eb24e5a-29a2-4d52-870c-a8346c4d

Case Management Society of America. (2022). *Standards of practice for case management*. Author.

eHealth Initiative. (n.d.). *The role of case management in value-based health care*. Author. https://www.ehidc.org/sites/default/files/resources/files/The_Role_of_Case_Management_in_Value-based_Health_Care.pdf

Health Affairs. (2022). *Value-based payment as a tool to address excess U.S. health spending*. Author. http://doi.org/10.1377/hpb20221014.526546

Institute of Medicine of the National Academies. (2013). *Principles and values of team-based care*. Author. https://www.pcpcc.org/sites/default/files/pcpcc_webinar_feb_28_2013.pdf

Middleton, T. (2022, January 25). The importance of teamwork (as proven by science). *Teamwork*. https://www.atlassian.com/blog/teamwork/the-importance-of-teamwork

Morkisch, N., Upegui-Arango, L. D., Cardona, M. I., van den Heuvel, D., Rimmele, M., Sieber, C. C., & Freiberger, E. (2019, July 29). Components of the transitional care model (TCM) to reduce readmission in geriatric patients: A systematic review. *BMC Geriat rics, 20*(345). https://doi.org/10.1186/s12877-020-01747-w

White, C. (2021, July 19). *Case management workforce needs are driven by supply and demand*. Case Management Society of America. https://cmsa.org/case-management-workforce-needs-are-driven-by-supply-and-demand/

CHAPTER 18

The Integrated Case Management Complexity Assessment Grid as an Outcome Measure

Rebecca Perez

OBJECTIVES

- Discover how risk in the four domains of health interact to create complexity
- Demonstrate risk scoring based on the criteria provided
- Demonstrate overall risk reduction with targeted care planning based on assessed risk

Introduction

Case management research, demonstrating improved outcomes, is not routinely published in the United States; however, regular research is conducted in other parts of the world. Demonstrating the impact of case management intervention is something every case manager and case management organization should prioritize. The phrase, "case managers are the best kept secret" is not a great way to promote the practice, nor does it help with establishing best practices that result in improved health outcomes.

Case Managers and Process Improvement

Case managers in the United States need to become inspired to participate in research and process improvement to highlight the good work being done and the many problems solved. A literature review performed by Buja et al. (2020) in Italy revealed strong evidence that case management improves adherence to treatment guidelines and patient satisfaction. The literature review also found that case management interventions, using standard clinical pathways customized to a particular patient, further demonstrated that patients received evidence-based treatment (Buja et al., 2020). Additional interventions recognized impactful support of adherence and adjustments in medication for multimorbid patients preventing complications (Buja et al., 2020). The conclusion of the review found an overwhelming increase in patient satisfaction and reduction in hospitalization rates for patients with high disease burden.

Use of Assessment Grids in Case Management

Of interest was the finding that greater efficacy in reducing secondary care services occurred when case managers used a risk tool rather than relying on clinical judgment alone (Buja et al., 2020). This last finding segues to the use of Case Management Society of America's (CMSA) Integrated Complexity Assessment Grid (ICM-CAG) and the Pediatric Integrated Management Complexity Assessment Grid (PIM-CAG) to identify and prioritize risk.

Both grids are used to systematically examine the risk of worsening health in four domains: biological, psychological, social, and health system. Assessment of social determinants of health are included in the assessment of risk associated with health stability and improvement. Use of these grids becomes quick and easy with practice, reducing the burden of "one more assessment." The results of the risk assessment can be utilized in the development of a targeted care plan that is simple to implement and meant to demonstrate risk reduction more efficiently.

Scoring risk is based on whatever comprehensive assessment is used by an individual's organization. Past work with the integrated Case Management (ICM) model has resulted in the recommendation to repeat the risk assessment every 90 days after the initial score is recorded and a targeted care plan has been developed. The risk score should decrease over time. Following is an example of how the risk score can demonstrate outcomes; for this we return to the case of Sam first introduced in Chapter 12.

CASE STUDY

Sam's uncontrolled diabetes has resulted in a nonhealing ulcer on the bottom of his foot. He has already had two admissions for infections and debridement of the ulcer. Sam lives alone, has a history of depression, has no close family or social ties, does not have a good relationship with his primary care provider, cannot always afford to buy healthy foods, and is unable to drive because the ulcer is on the bottom of his right foot. He has not been attending medical appointments and is ordering fast food delivery because he cannot get to the grocery store. He has not been regularly checking his blood sugar; his last A1c was over 6 months ago and at that time it was 9.2. He also has neuropathy in his feet and had been prescribed orthotic diabetic shoes, but he has not been wearing them. Sam has multiple risks and now his case manager must prioritize them to create a care plan that will result in the goal of a healed foot ulcer. Before putting that clinician hat back on, be sure to spend some time talking to Sam about what is important to him: What does he see are the barriers to better diabetes management? He tells his case manager that while he does not have any close family ties as most of his family is deceased, he does enjoy attending religious services and the socials that follow on Sundays at the church near his apartment. He does have a few former work acquaintances that he talks to every couple of months, but he does not engage further because he does not believe they want a "guy with bad diabetes hanging around." He is a retired copyright editor from the local newspaper and only has a modest pension in addition to his Social Security benefits. His health coverage is with a Medicare Advantage plan.

Date: **Grid No. 1**	**HEALTH RISKS AND HEALTH NEEDS**					
Name: Sam	**HISTORICAL**		**CURRENT STATE**		**VULNERABILITY**	
Total Score = 39	**Complexity Item**	**Score**	**Complexity Item**	**Score**	**Complexity Item**	**Score**
Biological domain	Persistent, sustained, medical conditions (PSMC)	**2**	Symptom severity/ impairment	**2**	Complications and life threat	**2**
	Diagnostic difficulty	**0**	Adherence ability	**3**		
Psychological domain	Barriers to coping	**1**	Treatment choice	**2**	Mental health threat	**3**
	Mental health history	**2**	Mental health symptoms	**2**		
Social domain	Work and leisure	**3**	Residential stability	**1**	Social vulnerability	**3**
	Relationships	**1**	Social support	**2**		

Date: **Grid No. 1**	**HEALTH RISKS AND HEALTH NEEDS**					
Name: Sam	**HISTORICAL**		**CURRENT STATE**		**VULNERABILITY**	
Total Score = 39	**Complexity Item**	**Score**	**Complexity Item**	**Score**	**Complexity Item**	**Score**
Health system domain	Reimbursement and provider access	**2**	Getting needed services	**3**	Health system deterrents	**2**
	Treatment experience	**1**	Provider collaboration	**2**		
Comments						
Enter pertinent information about the reason for the score of each complexity item here (e.g., poor patient adherence, death in family with stress to patient, nonevidence-based treatment of migraines).						

Scoring System:
0 = no need to act
1 = mild risk and need for monitoring or prevention
2 = moderate risk and need for action or development of intervention plan
3 = severe risk and need for immediate action or immediate intervention plan

Sam's total risk score is 39, indicating significant risk. Sam's greatest risk or health priority is the nonhealing foot ulcer. Clinicians understand where nonhealing diabetic ulcers and neuropathy lead—they lead to amputation. In Chapter 12, Sam's challenges, goals, and interventions were established. Healing of the foot ulcer will require that Sam start actively managing his diabetes, check his blood sugar regularly, eat a healthy diet, and take his medication. He will need ongoing wound care from a wound specialist and home skilled nursing. In addition to facilitating these clinical needs, his case manager will need to coordinate transportation to medical appointments, work with the home health provider for wound care, and facilitate proper nutrition by arranging a meal service like Meals on Wheels.

Sam's depression is likely interfering in his motivation to manage his diabetes. More care coordination regarding medication and counseling should be included in the case manager's interventions along with Sam's desire to reconnect with his church and former coworkers. In addition to counseling and medication, Sam's case manager will want to ask Sam to reach out to his church to see if there are volunteers willing to take him to church functions until he can drive again. Resuming socialization will hopefully support the mechanisms of counseling and antidepressants. If he is less depressed, his motivation to actively manage his diabetes will return. Here is a follow-up risk assessment after his case manager has implemented all of these interventions.

Date: Grid No. 2	**HEALTH RISKS AND HEALTH NEEDS**					
Name: Sam	**HISTORICAL**		**CURRENT STATE**		**VULNERABILITY**	
Total Score = 25	**Complexity Item**	**Score**	**Complexity Item**	**Score**	**Complexity Item**	**Score**
Biological domain	Persistent, sustained, medical conditions (PSMC)	**2**	Symptom severity/ impairment	**1**	Complications and life threat	**2**
	Diagnostic difficulty	**0**	Adherence ability	**1**		
Psychological domain	Barriers to coping	**1**	Treatment choice	**1**	Mental health threat	**2**
	Mental health history	**2**	Mental health symptoms	**1**		
Social domain	Work and leisure	**3**	Environmental stability	**1**	Social vulnerability	**1**
	Relationships	**0**	Social support	**1**		
Health system domain	Reimbursement and provider access	**1**	Getting needed services	**1**	Health system deterrents	**1**
	Treatment experience	**2**	Provider collaboration	**1**		
Comments						
Enter pertinent information about the reason for the score of each complexity item here (e.g., poor patient adherence, death in family with stress to patient, nonevidence-based treatment of migraines).						

Scoring System:
0 = no need to act
1 = mild risk and need for monitoring or prevention
2 = moderate risk and need for action or development of intervention plan
3 = severe risk and need for immediate action or immediate intervention plan

His case manager's interventions have resulted in a significant reduction in risk. Work with Sam is not concluded as there is a need to continue to monitor the sustainability of the improvements. But within 90 days his risk score went from 39 to 25. This is a measurable outcome.

CONCLUSION

As this textbook concludes, take advantage of the resources provided in the appendices. CMSA offers a Certificate of Training course for those that wish to hone the skills needed to work with complex populations and to discover how to implement the use of the adult and pediatric complexity assessment grids. CMSA's Integrated Case Management program not only offers an advanced skill set, but a means to demonstrate the impact of case management. Perhaps the "secret" will no longer be a secret.

REFERENCE

Buja, A., Francesconi, P., Bellini, I., Barletta, V., Girardi, G., Braga, M., Cosentino, M., Marvulli, M., Baldo, V., & Damiani, G. (2020). Health and health service usage outcomes of case management for patients with long-term conditions: A review of reviews. *Primary Health Care Research and Development*, *21*(e26), 1–21. https://doi.org/10.1017/S1463423620000080

Appendices

APPENDIX A

Case Management Society of America's Standards of Practice for Case Management Revised 2022

I. Introduction

The delivery of high-quality healthcare that yields cost-effective outcomes continues to be an overarching goal of any nation's healthcare system. In the United States, the cost of care remains high in many segments of the healthcare market, but the pursuit of quality healthcare has not diminished. Over the past decades, advances in technology, complex payer models, federal and state legislation, health care professional roles, and the American economy at large have added challenges to an already complex healthcare system. In 2019, the emergence of the SARS-CoV-2 virus and the subsequent coronavirus disease 2019 (COVID-19) incidence resulted in a global pandemic that placed unprecedented stress on the healthcare system as America and other countries managed an expensive and deadly infectious disease outbreak. In addition, since many people's healthcare insurance is tied to employment, the consequences of job loss and a slowed economy due to the pandemic expanded the cohort of uninsured or underinsured across the country. Despite the cost of healthcare, the complexity of the delivery system, and the unprecedented burdens of supply and demand placed on healthcare personnel, the patient care experience is the priority and must be timely, safe, and high quality. The case management practice by professional nurses, social workers, pharmacists, physicians, and other licensed personnel improves access to services, drives better health outcomes, lowers costs, and ensures safe transitions of care across the healthcare system. The delivery of high-quality healthcare that yields cost-effective outcomes continues to be an overarching goal of any nation's healthcare system.

This update to the Case Management Society of America's (CMSA) Standards of Practice (SOP) upholds the definition of case management and the vital role of advocating for the patient/client care experience. Additionally, this version of the SOP punctuates the global perspectives on equity in healthcare, the integration of mental and physical health, the impact of social determinants of health (SDH), and the importance of licensed healthcare professionals to provide case management services in this complex and complicated healthcare delivery system. The healthcare consumer needs someone who has the appropriate education and completion of a rigorous licensing process and is practicing against a set of standards, ethical principles, and a professional code of conduct. This version of the CMSA's SOP provides the foundational benchmarks and paradigms for consumers, health plans, payers, healthcare systems and organizations, employers, federal agencies, entrepreneurs, policy makers, and academicians to utilize for education, training, process improvement, program development, accountability, and scope of practice.

To reiterate the point that case management practice continues to be grounded in professional practice and advocacy, consider the description of case management from the first edition of this textbook. Professional case management fosters the careful shepherding of healthcare dollars while maintaining a primary and consistent focus on the quality of care, safe transitions, timely access, and availability of services. Most important is client self-determination and client-centered and culturally relevant care. These, without a doubt, enhance the health of individuals and communities. However, they also demand a professional case manager who (a) is academically prepared in a health or human services discipline; (b) possesses an unrestricted license or certification as required by the jurisdiction of employment; (c) can function independently and according to the scope of practice of the background health discipline; (d) demonstrates current knowledge, skills, and competence to provide holistic and client-centered care effectively; and (e) acts in a supervisory capacity of other personnel who are involved in the client's care but unable to function independently due to limitations of license and/or education.

A cadre of professional case management experts combined over 300 years of knowledge, skills, abilities, and experience to retool a set of standards that will meet the challenges of today's and tomorrow's healthcare system. The standards were written with the future in mind as this group of experts used predictive reasoning to anticipate the needs of consumers and providers of healthcare. The consensus of this diverse group of professionals on guiding principles, professional practice behaviors, a code of conduct, and the expectation for advancement on the body of knowledge is a validation of case management value to consumers and providers. In addition, the SOP reviewers further solidified the importance of the SOP and its utility for many stakeholders.

The end-user of these standards will find the same sections and categories but with enhancements in current perspectives, evidence-based sources, and criteria that support a comprehensive case management practice. Some of the terms have broader definitions, and these descriptions are located in the glossary. This version provides additional content and a comprehensive representation of the literature in the appendices. The SOPs apply to all healthcare settings and guide licensed clinicians who deliver case management services.

In some settings, case managers may be referred to as care managers, but the expectation is the practitioner is a professional. These SOPs are relevant for care managers if their practice and services are consistent with these principles, benchmarks, and codes of conduct. The term "care coordinator" is also used within this practice community, but case management and care management incorporate far more than care coordination. Care coordination is one aspect of case and care management, typically describing services related to care transitions. The CMSA's SOP are current, foundational, evidence-based, relevant and valid, comprehensive and aspirational for a modern, innovative, and futuristic application to the professional practice of case management now and into the future.

Note: Evolution of the SOP for Case Management is now included in the Appendices.

II. Definition of Case Management

The basic concept of case management involves the timely coordination of quality services to address a client's specific needs cost-effectively and safely to promote optimal outcomes. This can occur in a single healthcare setting or during the client's transitions of care throughout the care continuum. In addition, the professional case manager serves as an essential facilitator among the client, family, or caregiver, the interprofessional healthcare team, the payer, and the community. The definition has evolved since first drafted in 1993. More information can be found in the Reference section of this document.

In 2016, the CMSA Board of Directors included client safety in the updated definition, and this definition is still relevant:

"Case management is a collaborative process of assessment, planning, facilitation, care coordination, evaluation, and advocacy for options and services to meet an individual's and family's comprehensive health needs through communication and available resources to promote patient safety, quality of care, and cost-effective outcomes."

Explaining case management to clients and the public can sometimes be challenging. The following is a definition that can be used for clients and the public:

"Case managers are healthcare professionals who serve as patient advocates to support, guide and coordinate care for patients, families, and caregivers as they navigate their health and wellness journeys."

III. Philosophy and Guiding Principles

A. Statement of Philosophy

Philosophy is a statement of belief and values that sets forth principles to guide a program, its meaning, its context, and the role(s) of the individual(s) that exist in it. For example, the CMSA philosophy of case management articulates that:

The underlying premise of case management is based on the fact that, when an individual reaches the optimum level of wellness and functional capability, everyone benefits: the individual client being served, the client's family or family caregiver, the healthcare delivery system, the reimbursement source or payer, and other involved parties such as the employer and healthcare advocates.

Professional case management serves to achieve client wellness and autonomy through advocacy, ongoing communication, health education, identification of service resources, and service facilitation.

Professional case management services are best offered in a climate that advances client engagement and empowerment with direct communication among the case manager, the client, the client's family or support system, and appropriate service personnel to facilitate desired outcomes.

The philosophy of case management underscores the recommendation that at-risk individuals, especially those with complex medical, behavioral, and psychosocial needs, be evaluated for case management interventions. The key philosophical components of case management address holistic and client-centered care, with mutual goals, stewardship of resources for the client and the healthcare system, and diverse stakeholders. Through these efforts, case management focuses simultaneously on achieving optimal health and attaining wellness to the highest level possible for each client.

It is the philosophy of case management that when healthcare is effective and efficient, all parties benefit. Case management, provided as part of a collaborative and interprofessional healthcare team, identifies options and resources acceptable to the client and the client's family or support system. This then, in turn, increases the potential for effective client engagement in self-management, adherence to the plan of care, and the achievement of desired outcomes.

Case management interventions focus on improving care coordination and transitions and reducing the fragmentation of the services the recipients of care often experience, especially when multiple healthcare providers and different care settings are involved. Collectively, case management interventions enhance client safety, well-being, and quality of life.

These interventions carefully consider healthcare costs through the professional case manager's recommendations of cost-effective and efficient alternatives for care. Thus, effective case management directly and positively impacts the healthcare delivery system, especially in realizing the goals of the "Triple Aim," which include improving the health outcomes of individuals and populations, enhancing the experience of healthcare, and reducing the cost of care.

B. Guiding Principles

Guiding principles are relevant and meaningful concepts that clarify or guide practice. Guiding principles for case management practice provide those professional case managers:

- Use a client-centric, collaborative partnership approach that is responsive to the individual client's culture, preferences, needs, and values.
- Facilitate client's self-determination and self-management through the tenets of advocacy, shared and informed decision-making, counseling, and health education, whenever possible.
- Use a comprehensive, holistic, and compassionate approach to care delivery that integrates a client's medical, behavioral, social, psychological, functional, and other needs.

- Practice cultural and linguistic sensitivity and maintain current knowledge of the diverse populations served.
- Implement evidence-based care guidelines in the care of clients, as available and applicable to the practice setting, or client population served.
- Promote optimal client safety at the individual, organizational, and community levels.
- Promote behavioral change science and principles integration throughout the case management process.
- Facilitate awareness of and connections with community supports and resources.
- Foster safe and manageable navigation through the healthcare system to enhance the client's timely access to services and achieve desired outcomes.
- Pursue professional knowledge and practice excellence and maintain competence in case management and health and human service delivery.
- Support systematic approaches to quality management and health outcomes improvement, implementation of practice innovations, and dissemination of knowledge and practice to the healthcare community.
- Maintain compliance with federal, state, and local rules and regulations and organizational, accreditation, and certification standards.
- Demonstrate knowledge, skills, and competency in applying case management SOP and relevant codes of ethics and professional conduct.
- Support clients and their support systems with access to available and advancing technologies such as applications, patient portals, and telehealth services.

Case management guiding principles, interventions, and strategies target the achievement of optimal wellness, function, and autonomy for the client and client's family or family caregiver through advocacy, assessment, planning, communication, health education, resource management, care coordination, collaboration, and service facilitation.

The professional case manager applies these principles into practice based on the individualized needs and values of the client to assure, in collaboration with the interprofessional healthcare team, the provision of safe, appropriate, effective, client-centered, timely, efficient, and equitable care and services.

IV. Case Management Practice Settings

Professional case management practice spans all healthcare settings across the continuum of health and human services. This may include the payer, provider, government, employer, community, and client's home environment. The practice varies in degrees of complexity, intensity, urgency, and comprehensiveness based on the following four factors:

A. The care context includes wellness and prevention, acute, subacute and rehabilitative, skilled, serious, or life-limiting illness.

B. Health and behavioral health conditions, needs of the client population(s) served, and those of the client's family or caregivers.

C. Reimbursement methods applied, such as managed care, workers' compensation, Medicare, or Medicaid.

D. Professional disciplines of the designated case manager may include occupational therapist, pharmacist, physician, physical therapist, registered nurse, speech therapist, social worker.

The following is a representative, though not exhaustive, list of practice settings. However, it is a reflection of where professional case managers practice today, whether in-person or virtually:

- Ambulatory care clinics and community-based organizations
- Federally qualified health centers
- Student or university counseling and healthcare centers
- Medical and health homes
- Primary care practices
- Corporations
- Geriatric services including residential, senior centers, assisted living facilities, and continuing care retirement communities
- Government-sponsored programs such as correctional facilities, military health, and Veterans Administration, and public health
- Hospitals and integrated care delivery systems, including acute care, subacute care, long-term acute care (LTAC) facilities, skilled nursing facilities (SNFs), and rehabilitation facilities
- Independent and private case management companies
- Lifecare planning programs
- Long-term care services, including home, skilled, custodial, and community-based programs
- Population health, wellness and prevention programs, and disease and chronic care management companies
- Private health insurance programs including workers' compensation, occupational health, catastrophic and disability management, liability, casualty, automotive, accident and health, long-term care insurance, group health insurance, and managed care organizations
- Provider agencies and community-based facilities, including mental/behavioral health facilities, home health services, ambulatory and daycare facilities

- Public health insurance and benefit programs such as Medicare, Medicaid, and state-funded programs
- Primary care and specialty group practices, patient-centered medical homes (PCMH)
- Accountable care organizations (ACOs) and physician-hospital organizations (PHOs)
- Schools
- Serious illness, hospice, palliative, and respite care programs

V. Professional Case Management Roles and Responsibilities

The role of a professional case manager concerning the patient is that of advocacy. Advocacy is used to coordinate the influential factors that affect the patient or a group of patients' ability to achieve their optimum state of health. The contributing factors to well-being include financial, ethics and legal, social support, and providers of care. See Figure A1.

The professional case manager is responsible for being patient-centered and is held accountable to maintain the education and skills needed to deliver quality care. The professional case manager should demonstrate knowledge of health insurance and funding sources, healthcare services, human behavior dynamics, healthcare delivery and financing systems, community resources, ethical and evidence-based practice, applicable laws and

FIGURE A1 The continuum of healthcare and professional case management.

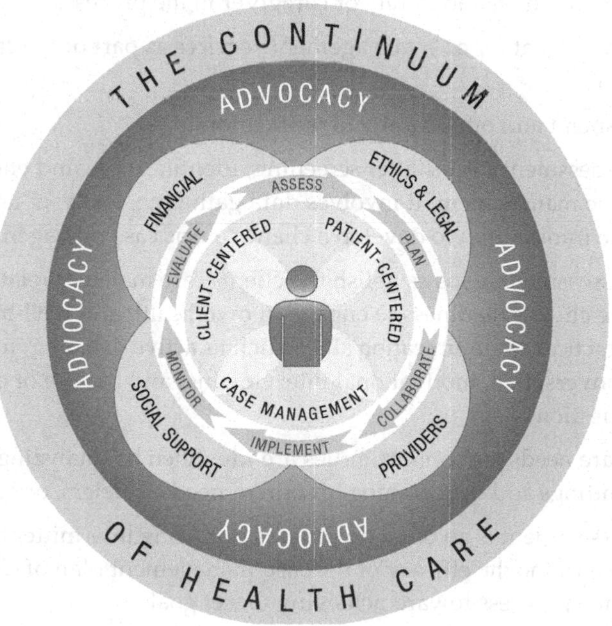

regulations, clinical standards and outcomes, and health information technology (HIT) and digital media for effective and competent performance.

As the professional case manager executes the case management process, the specific roles and responsibilities may vary based on their health discipline background and the environment or care setting in which they practice. A job description sums up each unique practice site's discrete tasks, functions, and responsibilities.

VI. Components of the Case Management Process

The case management process is carried out within the ethical and legal realms of a case manager's scope of practice, using critical thinking and evidence-based knowledge. The overarching themes in the case management process include the activities described in the following

Note that the case management process is cyclical and recurrent rather than linear and unidirectional. For example, critical functions of the professional case manager, such as communication, facilitation, coordination, collaboration, and advocacy, occur throughout all the steps of the case management process and in constant contact with the client, client's family or caregiver, and other members of the interprofessional healthcare team. Primary steps in the case management process include client identification, selection, and engagement in professional case management:

- Focus on screening clients identified or referred by other professionals for case management as appropriate for services and the potential benefit from services.
- Engage the client and family or caregiver in the process.
- Obtain consent for case management services as part of the case initiation process.
- Assessment and opportunity identification:
    - Assessment begins after screening, identification, and engagement in case management. It involves data gathering, analysis, and synthesis of the information to develop a client-centric case management plan of care.
    - Assessment helps establish the client/case manager relationship and the client's readiness to engage in own health and well-being. It requires practical communication skills such as active listening, meaningful conversation, motivational interviewing, and the use of open-ended questions.
    - Care needs and opportunities are identified by analyzing the assessment findings and determining identified needs, barriers, or gaps in care.
    - Assessment is an ongoing process occurring intermittently, as needed, to determine the efficacy of the case management plan of care and the client's progress toward achieving target goals.

    - Assessment should cover medical, behavioral health, substance use and abuse, and SDH.
- Development of the case management plan of care:
    - The case management plan of care is a structured, dynamic tool used to document the opportunities, interventions, and expected goals the professional case manager applies during the client's engagement in case management services. It includes:
    - Identified care needs, barriers, and opportunities for collaboration with the client, family or caregiver, and members of the interprofessional care team to provide more effective integrated care
    - Prioritized goals and outcomes to be achieved
    - Interventions or actions needed to reach the goals

Client and client's family or caregiver input and participation in developing the case management plan of care are essential to promote client-centered care and maximize the potential for achieving the target goals.

- Implementation and coordination of the case management plan of care:
    - The case management plan of care is implemented by coordinating care, services, resources, and health education specified in the planned interventions.
    - Effective care coordination requires ongoing communication and collaboration with the client and client's family or caregiver, the provider, and the interprofessional healthcare team.
- Monitoring and evaluation of the case management plan of care:
    - Ongoing follow-up with the client, family, and caregiver and evaluation of the client's status, goals, and outcomes.
    - Monitoring activities include assessing the client's progress with planned interventions.
    - Evaluating care goals and interventions to determine if they remain appropriate, relevant, and realistic.
    - Making any revisions or modifications needed to the care needs, goals, or interventions specified in the client's case management plan of care.
- Closure of the professional case management services:
    - Mutual decision to discontinue case management services.
    - Case closure focuses on discontinuing professional case management services when the client has attained the highest level of functioning and recovery, the best possible outcomes, or when the needs and desires of the client have changed.

VII. Standards of Professional Case Management Practice

A. Standard: Qualifications

The professional case manager should maintain competence in the area(s) of practice by having one of the following:

- A current, active, and unrestricted licensure or certification in a health or human services discipline allows the professional to conduct an assessment independently as permitted within the discipline's scope of practice.
- The individual who practices in a state that does not require licensure or certification must have a baccalaureate or graduate degree in social work or another health or human services field that promotes the physical, psychosocial, or vocational well-being of the persons being served. In addition, the degree must be from an institution that is fully accredited by a nationally recognized educational accreditation organization and
- The individual must have completed a supervised field experience in case management, health, or behavioral health as part of the degree requirements.

How Demonstrated:

- Possession of education, experience, and expertise required for the professional case manager's area(s) of practice.
- Compliance with national, state, and local laws and regulations that apply to the jurisdiction(s) and discipline(s) applicable to the professional case manager practice.
- Maintain competence through participation in relevant and ongoing continuing education, certification, academic study, and internship programs.
- Practice within the professional case manager's area(s) of expertise, making timely and appropriate referrals, and seeking consultation with other professionals when needed.
- Supervision: See the Appendices for more information.
- The professional case manager acts in a supervisory or leadership role of other personnel who cannot function independently due to limitations of license or education.
- Due to the variation in academic degrees and other educational requirements, it is recommended that individuals interested in pursuing a professional case management career seek guidance as to the appropriate educational preparation and academic degree necessary to practice case management. In addition, these interested individuals may seek the CMSA, American Nurses Association, Commission for Case Manager Certification, or other relevant professional organizations for further advice and guidance.
- See the Appendices for more information about Social Work.

B. Standard: Professional Responsibilities

The professional case manager should engage in scholarly activities such as contributing to curricula and maintaining familiarity with current knowledge, competencies, case management-related research, and evidence-supported care innovations. The professional case manager should also identify best practices in case management and healthcare service delivery and apply such in transforming practice, as appropriate. Finally, the professional case manager should provide the highest quality care by staying informed of the latest innovations and best practices in healthcare delivery.

How Demonstrated:

- Incorporate current and relevant research findings into one's practice, including policies, procedures, care protocols or guidelines, and workflow processes applicable to the care setting.
- Efficient retrieval and appraisal of research evidence of one's practice and client population served.
- Proficient in the application of research-related and evidence-based practice tools and terminologies.
- Ability to identify and review evidence-based and peer-reviewed materials (e.g., research results, publications) and incorporate them into a professional practice of case management as available and appropriate.
- Accountability and responsibility for one are professional development and advancement.
- Participation in ongoing training or educational opportunities (e.g., conferences, webinars, academic programs) to maintain and enhance one's knowledge, skills, and abilities relative to the professional practice of case management.
- Participate in research activities that support the quantification and definition of valid and reliable outcomes, especially those that demonstrate the value of case management services and their impact on the individual client and population health.
- Identify and evaluate best practices and innovative case management interventions.
- Leverage opportunities in the employment setting to conduct innovative performance improvement projects and formally report on their results.
- Publish or present at conferences, disseminate practice innovations, research findings, evidence-based practices, and quality or performance improvement efforts.
- Participate in professional case management-related associations and local, regional, or national committees and task forces.
- Mentor and coach less experienced case managers, interprofessional healthcare team members, and providers.

C. Standard: Legal

The professional case manager shall adhere to all applicable federal, state, and local laws and regulations, which have full force and effect of law, governing all aspects of case management practice including, but not limited to, client privacy and confidentiality rights. It is the responsibility of the professional case manager to work within the scope of their license or underlying profession.

NOTE: *If the professional case manager's employer policies or other entities conflict with applicable legal requirements, the case manager should understand that the law prevails. In these situations, case managers should seek clarification of questions or concerns from an appropriate and reliable expert resource, such as a legal counsel, compliance officer, or an appropriate government agency.*

Confidentiality and Client Privacy

The professional case manager should adhere to federal, state, and local laws and policies and procedures governing client privacy and confidentiality. In addition, the professional case manager should act in a manner consistent with the client's best interest in all aspects of communication and recordkeeping, whether through traditional paper records or electronic health records (EHR).

NOTE: *Federal law preempts (supersedes) state and local law and provides a minimum mandatory national standard; states may enlarge client rights but not reduce them. For those who work exclusively on federal enclaves or tribal lands, any issues of concern should direct them to the licensing authority or federal law.*

How Demonstrated:

- The professional case manager shall demonstrate up-to-date knowledge of and adherence to applicable laws and regulations concerning confidentiality, privacy, and protection of the client's medical information.
- Evidence of reasonable effort to obtain the "client's written acknowledgment they received notice of privacy rights and practices."
- The professional case manager should obtain appropriate informed consent before implementing case management services.
- Evidence that the client or client's caregiver or support system have been thoroughly informed concerning:
- Proposed case management process and services relating to the "client's health condition(s) and needs."
- Possible benefits and costs of such services.
- Alternatives to proposed services.
- Potential risks and consequences of proposed services and alternatives.
- The right to decline the proposed case management services and awareness of risks and consequences of such a decision.

- Evidence that the information was communicated in a client-sensitive manner permits the client to make voluntary and informed choices.
- Document informed consent where client consent is a prerequisite to case management services.

D. Standard: Ethics

The professional case manager should behave and practice ethically and adhere to the tenets of the code of ethics that underlie their professional discipline.

How Demonstrated:

- Documentation should reflect:
- Awareness of case management's five fundamental ethical principles and how they are applied. These are:
- Autonomy (to respect individuals' rights to make their own decisions)
- Beneficence (to do good)
- Fidelity (to follow-through and to keep promises)
- Justice (to treat others fairly)
- Nonmaleficence (to do no harm)

Recognition of obligations:

- First, to clients cared for
- Second, to engage in and maintain cooperative and respectful relationships with employers, coworkers, and other professionals
- Third, to maintain personal and occupational health, safety, and integrity
  - Laws, rules, policies, insurance benefits, and regulations may conflict with ethical principles. In such situations, the professional case manager must address the conflicts to the best of their abilities or seek appropriate consultation
  - View clients as unique individuals whom case managers should engage without regard to disability, familial preference, gender identity, sexual orientation, race or ethnicity, national origin, migration, background, religion, socioeconomic status, geographic location, or other cultural considerations
  - Enact policies to ensure universal respect of the integrity and worth of each person
  - The needs of society as a whole by recognizing the complexities and impact on health and well-being that inequity and disparity, bias, exclusion, racism, and injustice caused, but address individually

E. Standard: Advocacy

The professional case manager will seek creative ways to advocate for clients' best interests. For example, case managers will pursue education to further their knowledge base, skill set, and practice to provide clients with the most current information relevant to their health situation. The case manager will also advocate for high-quality care for the client that uses evidence-based practices in the appropriate delivery systems, including the following:

- Promote the client's self-determination, informed and shared decision-making, autonomy, growth, and self-advocacy.
- Educate other healthcare and service providers in recognizing and respecting the client's needs, strengths, and goals.
- Facilitate client access to necessary and appropriate services while educating the client, caregiver, and support system about resource availability within practice settings.
- Recognize, prevent, and eliminate disparities in accessing high-quality care.
- Promote optimal client healthcare outcomes as they relate to race, ethnicity, national origin, and migration background; sex and marital status; age, religion, and political belief; physical, mental, or cognitive disability; gender orientation; or other cultural factors.
- Advocate for appropriate levels of care, timely and well-coordinated transitions, and allocations of resources to optimize outcomes.
- Advocate for expansion or establishment of services and client-centered changes in organizational and governmental policy.
- Address the need for a diverse and inclusive workforce to improve SDH and inequities in the healthcare system.
- Ensure a safety culture by engagement in quality improvement initiatives in the workplace.
- Encourage the establishment of client, caregiver, and support system advisory councils to improve client-centered care standards within the organization.
- Join relevant professional organizations in call-to-action campaigns, whenever possible, to improve the quality of care and reduce health disparities.
- Recognize that client advocacy can sometimes involve a conflict with the need to balance cost constraints. Therefore, the role of case management includes balancing fiscal responsibility with advocacy.

F. Standard: Cultural Competency

The professional case manager should maintain sensitivity and awareness to cross-cultural differences and be responsive to the cultural and linguistic diversity of the demographics of their work setting and the specific client and caregiver needs.

How Demonstrated:

- Evidence of communicating in a practical, respectful, and sensitive manner and following the client's cultural and linguistic context.
- Complete assessments, set goals, and develop a case management plan to accommodate cultural and linguistic needs and services preferences.
- Identify appropriate resources to enhance the client's access to care and improve healthcare outcomes. These may include the use of interpreters and health educational materials which apply language and format demonstrative of understanding of the client's cultural and linguistic communication patterns, including but not limited to speech volume, context, tone, kinetics, space, and other similar verbal/nonverbal communication patterns.
- Pursue professional education to maintain and advance "one's cultural competence and effectiveness while working with diverse client populations."

G. Standard: Resource Management

The professional case manager should integrate factors compliant with requisite employer standards regarding patient access, choice, cost, health equity, quality, and safety; all should be aligned with CMSA's SOP.

The professional case manager should document evidence of aligning the most effective and efficient use of health and behavioral health services and financial resources when designing a plan of care.

How Demonstrated:

- Documentation of:
  - Evaluation of safety, effectiveness, cost, and target outcomes to promote ongoing care needs of the client.
  - Application of evidence-based guidelines and practices when recommending resource allocation and utilization options.
  - Provision of client, family, or caregiver connection to cultural and linguistically appropriate resources to meet the needs and goals identified in the plan of care.
  - Communication with client, family, or caregiver about the length of time for availability of identified resources.
  - Ensured transparency regarding patient financial responsibility associated with a resource, and the range of potential associated outcomes related to resource utilization.
  - Communication with the interdisciplinary healthcare team during care transitions or when a significant change in the client's situation occurs.
  - The intensity of the case management service corresponds with the client's needs.

H. Standard: Health Information Technology

Health information technology (HIT) is intended to improve communication, patient care, reduce costs, increase efficiency, and improve patient outcomes. The case manager will take responsibility for learning new technologies and participating in ongoing use, especially with predictive analytics and resource optimization.

How demonstrated:

- Adherence to standards, regulations, existing local municipal, state, and federal laws, and employer requirements.
- Assist clients and their support systems with access to available technologies such as applications, patient portals, telehealth services, and so on.
- Understand how information is used, where it goes, and who has access to that information.
- Inform, educate, teach, and guide clients on how to access technology and monitor outcomes.

I. Standard: Client Selection

How individuals are selected for case management intervention requires a process that appropriately identifies those who will reap the most benefit. Case management programs are most effective when clients have illnesses or conditions that benefit from case management interventions. The development of effective and efficient case management services and programs require expansion of focus, beginning with the acute care setting advancing to encompass the entire continuum of care. The care continuum includes but is not limited to care access, caregiver support, behavioral health, socioeconomic status, health literacy, cultural preference, and any other social determinant that could impact health.

Identification of individuals or populations appropriate for case management programs may include multiple methods, but the selection should be made with the intent of benefit. These methods include a referral from other professionals, diagnosis-based regression models, risk assessments, predictive algorithms, and claims and pharmacy data. Screening of clients should be conducted without bias and be guided by the intent of health equity and ethical decision-making processes. The individual case manager's profession or organization guides the evaluation of an individual's candidacy for professional case management services inclusive of the ethics and scope of practice specific to the case management professional.

How Demonstrated:

- Candidates for case management should be those with the greatest need.
- Use screening criteria as appropriate to select a client for inclusion in case management. Examples of screening criteria may include, but are not limited to the following:

  - High emergency department use
  - High outpatient utilization
  - Avoidable hospital admissions
  - Complex health needs
  - Multiple chronic conditions
  - Barriers to accessing care and services
  - Developmental disabilities are complicated by complex or chronic illnesses
  - History of mental illness, substance use, suicide risk, or crisis intervention
  - Impaired functional status or cognitive deficits
- Complex health conditions complicated by socioeconomic needs such as:
  - Housing and transportation needs
  - Food insecurity
  - Forms of abuse, neglect, or trauma
  - Financial concerns
  - Complex health needs with lack of adequate social support, including caregiver support
  - Complex health needs and low health literacy, reading literacy, or numeracy literacy levels
- Use analytics that demonstrate the risk of high utilization and cost expected in the next 1 to 5 years
- Best-practice guides documentation of the referral source and method. To improve the potential for health improvement, ensure screening of referrals is completed timely to improve client engagement while supporting the case manager's caseload in times of limited resources
- A client, family, or caregiver request for professional case management services

J. Standard: Client Assessment

The professional case manager should complete a thorough individualized client-centered assessment that considers the client's unique cultural and linguistic needs, including their support network as appropriate.

Client assessment is a process that focuses on the evolving needs of a client as identified by the case manager throughout the professional relationship and across the transitions of care. Client assessment involves each client and the client's family or support network as appropriate. It includes the physical, psychological, social, environmental, and spiritual domains as pertinent to the practice setting access care.

The case manager shall engage clients—and, when appropriate, other members of the client's support network in an ongoing information gathering and decision-making process to assess health needs.

Case management assessments are conducted to connect available care and resources to address the client's illness, conditions, or care complexity. Assessment is a complex function requiring openness to a wide variety of verbal and nonverbal information presented by the client—and, when appropriate, other members of the client's support system. Using empathy, client-centered interviewing skills, and methods appropriate to clients' capacity, the case manager engages clients in identifying their needs, strengths, and challenges about health improvement and self-management. Based on this discussion, the case manager supports the client in establishing priorities and goals. Because the assessment guides care coordination and implementation, the case manager needs to complete initial assessments promptly.

Assessment is an ongoing activity, not a one-time event. During the reassessment process, the case manager and client (and, if appropriate, other members of the client's support system) revisit the needs, assets, and priorities identified in the initial assessment and discuss the client's emerging concerns. Reassessment serves both monitoring and evaluative functions, enabling the case manager and the client to determine whether services have been effective in helping achieve the client's goals. Based on such reassessment, the case manager and the client may determine that case management goals or the care plan need to be adjusted.

Throughout the assessment and reassessment process, some case managers may find standardized (CMSA Best Practices) instruments helpful in identifying and responding to the client's concerns. Such instruments can be used as a starting point in developing and refining an individualized, comprehensive assessment. The purpose of any tool or instrument should be explained to the client in detail.

Case management assessments are rooted in the profession's priority of person-centered care and advocacy, ensuring the client is at the center of every initiative, action, plan, or intervention. Assessments may vary based on organizational setting and practice specialty and should reflect each client's individual needs and strengths. Likewise, it can vary from one practice setting to another. Its identifying characteristics depend on the discipline that uses it, the personnel and staff mix used, and the setting in which the model is implemented. Many commercially available and proprietary assessments are too numerous to list but may focus on a particular illness, diagnosis, condition, or disability. Throughout the assessment, the case manager should be tuned to the congruence between goals and expectations of the client, structure, and philosophy of the case management program.

How Demonstrated:

- Document the client assessments using standardized tools, both electronic and written, commercial or proprietary, when appropriate. The assessment may include, but is not limited to the following components:

- Complete an assessment of the total individual, including physical, psychological, social, environmental, and spiritual needs.

The following are examples of assessments based on the stated health domains. However, specific assessments required or recommended by organizations and institutions may not be included.

Physical domain assessments may include:

- Presenting health status and conditions
- Personal health history
- Medical history inclusive of diagnosed conditions or illnesses, prescribed treatment, response to treatment, symptomatology, medical interventions
- The current medication regimen includes prescribed or over-the-counter medications and herbal products or plant-based medicines
- Prognosis
- Nutritional status, including body mass index (BMI)
- Healthcare providers involved in client's care
- Diagnostic testing results are known or pending

Psychological assessments may include:

- Current mental health status
- History of substance use
- History of depression, anxiety, or trauma
- History of behavioral health treatment
- Cognitive functioning
- Capacity to make informed decisions
- Learning and technology capabilities

Social assessments may include:

- Family or caregiver dynamics
- Caregiver resources: availability and degree of involvement
- Current or former employment/work environment
- Client social, cultural, values, needs, and preferences
- Recreational and leisure pursuits
- History of neglect, abuse, violence, or trauma
- Advance directives planning and availability of documentation
- Pertinent legal situations (e.g., custody, marital discord, and immigration status)

Environmental assessments may include:

- Living environment, residence, financial circumstances
- Safety concerns and needs
- Access to healthy foods
- Health insurance status and availability of healthcare benefits
- Language and communication preferences, needs, or limitations
- Client priorities, care goals, strengths, and abilities
- Functional status
- Access to care and resources
- Health literacy and activation
- Self-management, and self-care
- Client's readiness to change or learn
- Vocational or educational interests
- Expressive disorders
- Reading and numerical literacy
- Transitional or discharge planning needs and services, if applicable
- Skilled nursing, home health aide, durable medical equipment (DME), or other relevant services
- Transportation capability and constraints
- Follow-up care (e.g., primary care, specialty care, and appointments)
- Use of assistive technology/devices
- Internet access
- Use of technology: applications, websites, electronic personal health records, e-mail, text

Spiritual assessments may include:

- Spiritual beliefs and practices

Case management process and documentation:

- Reassessment of the client's condition, response to the case management plan of care and interventions, and validated metrics shall be completed to quantify progress.
- Include resource utilization and cost management documentation, provider options, and general health and behavioral care benefits.

- Provide evidence of relevant information and data required for the client's thorough assessment and obtain from multiple sources including, but not limited to:
- Client interviews
- Initial and ongoing assessments and care summaries are available in the client's health record and across the care transitions
- Include the client's family caregivers or support network (as appropriate), physicians, providers, and other involved members of the interdisciplinary healthcare team
- Past medical records available as appropriate
- Claims and administrative data

K. Standard: Identifying Care Needs and Opportunities

Recognizing the client's strengths and abilities as noted in the initial screening and ongoing assessment, the professional case manager should identify and stratify the client's care needs and opportunities that would benefit from case management interventions. These interventions may include education, communication, care coordination, resource management, and collaboration. Next, the professional case manager prioritizes the client's care needs with input from the client, the client's family or support network, and providers to reduce risk, improve health, support self-management, and create client satisfaction.

How Demonstrated:

- Documented agreement among the client and client's family or support network and other providers and organizations regarding the care needs and opportunities identified.
- Documented identification of opportunities for intervention, such as, but not limited to:
- Overutilization or underutilization of services and resources
- Use of multiple providers or agencies
- Integrated care gaps or delays in care
- Use of inappropriate services or level of care
- Lack of a primary provider or any provider
- Polypharmacy
- Financial barriers to adherence to the case management plan of care
- High-cost injuries or illnesses
- Frequent transitions between care settings or providers/readmissions

- An immediate need for transition to the next level of care
- Need for better coordination of resources and care
- Lack of established, evidence-based plan of care with a specific goal
- Lack of support from the client's family or support network, especially when under stress
- Nonadherence to the established plan of care (e.g., medication adherence) may be associated with the following:
- SDH
- Low reading level
- Language proficiency
- Client beliefs or values
- Lack of education or understanding of:
- Illness course or disease process
- Current condition(s)
- The medication list
- Substance use and abuse

L. Standard: Planning

The professional case manager, in collaboration with the client, client's family or caregiver, and other members of the interdisciplinary healthcare team, where appropriate, should identify relevant care goals and interventions to manage the client's identified care needs and opportunities. The case manager should also document these in an individualized case management plan of care.

How Demonstrated:

- Documented relevant, comprehensive information and data using analysis of assessment findings, client and client's family or caregiver interviews, input from the client's interprofessional healthcare team, and other methods as needed to develop an individualized case management plan of care.
- Document the client and client's family or caregiver participation in developing the written case management plan of care.
- Document the client's agreement with the case management plan of care, including target goals, expected outcomes, and any changes or additions to the plan.
- Recognition of the client's needs, preferences, and desired role in decision-making concerning developing the case management care plan.

- Validation of the plan is evidence-based and incorporates clinical practice guidelines as available and applicable, and it continues to meet the client's changing needs and health condition.
- Measurable goals are defined, and outcome indicators are expected to be achieved within specified time frames. These measures could include clinical and nonclinical domains of outcomes management, such as access to care, cost-effective care, safety and quality of care, and client's experience of care.
- Evidence of supplying the client, client's family, or caregiver with information and resources necessary to make informed decisions.
- Promote awareness of client care goals, outcomes, resources, and services included in the case management care plan.
- Adherence to payer expectations concerning how often to contact and reevaluate the client, redefine long and short-term goals, or update the case management plan of care.

M. Standard: Facilitation, Coordination, and Collaboration

The professional case manager should demonstrate the skills needed to facilitate coordination, communication, collaboration with the client, support network, involved members of the interdisciplinary healthcare team, and other stakeholders to achieve target goals and maximize positive client care outcomes.

How Demonstrated:

- Recognize the professional case manager's role and practice setting with those of other providers and organizations that provide care and case management services to the client.
- Proactive client-centered relationships through open communication and active listening with the client, client support network, and other relevant stakeholders maximize outcomes and enhance patient safety and optimal care experience.
- Evidence of facilitation, coordination, and collaboration to support the transitions of care, including:
  - Transfers within a facility from one level of care to another.
  - Transfers of clients to the most appropriate healthcare provider or care setting are coordinated in a timely and complete manner.
- Document the collaborative and transparent communication between the professional case manager and other healthcare team members, especially during each transition to another level of care within or outside the client's current setting.

- The plan of care, target goals, and client's needs and preferences were used as a guide for facilitation and coordination of services and collaboration among members of the interdisciplinary healthcare team client and client support network.
- Evidence of collaboration that optimized client outcomes; may include work with the community, local and state resources, primary care providers, members of the interdisciplinary healthcare team, the payer, and other relevant stakeholders.
- Evidence of the use of problem-solving skills and techniques to reconcile potentially differing points of view.
- Documented adherence to client privacy and confidentiality mandates during all aspects of facilitation, coordination, communication, and collaboration within and outside the client's care setting.
- Documentation showed adherence to regulatory and accreditation standards within the professional case manager's practice and employment setting.

N. Standard: Monitoring

The professional case manager should employ ongoing assessment and documentation to measure the client's response to the plan of care. The case manager should employ ongoing assessment, bidirectional communication, and documentation to measure the response of the client and their support system to the plan of care.

How Demonstrated:

- Document ongoing collaboration with the client, family or caregiver, providers, and other pertinent stakeholders. The client's response to interventions is reviewed and incorporated into the case management care plan.
- Awareness of circumstances necessitating revisions to the case management plan of care, such as changes in the client's condition, lack of response to the case management interventions, change in the client's preferences, transitions across care settings and providers, and barriers to care and services.
- Evidence that the plan of care continues to be reviewed and is appropriately understood, accepted by the client and client's family or caregiver, and documented.
- Sustain collaboration with the client, family or caregiver, providers, and other pertinent stakeholders regarding any revisions to the plan of care.
- Monitoring activities include assessing client's progress with planned interventions and detecting and proposing resolutions if needed with clients with multiple conditions and multiple treatment plans.
- Evaluate if care goals and interventions remain appropriate, relevant, and realistic.

- Detect deviations from goals using available clinical guidelines and engage the interdisciplinary team in this process
- Determine any revisions or modifications needed to the care needs, goals, or interventions specified in the client's case management plan of care.

O. Standard: Outcomes

Through a thorough individualized client-centered assessment, the professional case manager should maximize the client's health, wellness, safety, physical functioning, adaptation, health knowledge, coping with chronic illness, engagement, and self-management abilities.

How Demonstrated:

- Create a case management plan based on the thorough individualized client-centered assessment.
- Achieved through quality and cost-efficient case management services, client's satisfaction with care experience, shared and informed decision-making, and engagement in own health and healthcare.
- Evaluate the extent to which the goals and target outcomes documented in the case management plan of care have been achieved.
- Demonstrate efficacy, efficiency, quality, safety, and cost-effectiveness of the professional case manager's interventions in achieving the goals documented in the case management plan of care and agreed upon with the client and client's caregiver.
- Measure and report the impact of the case management plan of care in the following:
  - Clinical
  - Financial
  - Quality of life
  - Patient satisfaction with care
  - Physical functioning
  - Psychosocial and emotional well-being
  - Engagement and self-management
- Apply evidence-based adherence guidelines, standardized tools, and proven care processes. These can be used to measure the client's preference for and understanding of:
  - The proposed case management plan of care and needed resources
  - Motivation to change and demonstrate healthy lifestyle caregiver
- Apply evidence-based guidelines that are relevant to the care of specific client populations

- Evaluate client and client's family or caregiver experience with case management services
- Use national performance measures for transitional care and care coordination such as those endorsed by the regulatory, accreditation, agencies, and health-related professional associations to enhance quality, efficiency, and optimal client experience
- Readmission rates
- Prevented readmissions
- Lower levels of care

P. Standard: Case Closure of Professional Case Management Services

The professional case manager should appropriately complete the closure of case management services based upon established case closure guidelines. The extent of applying these guidelines may differ in various case management practices and care settings.

How Demonstrated:

- Achieve care goals and target outcomes, including those self-identified by the client and client support network.
- Identify reasons for and appropriateness of closure of case management services, such as:
- Change of healthcare setting which warrants the transition of the client's care to another healthcare provider(s) or setting.
- The employer or purchaser of case management services requests the closure of case management.
- Services no longer meet program or benefit eligibility requirements.
- The client refuses further case management services.
- Determination by the professional case manager that they are no longer able to provide appropriate case management services because of a client's ongoing disengagement in self-management and unresolved nonadherence to the case management plan of care.
- Death of the client.
- There is a conflict of interest.
- When a dual relationship raises ethical concerns.
- Evidence of agreement for closure of case management services by the client, client support network, payer, professional case manager, or other appropriate parties.
- Evidence that when a barrier to the closure of professional case management services arises, the case manager has discussed the situation with the

appropriate stakeholders and has reached an agreement on a plan to resolve the barrier.

- Documented notice for closure of professional case management services and actual closure that is based **upon the facts and circumstances of each client's case and care outcomes** supporting case closure. Evidence should show verbal or written notice of case closure to the client and other directly involved healthcare professionals and support service providers.
- Closed cases include documentation stating the reason for the closure and a closure summary.
- Follows established Policies and Procedures that outline the criteria and protocol for case closures.
- Evidence of client education about service or funding resources provided by the professional case manager to address any further needs of the client upon case closure.
- Completed transition of care handover to healthcare providers at the next level of care, where appropriate, with permission from the client, and inclusive of verbal and timely communication of relevant client information and continuity of the case management plan of care to optimize client care outcomes.
- Best practices.
- Providers attempt to reconnect clients lost to care to service. These attempts may include home visits, written/electronic correspondence, or telephone calls and may require contact with a client's known medical and human service providers (with prior written consent).
- When services are terminated, an exit interview is conducted if appropriate.
- Case managers attempt to secure releases that will enable them to share pertinent information with a new provider.
- A management review is completed when an agency intends to terminate services related to a client who threatens, harasses, or harms staff.
- Any termination of case management services needs to be followed with resources for the client to prevent legal or ethical care breaches.

VIII. Acknowledgments

The CMSA Board of Directors extends our gratitude to all the professionals who graciously gave their time and expertise to revise and comment on the Standards of Practice for Case Management 2022.

We would especially like to thank those who participated in the various workgroups:

2022 Revision Taskforce:
Chair: Melanie Prince, MSS, MSN, RN, CCM, NEC-BC, FAAN
Executive Director, CMSA: Amy Black, CAE
Staff Liaison: Rebecca Perez, MSN, RN, CCM
Legal Review: Barbara Dunn, Partner, Barnes & Thornburg LLP

Revision Taskforce Members:
Sherry Aliotta, RN-BC
Alan Boardman, LMSW
Jody Luttrell, MSN, RN, CCM
Michelle Santos Martinez, MHA, MSN, RN
Joan McLeod, RN, CCM
Ellen Fink Samnick, MSW, LCSW, CCM
Nancy Skinner, RN-BC, CCM, ACM-RN, CMCN
Sonia Valdez, DNP, RN, CVRN-BC, GANP, PHN

Peer Review Members:
Michael Demoratz, PHD, LCSW, CCM
Sandra Lowry, BSN, RN, CCM, ANCC-BC
Suzanne Powell, MBA, BSN, RN, CCM, CPQH
Andrea Spiller, BSN, RN, CCM

CMSA Board of Directors 2021–2022:
Melanie A. Prince, MSS, MSN, RN, CCM, NEC-BC, FAAN; President
Colleen Morley, DNP, RN, CCM, CMAC, CMCN, ACM-RN; President-Elect
Patricia Noonan, MBA, RN, CCM; Treasurer
Nadine Carter, MBA, BSN, RN, CDMS, CCM; Secretary
Jenny Quigley-Stickney, RN, MSN, MA, CCM, ACM-RN; Member-at-Large
Mark, Evans, MA, CCM, CRC, CBIS; Director
Laura Ostrowsky, RN CCM; Director
Sonia Valdez, DNP, RN, ACNP, GANP, PHN, CVRN-BC; Director
Samantha Walker, DNP, RN, CCM; Director
Vivian Greenway, PhD, MSA, BSN, RN, PAHM, CCM; Chapter Presidents' Council Rep

IX. Glossary

Activity: A discrete action, behavior, or task a person performs to meet the assumed role expectations. For example, an acute care case manager "completes concurrent reviews" with a payer-based case manager.

Advocacy: The act of recommending, pleading the cause of another, to favorably speak or write.

Assessment: A systematic data collection and analysis process involving multiple elements and sources.

Care Coordination: According to the Agency for Healthcare Research and Quality (AHRQ), "Care coordination involves deliberately organizing patient care activities and sharing information among all of the participants concerned with a patient's care to achieve safer and more effective care. This means that the patient's needs and preferences are known ahead of time and communicated at the right time to the right people, and that this information is used to provide safe, appropriate, and effective care to the patient."

Care Management: According to the AHRQ, "Care management is a promising team-based, patient-centered approach "designed to assist patients and their support systems in managing medical conditions more effectively. It also encompasses those care coordination activities needed to help manage chronic illness."

Care Planning: The process of assessing an individual's health, social risks and needs to determine the level and type of support required to meet those needs and objectives, and to achieve potential outcomes.

Case Management: A collaborative process of assessment, planning, facilitation, care coordination, evaluation, and advocacy for options and services to meet an individual's and family's comprehensive health needs through communication and available resources to promote patient safety, quality of care, and cost-effective outcomes.

Case Management Plan of Care: A document or electronic record that represents the synthesis and reconciliation of the multiple plans of care produced by each provider to address a Consumer's specific health concerns. The Case Management Plan of Care serves as a blueprint shared by healthcare team participants to guide the Consumer's care. As such, it provides the structure required to coordinate care across multiple sites, providers, and episodes of care.

Case Management Process: How case management functions are performed, including client identification, selection, engagement, monitoring, and outcomes in case management; assessment and opportunity identification; development of the case management plan of care, including specification of care goals and target outcomes; implementation and coordination of the case management plan of care; monitoring and evaluation of the case management plan of care; closure of case management services.

Certification: A process by which a government or nongovernment agency grants recognition to those who have met predetermined qualifications set forth by a credentialing body.

Chronic Care Management: An approach to care that encompasses the oversight of health and human service provision and education activities conducted by healthcare professionals to assist individuals with one or more chronic illnesses, such as diabetes, asthma, high blood pressure, heart failure, end-stage renal disease, and HIV or AIDS, to understand their health condition and live productive lives. This approach involves motivating patients to become actively engaged in their health, adhere to necessary therapies and interventions, and achieve acceptable health outcomes, including reasonable quality of life and well-being.

Chronic Care Management Services: Reimbursable care coordination services provided to Medicare beneficiaries with two or more chronic conditions which place the beneficiary at significant risk for death, acute exacerbation, or functional decline; and require the implementation of comprehensive plans of care that are monitored over time. The services are accessible on a 24-hour-a-day, 7-day-a week basis and consist of at least 20 minutes of clinical staff time directed by a physician or another qualified healthcare professional during a calendar month. The services include systematic assessments of the beneficiary's medical, functional, and psychosocial needs; preventive services; a review of medication reconciliation, adherence, and self-management; and creation of client-centered care transitions.

Client: (a) An individual who is the recipient of case management services. This individual can be a patient, beneficiary, injured worker, claimant, enrollee, member, college student, resident, or healthcare consumer of any age group. In addition, the term client may also infer the inclusion of the client's support. (b) Client can also imply the business relationship with a company that contracts or pays for case management services.

Client Support System: The client's support system is defined by each client and may include biological relatives, a spouse, a partner, friends, neighbors, colleagues, a healthcare proxy, or any individual who supports the client.

Consumer: A person who is the direct or indirect recipient of the organization's services. Depending on the context, consumers may be identified by different names, such as "client," "member," "enrollee," "beneficiary," "patient," "injured worker," "claimant," "college student," or "resident." In addition, a consumer relationship may exist even when there is no direct relationship between the consumer and the organization. For example, suppose an individual is a member of a health plan that relies on the services of a utilization management organization. In that case, the individual is a consumer of the utilization management organization.

Cultural Competence: Cultural competence is defined as the ability of providers and organizations to effectively deliver healthcare services that meet the social, cultural, and linguistic needs of patients. A culturally competent healthcare system can help improve health outcomes and quality of care and can contribute to the elimination of racial and ethnic health disparities. Examples of strategies to move the healthcare system toward these goals include providing relevant training on cultural competence and cross-cultural issues to health professionals and creating policies that reduce administrative and linguistic barriers to patient care.

Culture: Culture can be defined as all the ways of life including arts, beliefs, and institutions of a population that are passed down from generation to generation. Culture has been called "the way of life for an entire society." As such, it includes codes of manners, dress, language, religion, rituals, art. Norms of behavior, such as law and morality, and systems of belief. Culture may include, but is not limited to, race, ethnicity, national origin, and migration background; sex, sexual orientation, and marital status; age, religion, and political belief; physical, mental, or cognitive disability; gender, gender identity, or gender expression.

Disease Management: A coordinated healthcare interventions and communications system for populations with conditions in which patient self-care efforts are significant. This system supports the physician or practitioner/client relationship and plan of care; emphasizes prevention of exacerbations and complications using evidence-based practice guidelines and patient empowerment strategies; and evaluates clinical, humanistic, and economic outcomes on an ongoing basis to improve overall health. Because of the presence of comorbidities or multiple conditions in most high-risk patients, this approach may become operationally challenging to execute, with patients being cared for by more than one program. Over time, the industry has moved more toward a whole-person model in which all the diseases a patient has are managed by a single disease management program.

Domains of Health: The World Health Organization defines health as "a state of complete physical, mental and social well-being." The University of Utah School of Medicine has identified seven domains of health and these domains impact quality of life. The identified domains are:

- Physical
- Emotional
- Environmental
- Social
- Intellectual
- Financial
- Spiritual

Domains of Healthcare Quality: The Institutes of Medicine (IOM) put forth a framework for the development of quality measures. The framework includes the following aims:

- Safe: Avoiding harm to patients from the care that is intended to help them.
- Effective: Providing services based on scientific knowledge to all who could benefit and refraining from providing services to those not likely to benefit (avoiding underuse and misuse, respectively).
- Patient-centered: Providing care that is respectful of and responsive to individual patient preferences, needs, and values and ensuring that patient values guide all clinical decisions.
- Timely: Reducing waits and sometimes harmful delays for both those who receive and those who give care.
- Efficient: Avoiding waste, including waste of equipment, supplies, ideas, and energy.
- Equitable: Providing care that does not vary in quality because of personal characteristics such as gender, ethnicity, geographic location, and socioeconomic status.

Dual Relationships: Occur when a case manager has multiple relationships with a client, whether professional, social, or business. It is understood across interprofessional codes of ethics that dual relationships can and will occur; at times they are unavoidable. The onus is always on involved professionals to act in accordance with state laws and professional codes for their discipline, as well as organizational policies. It might be acceptable for the case manager to maintain the assignment, but a contract and/or plan should be put in place to ensure appropriate professional boundaries are maintained.

Examples:

- An individual is employed as the only case manager for a small rural community hospital within the county where they also reside. The case manager must regularly engage with clients who are neighbors, friends, and family members.
- The case manager starts a business focused on professional mentoring, offering discounts to all colleagues who contract with them for at least 6 months.

- The case manager at a managed care organization is assigned a new client; they identify the client as their son's best friend.
- The case manager has multiple part-time roles: one for a hospital, the other for an agency offering palliative care at home. The case manager receives an annual incentive bonus for increased referrals to the program. Hospital staff are informed that all patients referred to the palliative care program will be prioritized.

Evidence-Based Criteria: Guidelines for clinical practice that incorporate current and validated research findings.

Family: Family members and those individuals designated by the client as the client's support system. Family members are not limited to blood relatives; they constitute any person the client wishes to designate as family or support system.

Family Caregiver (informal): Any relative, partner, friend, or neighbor who has a significant personal relationship with, and provides a broad range of assistance for, an older person or an adult with a chronic or disabling condition. These individuals may be primary or secondary caregivers and live with, or separately from, the person receiving care.

Formal Caregiver: A provider associated with a formal service system, whether a paid worker or a volunteer.

Function: A clinical operating system for the application of a patient-centered, systems biology approach to healthcare. Its focus is on understanding an individual's physiological, cognitive, emotional, and physical function, as well as on the design and implementation of a therapeutic program that is personalized to the functional needs of the patient. The functional assessment can be applied at many organizational levels derived from a systems network biology perspective ranging from the patient's social and spiritual functions to organ system, organ, tissue, cellular, or subcellular functional levels. The word function is aligned with the evolving understanding that disease is an endpoint and function is a process.

Handover: Sometimes referred to as handoff—the transfer of authority, responsibility, and accountability for something to another individual. In the context of professional case management, handover refers to the transfer of authority, responsibility, and accountability for the care of a client to another healthcare professional within or outside a healthcare setting as indicated based on the client's needs and care goals.

Health: The definition according to the Constitution of the World Health Organization:

- Health is a state of complete physical, mental, and social well-being and not merely the absence of disease or infirmity.
- The enjoyment of the highest attainable standard of health is one of the fundamental rights of every human being without distinction of race, religion, political belief, economic, or social condition.
- The health of all peoples is fundamental to the attainment of peace and security and is dependent on the fullest cooperation of individuals and states.
- The achievement of any state in the promotion and protection of health is of value to all.

- Unequal development in different countries in the promotion of health and control of diseases, especially communicable disease, is a common danger.
- Healthy development of the child is of basic importance; the ability to live harmoniously in a changing total environment is essential to such development.
- The extension to all peoples of the benefits of medical, psychological, and related knowledge is essential to the fullest attainment of health.
- Informed opinion and active co-operation on the part of the public are of the utmost importance in the improvement of the health of the people.
- Governments have a responsibility for the health of their peoples which can be fulfilled only by the provision of adequate health and social measures.

Health Literacy: The degree to which individuals can obtain, process, and understand basic health information needed to make appropriate health decisions.

Health Outcomes: Changes in current or future health status of individuals, groups, or communities that can be attributed to antecedent actions or measures. The change may result from a planned intervention or series of interventions, regardless of whether such an intervention was intended to change an individual's health status.

Health Services: Medical or health and human services.

Interdisciplinary Healthcare Team: Inter- or multidisciplinary teams include all members of healthcare teams, professional and nonprofessional. According to Nancarrow et al., interdisciplinary teamwork is, "a dynamic process involving two or more health professionals with complementary backgrounds and skills, sharing common health goals, and exercising concerted physical and mental effort in assessing, planning, or evaluating patient care. This is accomplished through interdependent collaboration, open communication, and shared decision-making. This in turn generates value-added patient, organizational and staff outcomes."

Interprofessional Healthcare Team: An interprofessional team is comprised of team members from two or more different professions (e.g., nurses and physicians, physicians and community health workers, social workers and psychologists, pharmacists, and respiratory therapists) who learn with, from, and about each other to enable effective collaboration and improve health outcomes.

Licensure: Licensure is a process by which a government agency grants permission to an individual to engage in each occupation, if person possesses the minimum degree of competency required to reasonably protect public health, safety, and welfare.

Managed Care: Services or strategies designed to improve access to care, quality of care, and the cost-effective use of health resources. Managed care services include, but are not limited to, case management, utilization management, peer review, disease management, and population health.

Medical Home: A medical home model provides accessible, continuous, coordinated, and comprehensive patient-centered care and is managed centrally by a primary care physician with the active involvement of nonphysician practice personnel. Providers deemed a medical home may receive supplemental payments to support operations expected of a medical home. In addition, physician practices may be encouraged or required to improve practice infrastructure and meet specific qualifications to achieve eligibility.

Outcomes: Measurable results of case management interventions, such as client knowledge, adherence, self-care, satisfaction, and attainment of a meaningful lifestyle.

Patient Activation: Patient activation refers to patients' knowledge, skills, and confidence in self-managing health conditions. In large cross-sectional studies, individuals with higher patient activation are observed to have better health outcomes with the assumption that they are more engaged in health self- management.

Patient Engagement: Patient engagement is both process and behavior and is shaped by the relationship between the patient and provider and the environment in which healthcare delivery takes place.

Payer: An individual or entity that funds related services, income, or products for an individual with health needs.

Predictive Modeling: Modeling is the process of mapping relationships among data elements that have a common thread. Data are "mined" with predictive modeling software to examine and recognize patterns and trends, potentially forecasting clinical and cost outcomes. This allows an organization to make better decisions regarding current/future staff and equipment expenditures, provider and client education needs, allocation of finances, and better risk stratifying population groups.

Provider: The individual, service organization, or vendor who provides healthcare services to the client.

Risk Stratification: The process of categorizing individuals and populations according to their likelihood of experiencing adverse outcomes, for example, high risk for hospitalization.

Role: A general and abstract term that refers to a set of behaviors and expected consequences associated with one's position in a social structure. A role consists of several functions which constitute what is commonly known as a "job description." Each function in a role is described through a list of specific and related activities. Usually, organizations and employers use a person's title as a proxy for their role, for example, "acute care case manager."

Standard: An authoritative statement agreed to and promulgated by the practice based on the quality of practice and service.

Stewardship: Responsible and fiscally thoughtful management of resources.

Transitional Care: Transitional care includes all the services required to facilitate the coordination and continuity of healthcare as the client moves between one healthcare service provider and another.

Transitions of Care: Transitions of care are the movement of patients from one healthcare practitioner or setting to another as their condition, and care needs change. Also known as "care transitions."

Value-Based Purchasing: A program provided by the Centers for Medicare & Medicaid Services as part of the Patient Protection and Affordable Care Act of 2010. This program rewards providers with incentive payments based on the quality of care delivered to Medicare beneficiaries, how closely best clinical practices are followed and enhances the patient experience.

X. Appendices

Appendix A

Standard A. Case Manager Qualifications: Social workers who are prepared at the Master's in Social Work (MSW) degree level and educated under a program that would preclude them from sitting for licensure (where required) or practice at the clinical level should consult with their state licensing board to determine if additional education and/or practicum hours are required.

Appendix B

Standard B. Client Assessment: A multitude of assessments are available including those that target specific conditions. These can include cognitive, food insecurity, disease-specific (i.e., diabetes), depression, anxiety or other mood disorders, physical function, and quality of life. Physical disease-specific assessments can be located using a simple internet search or accessing websites for specific conditions. Many organizations develop proprietary assessment tools based on customer requirements. For example, state Medicaid plans' required assessments will differ based on the needs identified in each state population.

Examples of specialty assessments:

- GAD-7 assesses anxiety
- PHQ-9 assesses depressive symptoms
- Patient Activation Measure (PAM): assesses client engagement
- Accountable Health Communities Health-Related Social Needs Screening Tool: Assesses social determinants of health
- Multidimensional Scale of Perceived Social Support (MSPSS)
- Pain rating or assessments of pain's impact on function examples
  - Words to describe the pain; Intensity; Location; Duration; and Aggravating and Alleviating factors (WILDA)
  - Numerical Rating Scale (NRS)
  - Defense and Veterans Pain Rating Scale (DVPRS)
  - Pediatric: Faces, Legs, Activity, Cry, and Consolability (FLACC)
  - Behavioral Pain Scale (BPS)
- Healthcare Quality of Life examples
  - Health-Related Quality of Life scale (HRQoL)
  - Patient-Reported Outcomes Measurement System (PROMIS)
- Spiritual Assessment examples
  - FICA Spiritual History Tool

- HOPE Questions for Spiritual Assessment

Appendix C

CASE MANAGEMENT MODEL ACT

Case Management is Essential to Population Health

1. Title Protection for Case Management—Case managers are licensed professionals with the experience to support consumers and their families. Several professional groups, including the Case Management Society of America (CMSA), develop and maintain professional standards of practice (SOP), along with several nationally recognized certification bodies. Using non-licensed/certified individuals for case management can jeopardize patient care and creates opportunities for fraud.
2. Promoting Clinical Outcomes—The Case Management Model Act addresses many of the key building blocks to improve clinical outcomes. Case management is a collaborative process of assessing, planning, facilitating, coordinating and evaluating, to meet a consumer and their family's comprehensive health needs.
3. Optimizing Value-Based Purchasing—The Model Act can be configured to be national in scope or more targeted to support a range of value-based purchasing initiatives. Case managers can serve as the lynchpin on many initiatives, including collaborative care, to improve quality while optimizing the healthcare dollar-spend.
4. Advancing Integration—By leveraging a wide range of resources and utilizing dynamic population health solutions, the Model Act creates a pathway to healthcare integration. Case management offers a unique and effective way to mobilize resources to promote transitions of care and reduce unnecessary readmissions in a variety of healthcare settings. One primary example is encouraging case managers to help integrate care for consumers who need both traditional medical/surgical services in conjunction with mental health and substance use disorders (MH/SUD) services.
5. Improving Quality— The Case Management Model Act promotes a systems approach to quality improvement and clearly delineates between the role of the case manager and other support personnel, such as a navigator or case manager extender. Case management provides services that are crucial to improving quality and saving costs in a healthcare system where the majority of healthcare dollars are spent on chronic illness.
    a. Facilitate Consumer Self Determination—Shared and informed decision-making, counseling, and health education. It is important to include the patient or consumer as the main decision maker.

The full document can be accessed at:
https://cmsa.org/wp-content/uploads/2020/09/2017-Model-Care-Act Final-9.27.pdf

Appendix D

Evolution of the SOP for Case Management

1. Standards of Practice for Case Management. In 1995, the President of the CMSA wrote a foreword in the 1995 CMSA SOP. In it he stated that the "development of national Standards represents a major step forward for case managers. The future of our practice lies in the quality of our performance, as well as our outcomes" (CMSA, 1995, p. 3). These first Standards included this definition of case management (CMSA, 1995, p. 8): "Case management is a collaborative process which assesses, plans, implements, coordinates, monitors and evaluates options and services to meet an individual's health needs through communication and available resources to promote quality cost-effective outcomes."

   The 1995 SOP were recognized as an anticipated tool that case management professionals would use within every case management practice arena. They were seen as a guide to move case management practice to excellence. The Standards explored the planning, monitoring, evaluating, and outcomes phases of the case management process, followed by Performance Standards for the practicing case manager. The Performance Standards addressed how the case manager worked within each of the established Standards and with other disciplines to follow all related legal and ethical requirements. Even at that first juncture, the Standards committee recognized the importance of the case managers basing their individual practice on valid research findings. The committee encouraged case managers to participate in the research process, programs, and development of specific tools for the effective practice of case management. This was evidenced by key sections that highlighted measurement criteria in the collaborative, ethical, and legal components of the Standards (CMSA, 1995).

2. Standards of Practice for Case Management (2002)

   The 2001 Board of Directors of CMSA identified the need for a careful and thorough review and, if appropriate, revision of the 1995 published Standards. The revised Standards of Practice for Case Management were then published in 2002. The previously articulated definition of case management was amended at the time to highlight the importance of the case manager's role in client advocacy (CMSA, 2002, p. 5): "Case management is a collaborative process of assessment, planning, facilitation and advocacy for options and services to meet an individual's health needs through communication and available resources to promote quality cost-effective outcomes."

   The section on Performance Indicators was also expanded to further define the case manager. The purpose of case management was revised to address quality, safety, and cost-effective care, as well as to focus upon facilitating the client's appropriate access to care and services.

   Primary case management functions in 2002 included both current and new skills and concepts: positive relationship-building; effective written and verbal communication; negotiation skills; knowledge of contractual and risk arrangements, the importance of obtaining consent, confidentiality, and client privacy; attention to cultural competency; ability to effect change and perform ongoing evaluation; use of critical thinking and analysis; ability to plan and organize effectively; promoting client autonomy and self-determination; and demonstrating knowledge of funding sources, healthcare services, human behavior dynamics, healthcare delivery and financing systems, and clinical standards and outcomes.

The Standards in 2002 indicated that case management work applied to individual clients or to groups of clients, such as in disease management or population health models. The facilitation section of the Standards included more detail about the importance of communication and collaboration on behalf of the client and the payer. The practice settings for case management were increased to capture the evolution of, and the increase in, the number of venues in which case managers practiced.

3. Standards of Practice for Case Management (2010)

The 2010 Standards of Practice for Case Management addressed topics that influenced the practice of case management in the dynamic healthcare environment while the definition of case management generally remained as that articulated in 2002. Included in the 2010 revision however were (CMSA, 2010):

- Addressing the total individual, inclusive of medical, psychosocial, behavioral, and spiritual needs.
- Collaborating efforts that focused upon moving the individual to self-care whenever possible.
- Increasing involvement of the individual and caregiver in the decision-making process.
- Minimizing fragmentation of care within the healthcare delivery system.
- Using evidence-based guidelines, as available, in the daily practice of case management.
- Focusing on transitions of care, which included a client's transfer to the next care setting or provider while assuring effective, safe, timely, and complete transition.
- Improving outcomes by using adherence guidelines, standardized tools, and proven processes to measure a client's understanding and acceptance of the proposed plans, his/her willingness to change, and his/her support to maintain health behavior change.
- Expanding the interdisciplinary team to include clients and/or their identified support system, health care providers, and community-based and facility-based professionals (i.e., pharmacists, nurse practitioners, holistic care providers, etc.).
- Expanding the case management role to collaborate within one's practice setting to support regulatory adherence.

- Moving clients to optimal levels of health and well-being.
- Improving client safety and satisfaction.
- Improving medication reconciliation for a client through collaborative efforts with medical staff.
- Improving adherence to the plan of care for the client, including medication adherence.

Those changes advanced case management credibility and complemented the trends and changes in the healthcare delivery system occurring at the time.

4. Standards of Practice for Case Management (2016)

During the 2010s revision of the SOP for Case Management, the team involved thought that future case management SOP would likely reflect the climate of health care and build upon the evidence-based guidelines that were to be proven successful in the coming years. That prediction was not far from becoming reality.

The impetus for the 2016 revision of the SOP for Case Management is the need to emphasize the professional nature of the practice and the role of the case manager. The maturity of the practice of case management, the importance of protecting the professional role of case managers, and the enactment of new laws and regulations including the Patient Protection and Affordable Care Act, all legitimize professional case management as an integral and necessary component of the healthcare delivery system in the United States.

It is important to note that the 2016 SOP for Case Management remain primarily like and aligned with those released in 2010 except for some modifications which are meant to communicate the value of professional case management practice and demonstrate adherence to relevant and recently enacted laws and regulations.

The revised Standards:

- Update the definition of case management to reflect recent changes in the practice.
- Clarify who the professional case manager is, and the qualifications expected of this professional.
- Emphasize the practice of professional case management in the ever-expanding care settings across the entire continuum of health and human services, and in constant collaboration with the client, client's family or caregiver, and members of the interprofessional healthcare team.
- Communicate practical expectations of professional case managers in the application of each Standard. These are found in the "how demonstrated" section that follows each Standard.
- Reflect legislative and regulatory changes affecting professional case management practice such as the need to include the client's family or caregiver in the provision of case management services and to the client's satisfaction.

- Replace the use of stigmatizing terms such as problems and issues with others that are empowering to the client such as care needs and opportunities.
- Communicate the closure of professional case management services and the case manager–client relationship instead of termination of services and/or the case management process. This subtle change is better reflective of the reality that despite case closure, a client may continue to receive healthcare services however not in a case management context.
- Emphasize the provision of client-centered and culturally and linguistically appropriate case management services.
- Highlight the value of professional case management practice and the role of the professional case manager.
- Recognize the need for professional case managers to engage in scholarly activities, including research, evidence-based practice, performance improvement and innovation, and life-long learning.

BIBLIOGRAPHY

Agency for Healthcare Research and Quality. (2018a, August). *Care coordination*. Author. https://www.ahrq.gov/ncepcr/care/coor- dination/mgmt.html

Agency for Healthcare Research and Quality. (2018b, August). *Care management: Implications for medical practice, health policy, and health services research*. Author. https://www.ahrq.gov/ncep- cr/care/coordination.html

Agency for Healthcare Research and Quality. (2018c, November). *Six domains of health care quality*. Author. https://www.ahrq.gov/talkingquality/measures/six-domains.html

Ashford, J. B., LeCroy, C. W., & Williams, L. R. (2017). *Human behavior in the social environment: A multi-dimensional perspective* (6th ed.). Cengage Learning.

Bland, J. (2017). Defining function in the functional medicine model. *Integrative Medicine (Encinitas Calif.)*, *16*(1), 22–25.

Bokarius, V. (2021). Bridging the gap from symptoms to disability: Returning to work from psychiatric illness . *Psychiatric Annals*, *51*(2), 64–69. http://doi.org/10.3928/00485713-20210106-01

Care planning. (n.d.). *Segen's Medical Dictionary 2011*. https://medical-dictionary.thefreedictionary.com/care+planning

Case Closure; NYS Department of Health. (2013). *Case closure*. www/health.ny.gov/

Case Management Model Act. (2017). *Case Management Society of America*. https://www.cmsa.org/wp-content/uploads/2020/09/2017- Model-Care-Act_Final-9.27.pdf

CCMC's Case Management Body of Knowledge. (2012–2021). http://cmbody of knowledge.com/

CLAS Standards. National Standards for Culturally and Linguistically Appropriate Services. https://thinkculturalhealth.hhs.gov/clas/standards

Code of Ethics. (2021). *National association of social workers*. https://www. socialworkers.org/About/Ethics/Code-of-Ethics/Code-of-Ethics-English

Cultural competence in healthcare: Is it important for people with chronic conditions? (n.d). *Health policy institute, Georgetown University*. https://hpi.georgetown.edu/cultural/

Definitions. (2022). *Family caregiver alliance*. https://www.caregiver.org/re- source/definitions-0/

Erturkmen, G. B. L., Yuksel, M., Sarigul, B., Arvanitis, T. N., Lindman, P., Chen, R., Zhao, L., Sadou, E., Bouaud, J., Traore, L., Teoman, A., Keung, S. N. L. C., Despotou, G., de Manuel, E., Verdoy, D., de Blas, A., Gonzalez, N., Lilja, M., von Tottleben, M., . . . Kalra, D. (2019). A collaborative platform for management of chronic diseases via guide-line-drives individual care plans. *Computational and Structural Biotechnology Journal, 17*, 869–885.

Fabbri, E., De Maria, M., & Bertolaccini, L. (2017). Case management: An up- to-date review of literature and a proposal of a county utilization. *Annals of Translational Medicine, 5*(20), 396. https://doi.org/10.21037/atm.2017.07.26

Gao, J., Arden, M., Hoo, Z. H., & Wildman, M. (2019). Understanding patient activation and adherence to nebulizer treatment in adults with cystic fibrosis: Responses to the UK version of PAM-13 and a think aloud study. *BMC Health Services Research, 19*, 420. https://doi.org/10.1186/s12913-019-4260-5

Higgins, T., Larson, E., & Schnall, R. (2017, January). Unraveling the meaning of patient engagement: A concept analysis. *Patient Education and Counseling, 100*(1), 30–36. https://doi.org/10.1016/j.pec.2016.09.002 . Epub 2016 Sep 3. PMID: 27665500.

Institute for Healthcare Improvement http://www.ihi.org/resources/Pages/ImprovementStories/AcrosstheChasm-SixAimsforChangingtheHealthCareSystem.aspx

Joo, J. Y., & Huber, D. L. (2019). Case management effectiveness on health care utilization outcomes: A systematic review of reviews. *Western Journal of Nursing Research, 41*(1), 111–133. https://doi.org/10.1177/0193945918762135

Nancarrow, S. A., Booth, A., Ariss, S., Smith, T., Enderby, P., & Roots, A. (2013). Ten principles of good interdisciplinary teamwork. *Human Resources for Health, 11*, 19. https://doi.org/10.1186/1478-4491-11-19

Nursing Scope and Standards of Practice, 2021, ANA, 4th ed

Powell, S. K., & Tahan, H. M. (2019). *Case management: A practical guide for education and practice* (4th ed.). Wolters Kluwer.

Six Domains of Health Care Quality as Defined by the Institute of Medicine. *Six domains of health care quality* . Agency for Healthcare Research and Quality. https://uo- fuhealth.utah.edu/coe-womens-health/seven-domains-health/

Thumboo, J., Ow, M. Y. L., Elenore Judy, B. U., Xin, X., Zi Ying, C. C., Sung, S. C., Bautista, D. C., & Cheung, Y. B. (2018). Developing a comprehensive, culturally sensitive conceptual framework of health domains in Singapore. *PLoS One, 13*(6), e0199881. https://doi.org/10.1371/journal.pone.0199881

What is an interprofessional team? (2021). *Accreditation council for con tinuing medical education.* https://www.accme.org/faq/what-interpro- fessional-team-described-engages-teams criterion#:~:text=An%20 inter- professional%20team%20is%20comprised,to%20enable%20effective%20 collaboration%20and

What is culture?. (2016). *Boston University School of public health.* https://sphweb.bumc.bu.edu/otlt/mph-modules/PH/CulturalAwareness/ CulturalAwareness2.html

APPENDIX B

Example of an Interdisciplinary Team

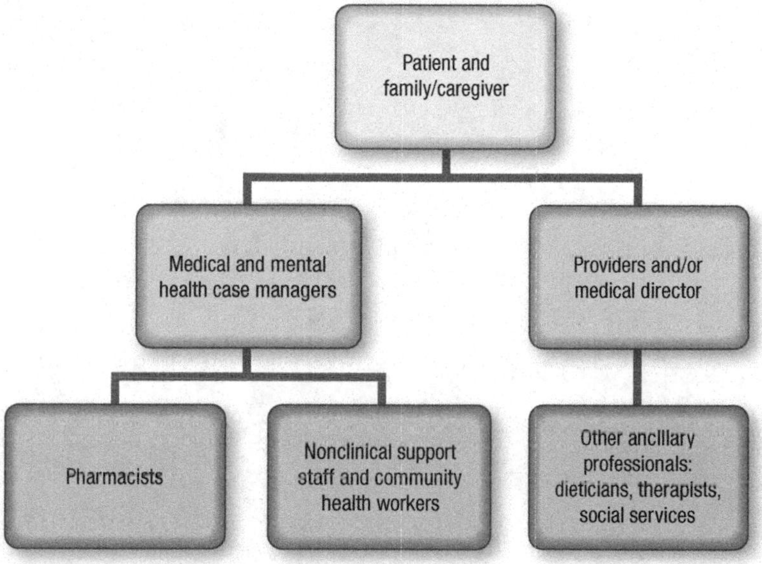

APPENDIX C

Triggers for Integrated Case Management Intervention

Sources

Data

- Predictive modeling
  - Determines future risk based on past utilization
  - Diagnoses
  - Population health categorization
  - Identification of missing preventive or needed services
- Utilization
  - Inpatient admissions
  - Length of stay
  - Emergency department visits
  - Medication adherence
    - Medications filled as ordered
  - Diagnoses
    - Medical conditions
    - Mental illness
    - Behavioral conditions
  - Reports

- State reporting of special needs populations
  - Long-term support services recipients
  - Individuals diagnosed with intellectual/developmental disabilities
  - Children in foster care
  - Waiver recipients
  - Other special needs populations

Screenings, Assessments, and Self-Reporting

- Self-assessment
- Comprehensive assessment conducted by professional case manager
- Family/caregiver referral
- Physician referral
- Other provider or community referral

APPENDIX D

Adult Integrated Case Management Complexity Assessment Grid

ICM-CAG

Date:	**HEALTH RISKS AND HEALTH NEEDS**					
Name:	**HISTORICAL**		**CURRENT STATE**		**VULNERABILITY**	
Total Score =	**Complexity Item**	**Score**	**Complexity Item**	**Score**	**Complexity Item**	**Score**
Biological domain	Persistent, sustained medical conditions		Symptom severity/impairment		Complications and life threat	
	Diagnostic dilemma		Diagnostic therapeutic challenge			
Psychological domain	Barriers to coping		Treatment choice		Mental health threat	
	Mental health history		Mental health symptoms			
Social domain	Work and leisure		Environmental stability		Social risk	
	Relationships		Social support			

(continued)

Date:	**HEALTH RISKS AND HEALTH NEEDS**					
Name:	**HISTORICAL**		**CURRENT STATE**		**VULNERABILITY**	
Total Score =	**Complexity Item**	**Score**	**Complexity Item**	**Score**	**Complexity Item**	**Score**
Health system domain	Reimbursement and provider access		Getting needed services		Health system deterrents	
	Treatment experience		Provider and patient collaboration			
Comments						
(Enter pertinent information about the reason for the score of each complexity item here. For example, poor patient adherence, death in family with stress to patient, nonevidence-based treatment of migraines, etc.)						

Scoring System:
0 = no need to act
1 = mild risk and need for monitoring or prevention
2 = moderate risk and need for action or development of intervention plan
3 = severe risk and need for immediate action or immediate intervention plan

Biological Domain Items		Psychological Domain Items	
Persistent, sustained medical conditions	In the last 5 years: Chronic conditions, persistent complaints, history of physical injury/trauma	Barriers to coping	In the last 5 years: Problems handling stress and/or problem solving (gambling, drinking, chronic complaining, feigning illness, participation in other risky behaviors)
Diagnostic dilemma	In the last 5 years: Historic problems in the diagnosis of physical illness; diagnostic effort	Mental health history	At any time in the patient's life: Diagnosis, treatment of, or admission for mental illness
Symptom severity/ impairment	In the last 30 days: Physical illness symptoms, severity, and presence of impairment	Treatment choice	In the last 30 days: Has the patient refused or resisted treatment; or have they made choices about whether or not to follow prescribed treatment, for various reasons
Adherence ability	In the last 30 days: What has been interfering with the ability to follow a treatment plan (finances, social determinants, behaviors, etc.)	Mental health symptoms	In the last 30 days: Is the patient experiencing mental health symptoms such as depressed mood, overexcitability, delusions, hallucinations, suicidal ideation, nervousness, etc.

(continued)

Date:	**HEALTH RISKS AND HEALTH NEEDS**					
Name:	**HISTORICAL**		**CURRENT STATE**		**VULNERABILITY**	
Total Score =	**Complexity Item**	**Score**	**Complexity Item**	**Score**	**Complexity Item**	**Score**
Complications and life threat	In the next 3–6 months: What are anticipated or expected difficulties in diagnosis, treatment, or response to treatment without case manager intervention		Mental health threat	In the next 3–6 months: Risk of persistent personal barriers or poor mental condition without case management intervention		
Social Domain Items			Health System Domain Items			
Work and leisure	In the last 5 years: Working actively, able to meet financial obligations; actively working but unable to meet financial obligations; retired from employment; full-time student, full-time parent, full-time, stay-at-home partner, caregiver, volunteer. Participation in hobbies, clubs, player on sports teams, regularly scheduled social events, family outings/events, entertaining, travel, etc.		Reimbursement and provider access	In the last 5 years: The patient has had a means to pay for healthcare (insurance, Medicare, Medicaid, etc.) and has choice in finding trusted providers		
Relationships	In the last 5 years: Able to make and maintain relationships		Treatment experience	In the last 5 years: Experiences with doctors or the health system; using emergency department or urgent care instead of a primary care physician		
Environmental stability	In the last 30 days: The patient is in a safe and healthy environment, able to meet financial obligations, without violence or abuse, has access to healthy food and outdoor activities		Getting needed services	In the last 30 days: Logistical ability to get needed care at service delivery level		
Social support	In the last 30 days: The patient has readily available social support		Provider and patient collaboration	In the last 30 days: Communication and collaboration between providers and between patient and providers		

(continued)

Date:	HEALTH RISKS AND HEALTH NEEDS					
Name:	HISTORICAL		CURRENT STATE		VULNERABILITY	
Total Score =	Complexity Item	Score	Complexity Item	Score	Complexity Item	Score
Social risk	In the next 3–6 months: The patient will not be able to work, support themselves or family, have social supports or a safe place to live without case manager intervention		Health system deterrents	In the next 3–6 months: Risk of continued poor access to and/or coordination of services if without case management intervention		

APPENDIX E

Adult Integrated Case Management Complexity Grid Elements and Rating Scales

Biological Domain Items		**Psychological Domain Items**	
Persistent, sustained medical conditions	Physical illness chronicity	Barriers to Coping	Problems handling stress and/or problem-solving
Diagnostic difficulty	Difficulty getting a condition diagnosed; multiple providers consulted; multiple diagnostic tests completed	Mental health history	Prior mental condition difficulties
Symptom severity	Physical illness symptom severity and impairment; does the severity of symptoms result in a disability, i.e., unable to care for self, unable to perform activities of daily living or instrumental activities of daily living, unable to work or go to school	Treatment choice	Resistance to treatment/ nonadherence; does not believe the treatment is right for them; not following a physician's treatment plan due to poor health literacy/ does not understand the goal of treatment; or a behavioral condition has interfered, i.e., depression, anxiety, poorly managed serious mental illness

(continued)

Biological Domain Items		**Psychological Domain Items**	
Adherence ability	Current difficulties in the ability to follow a physician's treatment plan	Mental health symptoms	Current mental condition symptom severity
Complications and life threat	Risk of physical complications and life threat if case management is stopped	Mental health threat	Risk of persistent personal barriers or poor mental condition care if case management is stopped
Social Domain Items		**Health System Domain Items**	
Work and leisure	Personal productivity and leisure activities; employed in the last 6 months; function as a caregiver, full-time parent, and/or homemaker; attend school; have leisure activities like hobbies, participation in social groups, regular outings with friends and family	Reimbursement and Provider Access	Access to care and services as they relate to insurance coverage, financial responsibility, language, culture, and geography; use of the emergency department instead of establishing a relationship with a physician(s) or another provider(s)
Relationships	Healthy relationships; relationship difficulties; ability to maintain relationships with spouse, family, neighbors, friends, coworkers; presence of dysfunctional relationships; physical altercations with others	Treatment experience	Experiences with doctors, hospitals, or health system

(continued)

Social Domain Items		**Health System Domain Items**	
Residential stability	Residential stability or suitability; ability to meet financial obligations (rent, mortgage, and utilities); access to food, clothing, etc.; housing is safe	Getting needed services	Logistical ability to get needed care: getting appointments, transportation to/from appointments; use of the emergency department instead of seeing outpatient providers; seeing providers who accept cultural practices and/or speak the patient's primary language
Social support	Availability of social support: have help available when needed or wanted from family, friends, coworkers, and other social contacts (e.g., church patients) or community supports (e.g., peer support, community health worker)	Provider collaboration	Communication among providers to ensure coordinated care
Social vulnerability	Risk of work, loss of income, home, and relational support needs if case management is stopped	Health system deterrents	Risk of continued poor access to and/or coordination of services if case management is stopped

TIMEFRAMES

- History
- Current status
- Future risk

BIOLOGICAL DOMAIN

Persistent Sustained Medical Conditions

0 = Less than 3 months of physical dysfunction and/or an acute condition

- No action required

1 = More than 3 months of physical dysfunction, or intermittent dysfunction for the last 3 months (i.e., pain, loss of appetite)

- Review with the patient their understanding of why this dysfunction has occurred; the cause of the dysfunction
- Will need to observe over time to see if the dysfunction becomes a chronic condition
- Ensure that patient is following up with the primary care or specialty provider

2 = Presence of a chronic disease/illness

- Review with the patient their understanding of the condition and treatment
- Assist the patient in simplifying management if it appears needed
- Ensure the patient is keeping medical appointments
- Evaluate control of the condition by reviewing any symptoms and what metrics are regularly completed (e.g., for patients with diabetes, when was the last HgA1c completed and the results; for a patient with hypertension, how often is blood pressure checked and what was the most recent reading)

3 = More than one chronic disease/illness

- Complete activities for Risk Level 2
- Customize any actions related to the results of the assessment, for example, the patient has not had an HgA1c in over a year—important to schedule as soon as possible; a patient with heart disease who states they have intermittent chest pain—schedule an appointment with the provider as soon as possible, or refer to the emergency department if having acute symptoms
- Evaluate the number of providers involved in the patient's care and report findings to the treating providers ensuring all are aware

Diagnostic Difficulty

0 = No difficulty with the diagnosis of a condition; diagnosis was made easily; for example, blood pressure has been elevated for 3 months

- No action needed

1 = A diagnosis was arrived at relatively quickly; for example, patient exhibiting flu-like symptoms and a localized rash—blood test revealed ehrlichiosis from a tick bite

- Observe for any changes in the patient's clinical status

2 = Diagnosis made but only after considerable diagnostic workup, for example, patient diagnosed with multiple sclerosis but only after blood work, MRI, and spinal tap

- Review with the patient their understanding of the condition(s), prescribed treatment, what improvements are expected, and over what time frame
- Assess how the patient managed the diagnostic period
- Discuss what we can do to support the patient to experience a positive outcome
- If the patient is having difficulty with the diagnosis, ask if they have discussed this with the physician(s) and would the patient like for us as the case manager to communicate their concerns

3 = After significant diagnostic workup, no firm diagnosis has been made

- Complete all actions under Risk Level 2 immediately
- Customize any interventions based on what we learn
- Ask the patient what concerns them the most about not reaching a diagnosis
- Offer to communicate these concerns to all involved providers

Symptom Severity and Impairment

0 = No physical symptoms or symptoms are resolved by treatment; for example, migraine headaches are controlled by regularly scheduled Botox injections

- No action required other than to observe efficacy of current treatment

1 = Mild symptoms, but do not interfere with daily function; for example, arthritic pain in hands but still able to knit and crochet, able to work in the garden

- Observe for worsening symptoms

2 = Moderate symptoms that interfere with daily functions; for example, chronic back pain that requires rest and analgesics; may miss 1 to 3 days of work

- Ensure primary care and other involved providers are aware of symptoms
- Ensure patient is following up with providers as required
- Be aware of any follow-up testing that may be ordered for worsening symptoms
- Make sure patient understands condition, what to report to providers, and when to seek immediate care
- If assistive interventions are required, assist in facilitation and coordination

3 = Severe symptoms that result in an inability to perform many daily functions; for example, patient with chronic obstructive pulmonary disease unable to climb the stairs to the second floor of their home, vacuum the floors, or walk one block to the market; a patient with multiple sclerosis is chairbound and requires assistance to bathe and use the toilet

- Update the patient's providers with any concerns or risks
- Customize other actions based on what was learned from the assessment
- Assess what current interventions help the patient most; what is working
- Assess what is not working; where challenges lie
- Evaluate the presence of social support that can aid with those activities too difficult for the patient to perform or complete
- Facilitate and coordinate, with collaboration from the treating physician, services that might result in comfort or improvement: rehabilitation, home care

Adherence Ability

0 = Ability to follow a treatment plan; the treatment plan is uncomplicated
1 = The treatment plan is slightly complicated but the patient can follow
2 = The treatment plan is slightly complicated but the patient has difficulty following. The patient needs support and motivation to adhere (support may be financial or social)
3 = The patient is unable to follow the prescribed treatment plan due to physical symptoms or has behavioral conditions that interfere with the ability to adhere

Vulnerability and Life Threat

0 = Little to no risk of worsening physical symptoms and/or limitations in activities of daily living

- No action required

1 = Mild risk of worsening physical symptoms and/or limitations in activities of daily living

- Encourage adherence to treatment and observe for any barriers that may appear
- Work with patient to remove barriers

2 = Moderate risk of worsening physical symptoms and/or substantial limitations in activities of daily living

- Work with the patient to address any causes for nonadherence
- If behavioral conditions are a cause, work to coordinate needed behavioral services
- Ensure patient and provider are communicating and each understands each other's goals and concerns
- Monitor appropriate clinical tests and utilization, for example, blood sugar, blood pressure, blood chemistries, scans, admissions, and emergency department visits
- Case management intervention may be intermittent or long term

3 = Severe risk of physical complications associated with permanent loss of function and/or risk of death

- Customize actions based on assessment
- Perform frequent reassessment of physical symptoms and response to prescribed treatment
- Case management intervention will need to continue until risks are reduced or mitigated
- If appropriate, coordinate long-term, palliative, or hospice care

PSYCHOLOGICAL DOMAIN

Barriers to Coping

0 = The ability to manage stress, life situations, and health concerns by seeking support or participating in activities that result in relaxation and satisfaction; for example, seeking medical advice, hobbies, and social activities

- No action required

1 = Limited coping skills, such as a need for control, denial of illness, and irritability

- Help the patient identify stressors and supports for stressful situations
- Encourage counseling to gain insight into positive coping strategies

2 = Impaired coping skills, such as chronic complaining, substance use (self-medication), or other unhealthy behaviors, but without serious impact on medical conditions, mental health, or social situation

- Encourage counseling to gain insight into positive coping strategies that may include specific stress-reduction techniques or conflict resolution training
- Recommend Employee Assistance Program (EAP) for any work-related stressors
- If living arrangements, work location, or social activities seem too stressful, discuss with patient strategies to change to reduce stressors

- Screen for alcohol abuse if needed
- Consider reaching out to the patient's primary care provider if substance/alcohol abuse is of concern or if the patient may benefit from a mental health professional referral

3 = Poor or absent coping skills manifested by destructive behavior like substance abuse/dependence, gambling, risky behaviors, psychiatric illness, self-mutilation, suicide attempts, and failed/failing social relationships

- Customize actions based on what was learned in the assessment
- Assist in the development of a crisis intervention plan that may include the patient's support system and providers
- Collaborate with providers for a mental health referral for assessment and treatment recommendations
- Support and encourage mental health treatment with the patient
- Collaborate with the primary care provider for a referral to substance/alcohol abuse treatment
- Support and encourage participation in substance/alcohol abuse treatment

Mental Health History

0 = No history of mental health problems or conditions

- No action required

1 = Mental health problems or conditions diagnosed, but managed or without clear effects on daily function

- Encourage regular primary care screenings for mental conditions with intervention, if appropriate
- Check for access to support from mental health professionals

2 = Mental health conditions diagnosed that have clear effects on daily function, the need for therapy, medication, day treatment, or a partial inpatient program

- Ensure the patient's understanding of potential for recurrence of mental health conditions by using lay language
- Understand the potential for medical and physical condition interactions, if indicated
- Facilitate and coordinate visits and regular follow-up with a psychiatrist and/or mental health team (psychologists, social workers, nurses, substance use disorder and other counselors) provide support when conditions destabilize
- Facilitate, coordinate, and support follow-up with the primary care provider
- Refer to a medical home, if available, to ensure all needed services are provided in one setting
- Monitor patient symptoms over time (e.g., PHQ-9, GAD-7)
- Assist with communication among physical and mental health–treating clinicians

3 = Psychiatric admissions and/or persistent effects on daily function due to mental illness

- Include customized actions based on interview
- Facilitate communication between the mental health team for mental conditions and with the primary care provider who care for concurrent physical illness
- Collaborate with providers to develop transition plans that will prevent readmissions
- Support, encourage, and assist the patient to make and keep appointments with providers, especially mental health providers

- Facilitate and coordinate any outpatient services ordered by the treating physician to help stabilize the patient's mental illness(es)
- Facilitate and coordinate appropriate social supports for the patient to prevent symptom exacerbation and readmission

Treatment Choice

0 = Interested in receiving treatment and willing to cooperate actively

- No action required

1 = Some ambivalence or hesitation, though willing to cooperate with prescribed treatment; choices about treatment are made based on the patient's situation

- Educate patient/family about illnesses
- Initiate discussions with patient about willingness to recognize conditions and prescribed treatments using motivational interviewing and problem-solving techniques to facilitate change
- Explore other barriers to treatment adherence
- Inform providers of adherence problems and work with them to consider alternative interventions, if needed

2 = Choices made due to misunderstanding of treatment, nonadherence; hostility or indifference toward healthcare professionals, diagnosed conditions, and/or treatments

- Actively explore and attempt to reverse other sources of resistance (e.g., family patient's negativism, religious objections, cultural influences, relationships with treating physician)

3 = Active resistance to important medical care

- Include customized actions based on interview
- Collaborate with treating clinicians in considering and instituting alternative interventions
- If needed, work with case management medical director to find second opinion practitioners
- If significant resistance exists and is pervasive, consider discontinuation of case management

Mental Health Symptoms

0 = No mental health symptoms

- No action needed

1 = Mild mental health symptoms, such as problems with concentration or feeling tense or nervous but do not interfere with current functioning

- Ensure the patient is receiving primary care treatment with access to support from mental health professionals
- Facilitate communication among all treating providers

2 = Moderate mental health symptoms, such as anxiety, depression, or mild cognitive impairment, that interfere with current functioning

- Encourage ongoing treatment by primary care providers with mental health support
- Facilitate primary maintenance and continuation treatment provided by primary care providers in a medical home if possible, with mental health specialist assistance—that is, a psychiatrist and mental health team (psychologists, social workers, nurses, substance abuse

counselors, etc.)—when condition destabilizes, becomes complicated, or demonstrates treatment resistance

- Evaluate and assess symptoms and document using the PHQ-9, GAD-7, and patient report; report concerns to providers
- Develop a crisis plan with the patient and with provider input

3 = Severe psychiatric symptoms and/or behavioral disturbances, such as violence, self-inflicted harm, delirium, criminal behavior, psychosis, or mania

- Include customized actions based on interview
- Support active and aggressive treatment for mental conditions by a mental health team working in close collaboration with primary care providers, who care for concurrent physical illness
- When possible, encourage geographically collocated physical and mental health personnel to facilitate ease of coordinating treatment; for example, medical home or practices in the same vicinity
- Evaluate and assess symptoms and document using the PHQ-9, GAD-7, and patient report; report any concerns immediately to providers

Mental Health Risk and Vulnerability

0 = No evidence of risk
1 = Mild risk of worsening mental health/behavioral symptoms

- Facilitate and coordinate access to appropriate mental health supports and services
- Support and encourage follow-up care with providers and perform intermittent mental health assessments, to monitor symptoms; that is, PHQ-9 and GAD-7
- Encourage and support coping and stress-reduction activates; can be formal or informal

2 = Moderate risk of worsening mental health symptoms

- Assist the patient in knowing where and from whom to get assistance: primary care provider, psychiatrist, counselor, and so on.
- Assess symptoms related to depression and anxiety by using tools, such as PHQ-9 and GAD-7
- Facilitate communication between medical and behavioral providers as necessary; facilitate access to an integrated medical home if possible
- Promote and encourage adherence to prescribed treatment
- Involve caregivers of the patient if agreeable and consent received, in all activities

3 = Severe and persistent risk of psychiatric disorder with frequent health service use

- Include interventions that are specific to the patient's prescribed treatment: medication, therapy, or other more aggressive interventions
- Work with the patient's clinicians to understand the clinical goals and assist the patient with understanding and with removal of barriers to achieve goals
- Patient may need long-term case management involvement

SOCIAL DOMAIN

Work and Leisure

0 = Patient is actively engaged in work or has a job which includes employment, furthering education, stay-at-home parent, or homemaker, and includes individuals who are retired; leisure activates that include clubs, hobbies, travel, and sports

- No action required.

1 = Patient has work or a job (as just described) but without leisure activities

- Discuss with the patient past experiences with leisure activity

2 = Patient has leisure activates but does not have work or a job now or for the last 6 months

- Discuss with patient their ability to work, willingness to work, or go to school
- Make referrals to appropriate resources; social security for disability, social services for educational and vocational resources
- If unable to return to work, provide information on how to access public assistance programs
- Follow-up timely to ensure the patient has been able to access any needed resources and assist as necessary
- Encourage any interest in leisure activities

3 = No work or job for more than 6 months and without leisure activities

- Perform activities under Risk Levels 1 and 2
- Explore the impact of not having a job and income in ability to access health services
- Access to public assistance may be more of an urgency; look for community resources that could assist in the interim

Relationships

0 = No social disruptions; no dysfunctional relationships
1 = Mild social disruptions or interpersonal problems; argues with family or friends but usually resolve differences with time

- If possible, observe the patient's interactions with family or providers

2 = Moderate social dysfunction, social relationships are tenuous, no strong friendships or family ties, would rather be alone

- Encourage the patient to include family or other supporting acquaintances to be involved in care
- Assess if social issues have any impact on the patient's health; for example, has no one to call when sick
- Assess if the patient is open to work with a counselor to improve social skills
- Explore with patient if there are social activities in which they might be willing to participate

3 = Severe social dysfunction, social isolation, unable to "get along" with family, friends, coworkers, or neighbors; argumentative, hostile

- Facilitate behavioral health assessment due to disruptive and/or destructive behaviors

Residential Stability

0 = Stable housing, stable living arrangements, able to live independently and afford all related expenses

- No action required

1 = Stable housing with support of others, for example, family available to assist, receiving home care or home and community-based services, or living in an institutional setting like assisted living, group home, or long-term care facility

- Facilitate and coordinate additional support where and when needed; this may require looking for community supports when services are not reimbursed, for example, church volunteers, extended family, friends, or coworkers willing to provide support
- Frequent assessments for potential changes in the patient's needs

2 = Unstable housing, for example, no support at home or living in a shelter; inability to meet financial obligations related to housing; housing is unsafe due to vectors, abuse; there is a need to change the current housing situation

- Consult with social services or community housing resources to explore housing options
- Consult with social services or community resources to assist with meeting financial obligations; explore with patient the willingness to include family and friends in proving more support
- Be timely with follow-up on availability and coordination of needed resources

3 = No current satisfactory or safe housing, for example, homeless, transient housing (couch surfing), or dangerous environment; an immediate change is required

- Immediately connect the patient with safe housing (e.g., emergency shelter or shelter with trusted individual)
- Follow-up with options as soon as the patient is safe for safe housing: consult with social services and/or community housing resources
- Follow-up on coordination of safe housing is a prioritized action
- If appropriate, contact housing authority for needed repairs or mitigation of other unsafe living situations unrelated to violence (e.g., vermin or insect infestations, unsafe structures)

Social Support

0 = Assistance is readily available from family, friends, coworkers, or acquaintances (e.g., church or club patients), always

- No action required

1 = Assistance is generally available from family, friends, coworkers, or acquaintances; assistance may be sporadic and not always available when needed

- Assess what assistance is needed
- Discuss with patient and social supports, who can assist and when
- Develop contingency plan for assistance when no one is available; for example, transportation to appointments, what to do in an emergency

2 = Limited assistance from family, friends, coworkers, or acquaintances (e.g., family does not live close, patient has a limited social circle)

- Discuss with patient and social supports, who can assist and when
- Develop contingency plan for assistance when no one is available; for example, transportation to appointments, what to do in an emergency.
- Assess for in-home support by home health agencies or volunteer organizations if appropriate

3 = No assistance is available from family, friends, coworkers, or acquaintances at any time

- Assess for the need and availability of in-home supports, for example, home- and community-based services
- Coordinate needed transportation, access to food

- Discuss with patient and providers the need for transfer to a setting that will provide more safety and support (e.g., assisted living, group home)

Social Vulnerability

0 = No risk present that warrants the need to change the living situation; social supports are present; and the patient can meet financial obligations

- No action required

1 = Some assistance might be needed to ensure social supports are available when needed

- Work with the patient to determine if current supports will be available in the future
- If in-home supports are needed, determine the length of time needed and availability of the services for that period
- Make sure contingency plan is developed for long term

2 = Risks exist that would result in the patient having little to no social support, will be unable to meet financial obligations, and keep medical appointments

- Work with the patient and support system to determine if support will continue regardless of how limited
- Explore availability of community and social resources to assist with financial obligations, access to food: Is there a limit to what can be accessed?
- Review benefits/reimbursement to ensure any coordinated services can be extended long term
- If unable to extend in-home services, community resources, and social support, explore placement options

3 = Immediate, and into the next few months, need for placement of supports, assistance with meeting financial obligations, emergency planning, and/or placement in a safe environment

- Expedite placement to a safe environment if home-based options are not feasible

HEALTH SYSTEM DOMAIN

Reimbursement and Provider Access

0 = Adequate access to care: no issues with insurance, reasonable premiums, coinsurance, co-pays; providers are available near the patient, the patient can make and keep appointments

- No action required

1 = Some difficulty accessing care; long travel to providers; limited access to specialists like psychiatrists; long waits to get appointments; high pharmacy co-pays; providers who meet preferred cultural practice or language or not available

- Assist the patient in researching providers who meet their preferences for culture or language
- Assist patients in making appointments
- Discuss medications with high co-pays with pharmacy staff or medical director to see if peer-to-peer could result in more affordable medication

2 = Difficulty accessing care due to geography, language, culture, insurance coverage, or premiums (see details in No.1)

- Speak with provider offices to facilitate expedited appointments or coordinate multiple appointments in 1 day so that travel is reduced

- Assist with filling gaps in care (e.g., lack of counselors: facilitate telephone, virtual meeting software, or other telecommunications for access to counseling services)
- If insurance costs are too high, explore what other options may be available to the patient

3 = No adequate access to care due to geography, language, culture, insurance coverage, or premiums (see details in No. 1)

- Contact social services to see if the patient might qualify for access to specialty clinics

Treatment Experience

0 = No problems with healthcare providers

- No action required

1 = Negative experiences with healthcare providers

- Ask the patient to describe the experiences
- Ask the patient if they could follow recommended treatment plans
- Ask the patient to describe what kind of provider they would like to see
- Help the patient better prepare for provider visits by helping the patient develop questions to ask the provider; recommend the patient write down the questions to take to appointments

2 = Multiple providers; has changed providers many times due to dissatisfaction or sees multiple providers

- Have the patient describe the conflicts and then assist the patient in resolving conflicts with practitioners if possible by communicating the patient's concerns to the provider
- Review the recommended treatment plan with the patient, ask if this is a plan he or she can follow; if not, why not; and to facilitate communication of those concerns with the provider
- If conflicts do not seem to be resolved, ask the medical director to speak with the provider
- If the patient is still not happy with provider, help the patient find a new provider

3 = Repeated provider conflicts and or emergency department use

- Speak with providers to see if a mental health evaluation is warranted
- Offer to coordinate conflict resolution training and strategies for the patients

Provider Collaboration

0 = Patient able to communicate effectively with all practitioners and practitioners communicate with each other; there are no problems with coordination of care

- No action required

1 = Primary care practitioner coordinates all care including mental health services; limited communication if patient has more than one practitioner; patient not confident in speaking with providers

- Review with patient if mental health practitioner or other is needed
- Communicate with primary care provider that mental health professional services can be coordinated
- Make the patient aware that integrated practices are available: patient-centered medical home or health home

- Facilitate communication between practitioners, coach patient on how to ask questions, provide medication lists, appointment dates, and so on

2 = Lack of communication between patient and provider(s), and or among providers related to a patient's conditions and ordered treatment

- Help the patient schedule same-day appointments for different problems. Patient can be instructed to bring summary of each visit to the next
- Communicate with all practitioners that you can facilitate coordination of needed care and services
- Suggest accessing care at an integrated clinic (patient-centered medical home or health home)

3 = No communication between patient and provider(s) and or among providers and no responsible party for care coordination

- Attend provider visits with the patient if possible
- Speak with treating practitioners on behalf of the patient, with the patient's permission (may need to have written consent)

Health System Deterrents/Vulnerability

0 = No risk or concern that care between medical and behavioral is not coordinated, no issues with insurance or financial

- No action required

1 = Mild risk of health system challenges such as insurance coverage restrictions, geographical access to care, inconsistent or limited communication between providers, or inconsistent coordination of care

- Examine with the patient any insurance coverage restrictions or deterrents like high deductible, or coinsurance, exclusions
- Investigate community resources for services not covered by insurance (e.g., counseling, other mental health services)
- Determine with the patient if they have the resources to maintain insurance coverage
- If there is a threat to maintaining coverage, strategize how to mitigate that threat
- Is it possible for the patient to continue to see providers who are not geographically convenient?
- Continue to facilitate communication between providers

2 = Moderate risk of health system challenges related to insurance coverage restrictions, potential loss of insurance coverage, geographical access to care, poor communication among providers, and poor care coordination

- Assist with finding resources to continue affordable health insurance coverage if unable to maintain current coverage
- Facilitate care in a medical home to improve communication and care coordination

3 = Severe risk of health system challenges such as no health insurance, limited coverage, providers resistant to communication, and no obvious coordination of care

- Immediately implement previous interventions as they apply to the patient's needs

APPENDIX F

Pediatric Integrated Case Management Complexity Grid

PIM-CAG

Date:	HEALTH RISKS AND HEALTH NEEDS					
Name:	**HISTORICAL**		**CURRENT STATE**		**VULNERABILITY**	
Total Score =	**Complexity Item**	**Score**	**Complexity Item**	**Score**	**Complexity Item**	**Score**
Biological	Persistent, sustained medical condition		Symptom severity/ impairment		Complications and life threat	
	Diagnostic difficulty		Adherence ability			
Psychological	Barriers to coping		Treatment choice		Learning and/or mental health threat	
	Mental health history		Mental health symptoms			
	Cognitive development					
	Adverse developmental events					

(continued)

Date:	**HEALTH RISKS AND HEALTH NEEDS**					
Name:	**HISTORICAL**		**CURRENT STATE**		**VULNERABILITY**	
Total Score =	**Complexity Item**	**Score**	**Complexity Item**	**Score**	**Complexity Item**	**Score**
Social	Learning ability		Residential stability		Family/school/ social system risk	
	Family and social relationships		Child/adolescent support system			
	Caregiver/parent health and function		Caregiver/family support			
			School and community participation			
Health system	Reimbursement and provider access		Getting needed services		Health system deterrents	
	Treatment experience		Provider and patient collaboration			

Scoring System:
0 = no vulnerability or need to act
1 = mild vulnerability and need for monitoring or prevention
2 = moderate vulnerability and need for action or development of intervention plan
3 = severe vulnerability and need for immediate action or immediate intervention plan

APPENDIX G

Pediatric Integrated Case Management Complexity Grid Elements and Rating Scales

Biological Domain Items		**Psychological Domain Items**	
Persistent, sustained medical condition	Physical illness chronicity	Barriers to coping	Problems handling stress or engaging in problem-solving
		Mental health history	Prior mental condition
Diagnostic difficulty	Difficulty getting a condition diagnosed; multiple providers have been consulted; multiple diagnostic tests completed	Cognitive development	Cognitive level and capabilities
		Adverse developmental events	Early adverse physical and mental health events: Complications during pregnancy; other adverse event that took place early in childhood resulting in interrupting cognitive or behavioral development; trauma
Symptom severity/ impairment	Physical illness symptom severity and impairment; do the physical symptoms result in a disability; e.g., unable to care for self, activities of daily living, and instrumental activities of daily living; unable to attend school or participate in any school-related activity, e.g., physical education	Treatment choice	Resistance to treatment; nonadherence; encompasses the parent/guardian and/or the child/adolescent: does not believe the treatment is right for them; not following a physician's treatment plan due to poor health, poor health literacy, lack of understanding related to the goal of treatment; a behavioral condition has interfered, e.g., depression, anxiety, poorly managed serious mental illness, or financial concerns

(continued)

Biological Domain Items		Psychological Domain Items	
Adherence ability	Current difficulties in the ability to follow a physician's treatment plan by the parent/ guardian or the child	Mental health symptoms	Current mental conditions with symptom severity; presence of mental health symptoms or challenging behaviors
Complications and life threat	Risk of physical complications and life threat if case management is stopped	Learning and/or mental health threat	Risk of persistent personal barriers, cognitive deficits, or poor mental condition care if case management is stopped
Social Domain Items		**Health System Domain Items**	
Learning ability	History/presence of learning difficulties, ability to participate in learning activities	Reimbursement and provider access	Access to care and services as they relate to insurance coverage, financial responsibility, language, and geography; use of the emergency department instead of establishing a relationship with a physician or other provider
Family and social relationships	Stability in parent/guardian relationships; ability to make friends, socialize with peers		
Caregiver health and function	Caregiver/parent physical and mental health condition and function; ability to support the health and well-being of the child/adolescent	Treatment experience	Experience with doctors, hospitals, or other areas of the health system
Residential stability	Food and housing situation; safe place to live, free from abuse, neglect; resources are available to support safe living, financial resources for food, utilities, rent, and mortgage	Getting needed services	Logistical ability to get needed care: getting appointments, use of the emergency department instead of seeking outpatient care
Child/ adolescent support system	Child/youth support system; who is available to support the child?		
Caregiver/ family support system	Caregiver/parent support system; who provides social support to family/caregiver?	Provider and patient collaboration	Communication among providers to ensure coordinated care
School and community participation	Attendance, achievement, and behavior at school		

(*continued*)

Biological Domain Items		Psychological Domain Items	
Family/school/social risk	Risk for home/school support or supervision needs if case management is stopped	Health system deterrents	Risk of continued poor access to and/or coordination of services if case management is stopped

TIMEFRAMES

- History
- Current status
- Future risk

When using the Pediatric Integrated Case Management Complexity Grid (PIM-CAG), assessment is conducted in the four domains but with additional risk elements. Those additional elements are detailed here.

PSYCHOLOGICAL DOMAIN

Cognitive Development

0 = No cognitive impairment

- No action required

1 = Possible developmental delay or immaturity; low IQ

- Assist in establishing level of impairment, including capacity of child/youth to communicate physical needs and symptoms by coordinating referrals for appropriate testing
- Discuss level of impairment and needs with caregivers, educator, and the pediatrician to ensure appropriate placement in school system
- Assess need for remedial educational assistance and home support; facilitate completion of an individual educational plan (IEP) to meet the child's/youth's educational needs
- Maintain communication with the school system and medical providers regarding the child's/youth's progress with learning

2 = Delayed development; mild or moderate cognitive impairment

- Review performance/adjustment issues with school facility; involve social services if needed if there is a lack of improvement
- Assess and assist with home support for child/youth based on functional capabilities and respite for caregivers/parents related to assimilation of social skills; provide relief for parents/guardians from day-to-day caregiving
- Assess and share child's/youth's ability to communicate

3 = Severe and pervasive developmental delays or profound cognitive impairment

- Ensure parents/guardians have access to needed resources and supports to deal with severe developmental delays
- In extreme circumstances, placement may be required. Work with providers and parents/guardian to facilitate such a difficult transition

Adverse Developmental Events

0 = No identified developmental traumas or injuries (e.g., physical or sexual abuse, meningitis, lead exposure, drug abuse, exposure to infection, or other untoward prenatal exposures)

- No action required

1 = Traumatic prior experiences or injuries with no apparent or stated impact on child/youth

- While at the time of assessment, there may appear to be no untoward effects of early trauma or exposure, observation is warranted as the child/youth grows and develops

2 = Traumatic prior experiences or injuries with potential relationship to impairment in child/youth

- Facilitate needed testing and evaluation to the extent that the trauma or exposure has affected the child/youth
- Facilitate appropriate interventions to reduce the resulting effects of the trauma or exposure

3 = Traumatic prior experiences with apparent and significant direct relationship to impairment in child/youth

- Urgently coordinate needed services to address the impairments experienced due to trauma and exposures

SOCIAL DOMAIN

Learning Ability

0 = Performing well in school with good achievement, attendance, and behavior

- No action required

1 = Performing adequately in school although there are some achievement, attendance, and behavioral problems (e.g., missed classes, pranks)

- Encourage parents/caregivers to become more closely involved with the child's teachers and administrators

2 = Experiencing moderate problems with school achievement, attendance, and/or behavior (e.g., school disciplinary action, few school-related peer relationships, academic probation)

- Recommend parents/guardians closely work with teachers and counselors to determine strategies to improve achievement, attendance, and reduce disruptive behavior
- May need to refer to additional counseling or tutoring resources outside of school

3 = Experiencing severe problems with school achievement, attendance, and/or behavior (e.g., homebound education, school suspension, violence, illegal activities at school, academic failure, school dropout, disruptive peer group activity)

- Urgently assist with facilitation of additional resources and referrals for counseling, tutoring

Family and Social Relationships

0 = Stable nurturing home, good social, and peer relationships

- No action is required

1 = Mild family problems, minor problems with social and peer relationships (e.g., parent/child conflict, frequent fights, marital discord, lacking close friends)

- Offer to facilitate counseling to address family problems or the child's/youth's challenges with making friends

2 = Moderate level of family problems, inability to initiate and maintain social and peer relationships (e.g., parental neglect, difficult separation/divorce, alcohol abuse, hostile caregiver, difficulties in maintaining same-age peer relationships)

- Collaborate with providers and school to encourage family counseling or counseling for the child's/youth's inability to maintain relationships
- Involve social services to assess family dysfunction and risk to child's/youth's safety

3 = Severe family problems with disruptive social and peer relationships (e.g., significant abuse, hostile child custody battles, addiction issues, parental criminality, complete social isolation, little or no association with peers)

- Immediately notify social services or appropriate authorities if there is a risk of danger to the welfare of your patient or other family member
- Notify the patient's providers of concerns with social isolation, facilitate referral to appropriate mental health providers

Caregiver/Parent Health and Function

0 = All caregivers healthy

- No action required

1 = Physical and/or mental health issues, including poor coping skills, and/or permanent disability, present in one or more caregiver that do not impact parenting

- Discuss with parent/guardian the challenges and contributors to difficulty coping and what, if any, resources are available to assist with coping
- Assess any needed assistance related to existing disabilities
- Provide resources to the parent/guardian to obtain defined assistance

2 = Physical and/or mental health conditions, including disrupted coping resources, and/or permanent disability, present in one or more caregiver that interfere with parenting

- Assist parent/guardian in making needed appointments for counseling and other mental health services
- Provide information on resources that may assist the parent/guardian with compensation of any physical disability

3 = Physical and/or mental health conditions, including disrupted coping styles, and/or permanent disability, present in one or more caregiver that prevent effective parenting and/or create a dangerous situation for the child/youth

- Immediately contact the patient's providers to advise of a dangerous situation
- Work with social services to ensure the patient has a safe environment even if just temporary
- Reassure the parent/caregiver that you will assist in making sure there is no interruption in the care and services received by the patient

Child/Adolescent Support

0 = Supervision and/or assistance readily available from family/caregiver, friends/peers, teachers, and/or community social networks (e.g., spiritual/religious groups) at all times

- No action required

1 = Supervision and/or assistance generally available from family/caregiver, friends/peers, teachers, and/or community social networks; but possible delays

- Ascertain who, besides parent/guardian, are able to provide support caring and supervision like friends or teachers
- Create a plan with the parent/caregiver that these supports are available when needed

2 = Limited supervision and/or assistance available from family/caregiver, friends/peers, teachers, and/or community social networks

- Complete actions under Risk Level 1
- Look for alternative supports like after-school care or community activities

3 = No effective supervision and/or assistance available from family/caregiver, friends/peers, teachers, and/or community social networks at any time

- Get permission to speak with extended family to ascertain their ability to support the patient
- Work with school and social services to see what programs might be available to address the patient's need for additional emotional support

School and Community Participation

0 = Attending school regularly, achieving and participating well, and actively engaged in extracurricular school or community activities (e.g., sports, clubs, hobbies, religious groups)

- No action required

1 = Average of 1 day of school missed/week and/or minor disruptions in achievement and behavior with few extracurricular activities

- Discover the reason for missed school days
- Strategize with parent/caregiver on how to prevent missed school days
- Work with parent/guardian and patient to learn what the child is interested in—hobbies, sports, games, and so on
- Encourage parent/guardian to connect patient to activities

2 = Average of 2 days or more of school missed per week and/or moderate disruption in achievement or behavior with resistance to extracurricular activities

- Contact patient's school to help facilitate parent/guardian communication with teachers and school counselors to develop plan to improve attendance, performance, and participation

3 = Truant or school nonattendance with no extracurricular activities and no community connections

- Complete actions under Risk Levels 1 and 2 with plan for urgent implementation

APPENDIX H

Integrated Case Management Complexity Assessment Grid Scoring Sheet

Date:	HEALTH RISKS AND HEALTH NEEDS					
Name:	HISTORICAL		CURRENT STATE		VULNERABILITY	
Total Score =	Complexity Item	Score	Complexity Item	Score	Complexity Item	Score
Biological domain	Persistent, sustained medical condition		Symptom severity/ impairment		Complications and life threat	
	Diagnostic difficulty		Adherence ability			
Psychological domain	Barriers to coping		Treatment choice		Mental health threat	
	Mental health history		Mental health symptoms			
Social domain	Work and leisure		Residential stability		Social vulnerability	
	Relationships		Social support			
Health system domain	Reimbursement and access to care		Getting needed services		Health system deterrents	
	Treatment experience		Provider collaboration			

(continued)

Date:	**HEALTH RISKS AND HEALTH NEEDS**					
Name:	**HISTORICAL**		**CURRENT STATE**		**VULNERABILITY**	
Total Score =	**Complexity Item**	**Score**	**Complexity Item**	**Score**	**Complexity Item**	**Score**
Comments						
(Enter pertinent information about the reason for the score of each complexity item here (e.g., poor patient adherence, death in family with stress to patient, nonevidence-based treatment of migraines)						
Scoring System: **0** = no need to act. **1** = mild risk and need for monitoring or prevention. **2** = moderate risk and need for action or development of intervention plan. **3** = severe risk and need for immediate action or immediate intervention plan.						

Note: Permission for reuse must be obtained from the authors by contacting ICM@cmsa.org.

APPENDIX

Pediatric Integrated Case Management Complexity Grid Scoring Sheet

Date:	**HEALTH RISKS AND HEALTH NEEDS**					
Name:	**HISTORICAL**		**CURRENT STATE**		**VULNERABILITY**	
Total Score =	**Complexity Item**	**Score**	**Complexity Item**	**Score**	**Complexity Item**	**Score**
Biological domain	Persistent, sustained medical conditions		Symptom severity/ impairment		Complications and life threat	
	Diagnostic difficulty		Adherence ability			
Psychological domain	Barriers to coping		Treatment choice		Learning and/or mental health threat	
	Mental health history		Mental health symptoms			
	Cognitive development					
	Adverse developmental events					

(*continued*)

Date:	**HEALTH RISKS AND HEALTH NEEDS**					
Name:	**HISTORICAL**		**CURRENT STATE**		**VULNERABILITY**	
Total Score =	**Complexity Item**	**Score**	**Complexity Item**	**Score**	**Complexity Item**	**Score**
Social domain	Learning ability		Residential stability		Family/school/ social system vulnerability	
	Family and social relationships		Child/adolescent support system			
	Caregiver/parent health and function		Caregiver/family support			
			School and community participation			
Health system domain	Reimbursement and access to care		Getting needed services		Health system deterrents	
	Treatment experience		Provider collaboration			
Comments						

Scoring System:
0 = no need to act
1 = mild risk and need for monitoring or prevention
2 = moderate risk and need for action or development of intervention plan
3 = severe risk and need for immediate action or immediate intervention plan

Note: Permission for reuse must be obtained from the authors by contacting ICM@cmsa.org.

APPENDIX J

Definition of Terms

Acuity: Related to the recentness with which an illness has shown presentation or increase in symptoms.

Age of consent: The minimum age at which a person is considered to be legally competent of consenting to sexual acts.

Care management: For purposes of this textbook, this term is intended to encompass all forms of management activity, including health coaching (wellness), employee assistance, disability management and workers' compensation management, disease management, and case management. It is considered synonymous with "health management."

Case management extender: Nonclinical staff who support case managers in completing care coordination activities that do not require clinical intervention as well as working directly with patients who may need only social support and do not need clinical interventions, and can encourage, support, and coordinate preventative services for patients needing to complete.

Child abuse and neglect: Any type of cruelty inflicted on a child, including mental abuse, physical harm, neglect, and sexual abuse or exploitation.

Clinician: Any clinical-based healthcare professional who assists the patient in receiving interventions that will lead to better clinical outcomes, such as nurse, social worker, counselor, pharmacist, doctor, and so on; or in a clinical helper role, such as treating practitioner, case or disease manager, therapy provider, medication advisors, and so on. Hospital or health plan administrators are not clinicians since they are not clinical-based healthcare professionals. Utilization managers, even though they are most often clinical-based healthcare professionals, are not clinicians since they are not functioning in a helper role.

Comorbidity: The occurrence of two or more illnesses or conditions in the same patient.

Complexity: The combination of biological, psychological, social, and health system circumstances that creates barriers to improvement, making it difficult for a person with illness to regain or stabilize health.

Cross-disciplinary roles: The primary case manager works with the member in all areas that impact health by becoming familiar with conditions less familiar.

Department of Veteran Affairs: Provides a range of benefits to men and women who served on active duty in the military, including health and medical care.

Emotional intelligence: The ability to manage one's emotions and understand the emotions of others.

Empathy: Seek to understand the emotions and feelings of others.

Evidence-based practice (EBP): Integrating clinical expertise with the best available external clinical evidence from systematic research.

Generalized Anxiety Disorder-7 (GAD-7): Standardized symptom scale for anxiety.

Health complexity: May include the presence of both medical and behavioral conditions, multiple chronic illnesses, the presence of social concerns, poor access to needed care and services, impairments or disabilities, and financial concerns.

Individualized care: Connecting a health professional with a general understanding of illnesses, treatments, the health system, and factors that create barriers to improvement, such as a case manager, to a patient/client with persistent health problems in an attempt to actively and personally assist them to stabilize or return to health over a period of days to years. This form of care is patient-centered, focusing on all complexity domains, with an outcome orientation.

Integrated behavioral health benefits: In the context of this textbook, it refers to the process by which a medical health plan not only owns behavioral health management and payment, but also makes it a part of the physical health benefits and adjudication process.

Integrated care: For the purpose of this textbook, this term applies to the availability of coordinated health services from all complexity domains (biological, psychological, social, and health system) without hassle or impediment.

Integrated case management: Follows Case Management Society of America's (CMSA) Standards of Practice for guidance and accountability in case management practice and is designed to impact individuals with health complexity by a single point of contact, or primary case manager through a multidimensional approach.

Long-term disability: Generally employees with permanent conditions, requiring time away from work for more than 6 months and little likelihood of improvement; when long-term disability is supported by a documentable medical condition, (a) the disabled person is paid a percentage of their prior salary, (b) they must document persistence of disabling signs and symptoms over time, and (c) the employer has no obligation to take the person back to their prior position (unemployed—disabled).

Maternal health: The health of a mother during pregnancy, childbirth, and the postpartum period.

Mental Health Parity: Under the Affordable Care Act (ACA) passed in 2010, behavioral health services were included as one of the 10 essential benefits, meaning insurers were required to cover mental health services equally to that of medical services.

Motivational interviewing: A person-centered counseling style for addressing the common problem of ambivalence about change.

Patient-centered care: A holistic approach oriented around an individual's goals and preferences and is essential to the delivery of high-quality care.

Patient Health Questionnaire-9 (PHQ-9): Standardized symptom scale for depression.

Population health management: The health outcomes of a group of individuals including the distribution of such outcomes within the group to improve the health of an entire human population by reducing health inequities or disparities due to social determinants of health.

Professional case manager: Performs the primary functions of assessment, planning, facilitation, coordination, monitoring, evaluation, and advocacy.

Severity: The seriousness of an illness; this is a component of complexity.

Shared decision-making: A process by which a healthcare choice is made by the patient (or significant others, or both) together with one or more healthcare professionals.

Short-term disability (STD): Time-limited illness in an employee that prevents their ability to work (usually 6 months or less); during this time, the employee retains their job, is paid during the time away from work, and cannot be fired or permanently replaced (employed—disabled).

Social determinants of health (SDH): The conditions in the environment where people are born, live, learn, work, play, worship, and age that affect a wide range of health, functioning, and quality of life outcomes and risks.

Telehealth: Telephonic consultation with a patient.

The Triple Aim: Comprised of three dimensions: improving the patient experience of care, improving the health of populations, and reducing the per capita cost of healthcare.

Transference: The patient's emotional reaction to a clinician, which is hypothesized to emanate from relationships with others (psychiatric jargon).

Transitions of care: The movement of patients from one healthcare practitioner, level of care, and/or a different setting to another, as their condition and care needs change.

Trauma-informed care: Strengths-based framework that is grounded in an understanding of and responsiveness to the impact of trauma, that emphasizes physical, psychological, and emotional safety for both providers and survivors.

Utilization management: The practice of approving or denying payment for services based on the presence of covered benefit or medical necessity; this is *not* considered a form.

Value-based care: Providers are reimbursed based on the quality of care provided versus the volume of services provided.

Veteran: A person who served in the active military, naval, air, or space service, and who was discharged or released therefrom under conditions other than dishonorable.

Warm transfer: The enrollment specialist keeps the patient on the line while the case manager who will be assuming responsibility for the case is brought on the line, personally introduced, and a short summary of the situation is given.

APPENDIX **K**

Abbreviations

AA	Alcoholics Anonymous
ABI/TBI	acute brain injury/traumatic brain injury
ACE	angiotensin-converting enzyme
ADHD	attention-deficit/hyperactivity disorder
ADL	activities of daily living
AFLS	Awareness, feelings, listen, solve
AIAN	American Indians and Alaska Natives
BI	brain injury
CAG	Complexity Assessment Grid
CBT	cognitive behavioral therapy
CCM	certified case manager
CHF	congestive heart failure
CM	case management
CMSA	Case Management Society of America
CNS	central nervous system
COPD	chronic obstructive pulmonary disease
CPT	current procedural terminology
CT	computed tomography
CVD	cardiovascular disease
DM	disease management
DME	durable medical equipment

(continued)

DOD	Department of Defense
DSM-5	*Diagnostic and Statistical Manual of Mental Disorders*, Fifth Edition
Dx	diagnosis
ED	emergency department
EEG	electroencephalogram
EKG	electrocardiogram
FEV1	forced expiratory volume in 1 second
GAD-7	Generalized Anxiety Disorder Symptom Scale
GP	general practitioner
HbA1c	hemoglobin A1c
HEDIS	Healthcare Effectiveness Data and Information Set
HIV	human immunodeficiency virus
HTN	hypertension
IADL	instrumental activities of daily living
ICD-10	*International Classification of Disease*, 10th edition
ICM	Integrated Case Management
ICM-CAG	Integrated Case Management Complexity Assessment Grid
IM-CAG	INTERMED-Complexity Assessment Grid
INF	infection
INTERMED	original name for the European version of the IM-CAG
IT	information technology
LOS	length of stay
MH	mental health
MH/SUD	mental health/substance use disorder
MHS	Military Health System
MI	motivational interviewing
NAMI	National Alliance for Mental Illness
NCQA	National Committee for Quality Assurance

(*continued*)

NIH	National Institutes of Health
NQF	National Quality Forum
ODD	oppositional defiant disorder
PC	primary care
PCC	patient-centered care
PCMH	patient-centered medical home
PCP	primary care physician
PH	physical health
PHI	personal health information
PHQ-2	Patient Health Questionnaire-2
PHQ-9	Patient Health Questionnaire-9
PIM-CAG	pediatric version of the INTERMED-Complexity Assessment Grid
PTSD	posttraumatic stress disorder
Rx	prescription
SDM	shared decision-making
SDH	social determinants of health
SMI	serious mental illness
SNRI	serotonin–norepinephrine reuptake inhibitor
SPMI	serious and persistent mental illness
SSRI	selective serotonin reuptake inhibitor (class of antidepressant and antianxiety agents)
SUD	substance use disorder
TIC	trauma-informed care
TTM	transtheoretical model
UM	utilization management
URAC	Utilization Review Accreditation Commission
VA	Department of Veterans Affairs

APPENDIX L

Suggested Scripted Interview Questions

Introduction and General Life Questions

"Hello Mr./Mrs./Ms. ____________, my name is __________ and I am a nurse/social worker case manager from __________. I am reaching out to see if I can be of any assistance to you."

"Is it alright to ask a few questions so that I can get to know you before we focus on your current health situation?"

If the patient answers yes, "Are you comfortable telling me a little about yourself? I'm interested in knowing how you spend your days; do have any hobbies or interests?"

If the patient is hesitant, try these questions:

"Do you work outside the home? If so, what kind of work do you do?"

"Do you have any difficulties meeting your financial obligations like rent, mortgage, utilities, food, medications, and so on?"

"Do you take care of anyone besides yourself? Children, parents, other relatives, neighbors, and so on?"

"Do you have any difficulties taking care of yourself (bathing, cooking, and housekeeping)? If so, who helps you?"

"Who are the people who support you when you need help?"

"Whom do you call when a crisis occurs?"

"How do you like to spend your free time?"

Physical Health Questions

"Tell me how your ______________ is affecting you today."

"Tell me about the physical illnesses you have had and how they have affected your life."

"What kind of symptoms are you having?"

"Were they difficult to diagnose? If so, how long did it take? Were many tests done?"

"What kind of treatment has the doctor prescribed? Has the treatment been helpful, effective?"

"Is it difficult for you to follow the doctor's orders? If so, why?"

"Do the symptoms interfere with your life? If so, how?"

Emotional Health Questions

"Do you ever feel worried, tense, and/or forgetful?"

"If yes, how often?"

"Has your physical health affected your emotions?"

"Have you had any mental health problems in the past? If so, tell me about them."

"Have you ever been hospitalized for a mental health condition? If so, why and for how long?"

"Have you ever received treatment for a mental or behavioral condition? If so, what kind of treatment?"

"Have you ever had difficulty following prescribed treatment for a mental or behavioral condition? If so, what kind of difficulty?"

"Are you receiving any treatment at present? If so, what has been prescribed and is it helping?"

"Do any emotional feelings interfere with your ability to work or do the things you like to do?"

Health System Questions

"Do you ever have trouble getting the care you need?"

"Do you have adequate coverage for your healthcare needs? If not, what care are you unable to access?"

"Do you have a primary doctor? Are you able to get appointments when you need them?"

"If no, have you had difficulty finding a trusted doctor? If so, is that something I can help with?"

"Do you see any specialists? If so, for what reasons?"

"Do you prefer a doctor who speaks your first language? Have you been able to find such a doctor?"

"If no, would you like to have a translator present for your appointments?"

"Do you have any cultural or religious practices that interfere with the prescribed treatment? If so, can you tell me about them?"

"Do you have any trouble paying for medical care?"

"Are you able to get to your appointments? Do you need assistance with transportation?"

"Do you live some distance from your providers? Would you like help in finding providers closer to where you live?"

"If you see multiple doctors, do you know if they communicate regarding your care?"

Personal Information Questions

"Do you smoke or use any tobacco products?"

"Are you interested in quitting?"

"Do you use any prescription painkillers? If yes, what kind and how often do you take them?"

"Do you use any illegal substances? If so, which ones and how often do you use them? Are you interested in treatment for substance use?"

"Do you drink alcohol? If yes, how often? Do you believe that alcohol is a problem for you? If yes, are you interested in treatment?"

"What are your biggest concerns right now?"

"In the next 3 months, what would you like to work on related to your health?"

"What would you like to be able to do that you cannot do right now (exercise, go to church, play with grandchildren, etc.)?

"What things are important to you that we did not discuss?"

APPENDIX M

Integrated Case Management Standards of Practice

1. **REASON FOR ISSUE:** This Veterans Health Administration (VHA) revised directive establishes a new policy that introduces integrated case management (ICM) in the Department of Veterans Affairs (VA). The directive brings an innovative approach to VHA by making case management (CM) services coordinated, collaborative, and Veteran-centric throughout VHA. This VHA directive defines CM services within VHA and sets forth practice framework, standards, competencies, and training requirements for the two largest providers of CM, Nurses, and Social Workers.
2. **SUMMARY OF MAJOR CHANGES:**
   a. Revised definitions for care coordination, care management, and CM to align with basic, moderate, and complex Levels of Care Coordination terminology.
   b. Addition of practice standards and staff responsibilities related to Care Coordination, Care Management, and CM activities.
   c. Addition of resources related to caseload sizes, CM Process Flow, and CM certification.
   d. Amendment dated May 18, 2020 includes:
      1. Addition of links to guidance on a phased approach to Care Coordination and Integrated Case Management (CC&ICM) model components.
      2. Update of VA Pulse links to VA SharePoint links.

This text sourced from VHA Directive 1110.04(1), amended May 18, 2020. Department of Veterans Affairs, Veterans Health Administration, Washington, DC 20420.

3. **RELATED ISSUES:** VHA Directive 1010, Transition and Care Management (TCM) of Ill or Injured Servicemembers and New Veterans, dated November 21, 2016; VHA Directive 1011, Department of Veterans Affairs Liaison for Healthcare Stationed at Military Treatment Facilities, dated January 27, 2017; VHA Directive 1110.02, Social Work Professional Practice, dated July 26, 2019; VHA Directive 1162.05(1), Housing and Urban Development Department of Veterans Affairs Supportive Housing (HUD-VASH) Program, dated June 29, 2017; VHA Handbook 1172.01, Polytrauma System of Care, dated March 20, 2013.
4. **RESPONSIBLE OFFICE:** The Office of Care Management and Social Work (CMSW; 10P4C) is responsible for the contents of this directive. Questions may be referred to 202-461-6780.
5. **RESCISSIONS:** VHA Handbook 1110.04, Case Management Standards of Practice, dated May 20, 2013, is rescinded.
6. **RECERTIFICATION:** This VHA directive is scheduled for recertification on or before the last working day of September 2024. This VHA directive will continue to serve as national VHA policy until it is recertified or rescinded.

BY DIRECTION OF THE OFFICE OF THE UNDER SECRETARY FOR HEALTH:

/s/ Lucille B. Beck
Deputy Under Secretary for Health for Policy and Services

NOTE: *All references herein to VA and VHA documents incorporate by reference subsequent VA and VHA documents on the same or similar subject matter.*

DISTRIBUTION: Emailed to the VHA Publications Distribution List on September 10, 2019.

Integrated Case Management Standards of Practice

1. Purpose

This VHA directive establishes the policy to ensure Veterans and Service members accessing care through VHA receive high quality, coordinated care that is delivered in a consistent manner, by a well-trained and responsive network of Case Managers. This VHA directive sets forth integrated CM standards and processes, establishes a formal structure for nursing and social work partnership, and describes how CM fits into a care coordination system. This directive also underscores that the Offices of Nursing Services (ONS) and CMSW have a dual responsibility for CMCM service implementation at all levels of the organization. **AUTHORITY:** Title 38 United States Code (U.S.C.) §1706 and 1710.

2. Background

a. VHA provides CM services to assist eligible Service members and Veterans, who have complex chronic care needs and socioeconomic vulnerabilities, with system navigation, care coordination, and biopsychosocial rehabilitation. CM services are delivered within specific clinical programs and service areas, and eligibility is determined by population- and condition-based criteria. As a growing number of VHA- enrolled Veterans seek care in the community, it is vital that VHA strengthens and integrates its care coordination services and resources. Care coordination services, including CM, must be synchronized along the healthcare continuum wherein Veterans needs are stratified, per their complexity, across levels of care. This approach promotes optimal health outcomes and effective utilization of VHA resources.

b. In FY2016, the Offices of CMSW and Nursing Services partnered and cosponsored a CM initiative that aimed to define, transform, and integrate VHA CM. The initiative's work identified and expanded upon internal, program-specific, and private sector CM best practices as well as contextualized CM within a broader Levels of Care Coordination framework. The result of this nation-wide effort is a National CC&ICM model (see paragraph 11, References). The model contains promising and best practices in the areas of care coordination and CM and is designed to keep pace with breakthroughs in these areas that emerge from continual process improvements.

3. Definitions

a. **Care Coordination.** Care coordination is a system-wide approach to the deliberate organization of all Veteran care activities between two or more participants or systems to facilitate the appropriate delivery of healthcare services. It can include, but is not limited to, care management and CM. Within the VHA level of care coordination framework, care coordination falls within the basic level.

b. **Care Management.** Care management is a population health approach to longitudinal care coordination focused on primary or secondary prevention of chronic disease and acute condition management. It applies a systems approach to collaboration and the linkage of Veterans, their families, and caregivers to needed services and resources. Care management manages and maintains oversight of a comprehensive plan for a specific cohort of Veterans. Within the VHA level of care coordination framework, care management falls within the moderate level.

c. **CM.** CM is a proactive and collaborative population health approach to longitudinal care coordination focused on chronic disease and acute condition management. CM includes systems collaboration and the linking of Veterans, families, and caregivers with needed services and resources, including wellness opportunities. CM includes responsibility for the oversight and management of a comprehensive plan for Veterans with complex care needs. Within the VHA level of care coordination framework, CM falls within the complex level.

d. **Disease Management.** A system of coordinated healthcare interventions for defined Veteran patient populations with conditions where evidence-based, standardized self-care efforts can be implemented. Disease management empowers individuals, working with other healthcare providers, to manage their disease and prevent complications through secondary or tertiary prevention efforts.

e. **Electronic Health Record (EHR).** EHR is the digital collection of patient health information resulting from clinical patient care, medical testing, and other care-related activities. Authorized VA healthcare providers may access EHR to facilitate and document medical care. EHR comprises existing and forthcoming VA software including CPRS, VistA, and Cerner platforms. ***NOTE:*** *The purpose of this definition is to adopt a short, general term (EHR) to use in VHA national policy in place of software-specific terms while VA transitions platforms.*

f. **Integrated Case Management (ICM).** A specialized, collaborative practice among multiple interprofessional healthcare teams. ICM provides structure and standards to support collaboration throughout the continuum of care and optimal utilization of healthcare resources. Its focus is on program intersections, care transitions, and provider and patient match. ICM emphasizes the importance of patient stratification by acuity, risk, and intensity into an appropriate level of care coordination. Within the VHA CC&ICM framework, ICM services correspond with a complex level of care coordination. Because of this, ICM services are higher in intensity and frequency, and delivered to Veterans with greater complexity, as compared with basic and moderate levels of care coordination. A comprehensive description of the CC&ICM framework is contained within the CC&ICM Portal on VA SharePoint and is beyond the scope of this directive. ***NOTE:*** *See the Care Coordination and ICM Portal on VA SharePoint:* https://dvagov.sharepoint.com/sites/VHACMSWS/CMI_Taskforce/ICM_Toolkit/GovernanceCouncil/Communications. *This is an internal VA website that is not available to the public.* Key components of the CC&ICM model are:

1. **CC&ICM Co-Champions.** CC&ICM Co-champions are care coordination, care management, or CM leaders (i.e., one Nurse and Social Worker) who are appointed by VA medical facility Executive Leadership and have expertise in coordinated care. CC&ICM Co-Champions serve as the integration liaison(s) between Executive Leadership and CM staff. Their role includes but is not limited to

a. Facilitating CM staff access to CM training and education.

b. Tracking performance metric reporting.

c. Monitoring quality of documentation and workload productivity.

d. Validating accuracy of coding and labor mapping (see paragraph 5.l).

***NOTE**: For implementation guidance related to CC&ICM Co-Champions, please see* https://dvagov.sharepoint.com/sites/VHACMSWS/CMI_Taskforce/ICM_Toolkit/GovernanceCouncil/Communications/SitePages/Start-your-CC&ICM-Journey.aspx. *This is an internal VA website that is not available to the public.*

2. **Care Coordination Review Team (CCRT).** CCRT is an interprofessional and interdepartmental team comprised of specialty CM program, primary care, and mental health staff with experience in care coordination that conducts high-level reviews of cases needing special attention. Veterans may be identified through self or provider referral, predictive analytics triggers, or screening/complexity tool. The CCRT assesses Veterans' clinical eligibility and utilizes mutually agreed upon stratification methodologies to determine the most appropriate care coordination level and Lead Coordinator (LC) recommendation. A transition of care or LC assignment is guided by the Veteran's predominant need and their location within the system. This information is applied to match the Veteran's acuity and complexity with the type and intensity of the intervention(s). ***NOTE**: For implementation guidance related to CCRT, please see* https://dvagov.sharepoint.com/sites/VHACMSWS/CMI_Taskforce/ICM_Toolkit/GovernanceCouncil/Communications/SitePages/Start-your-CC&ICM-Journey.aspx. *This is an internal VA website that is not available to the public.*

3. **LC.** A LC is a single, readily accessible, and clearly identifiable point of contact for a Service member or Veteran, their family and caregiver, and care team members. The LC has primary responsibility for ensuring the Veteran's care is coordinated across settings, services, and episodes of care, and the care plan is delivered as clinically indicated. While other care team members will provide direct services to the Veteran, having an LC who oversees care coordination and facilitates interprofessional team communication, reduces task and intervention duplication and improves the quality of care plan delivery. The LC role is a critical component of the CC&ICM framework (see paragraph 5.m). Additionally, the LC role is an expansion of the joint Department of Defense (DoD)/VA LC Model for transitioning Post 9/11-era Active Duty Service members to all service era Veterans. ***NOTE:** See VHA Directive 1010, TCM of Ill or Injured Service members and New Veterans, dated November 21, 2016, for further elaboration of the LC role.* ***NOTE**: For implementation guidance related to LC, please see* https://dvagov.sharepoint.com/sites/VHACMSWS/CMI_Taskforc

e/ICM_Toolkit/Governa *nceCouncil/Communications/SitePages/Start-your-CC&ICM-Journey.aspx. This is an internal VA website that is not available to the public.*

g. **Self-Management**. Self-management is the ability to manage the mental and medical aspects as well as the functions, roles, and emotions associated with having an acute or chronic condition.

h. **Shared Decision-Making.** Shared decision-making is defined as a collaborative process that allows patients and their providers to make healthcare decisions together, taking into account the best scientific evidence available, as well as the Veteran's values and preferences.

i. **Stratification.** Within the healthcare setting, stratification is the process or result of separating and arranging patient populations into categorical groups (i.e., basic, moderate, complex) per specified criteria (i.e., acuity, risk, intensity). Veteran stratification is based on measures of key prognostic factors (i.e., clinical, psychosocial, timing) obtained by a validated evaluation instrument. Its purpose is to match the right patients to the right level of care coordination and improve health outcomes. ***NOTE:*** *See paragraph 8 for elaboration of VHA's complexity and level of care coordination stratification methodology.*

j. **Population Health.** Population health is the health outcomes of a group of individuals, including the distribution of such outcomes within the group. It is an approach to healthcare that aims to improve the wellness of an entire population.

k. **VHA Case Manager.** VHA Case Managers are specially trained clinical staff with expertise in CM (e.g., complex care coordination). Case Managers are required to follow CM standards of practice (paragraph 6) and CM processes (paragraph 7).

l. **Whole Health.** Whole health is personalized, proactive, integrative, Veteran-centric care that affirms the importance of the relationship and partnership between Veterans and their community of providers. The focus is on self-care strategies, integrative health coaching, appropriate therapeutic approaches, and the components of health and well-being.

4. Policy

It is VHA policy that all Veterans and Service members accessing care through VHA will receive coordinated care. In addition, Veterans and Service members with complex care coordination needs will have access to CM services that follow evidence-based CM practice standards within an evidence-based CM model.

5. Responsibilities

a. **Under Secretary for Health.** The Under Secretary for Health is responsible for ensuring that

1. CM services are integrated and implemented at every level of VHA in accordance with this directive.
2. Care coordination is an enterprise-wide, corporate activity supported by all leaders and staff.

b. **Deputy Under Secretary for Health for Operations and Management.** The Deputy Under Secretary for Health for Operations and Management is responsible for

1. Communicating the contents of this directive to each Veterans Integrated Service Network (VISN).
2. Ensuring that each VA medical facility Director has the sufficient resources to fulfill the terms of this directive in all VA medical facilities within their VISN.
3. Providing oversight to VISNs to ensure compliance with this directive.

c. **Deputy Under Secretary for Health for Policy and Services.** The Deputy Under Secretary for Health for Policy and Services is responsible for ensuring implementation of this directive and quality of CM across VA.

d. **Deputy Under Secretary for Health for Community Care.** The Deputy Under Secretary for Health for Community Care is responsible for ensuring implementation of standards of CM for care provided through community providers.

e. **Deputy Chief Patient Care Services Officer for CMSW.** The Deputy Chief Patient Care Services Officer for CMSW is responsible for

1. Designating a full-time master's prepared social worker or nurse within the Office of CMSW to serve as the National TCM Program Manager.
2. Ensuring the implementation of integrated CM practice and process standards is a highly collaborative and coordinated effort with VHA program offices and specialty care management programs including but not limited to: the Office of Nursing Services (ONS), Office of Community Care (OCC), Office of Primary Care Services, Geriatrics and Extended Care (GEC), Office of Mental Health Services, Homeless Program Office, and other specialty CM programs (e.g., Polytrauma, VIST, Spinal Cord Injury/Disorder [SCI/D]), and other VA Central Office service areas that are impacted by CM integration.

f. **National TCM Program Manager.** The Office of CMSW, National TCM Program Manager is responsible for

1. Overseeing the development and implementation of CC&ICM in conjunction with the Offices of Nursing and Community Care.
2. Providing ongoing policy development and guidance as well as responding to internal and external inquiries.

g. **ONS.** The ONS is responsible for ensuring the implementation of the CC&ICM framework is a highly collaborative and coordinated effort with VHA program offices and specialty CM programs including, but not limited to: Office of CMSW, OCC, Office of Primary Care Services, GEC, Office of Mental Health Services, Homeless Program Office and all other specialty CM programs (e.g., Polytrauma, VIST, SCI/D), and other VA Central Office service areas that are impacted by CM integration.

h. **VISN Director.** Each VISN Director is responsible for ensuring that all VA medical facilities within the VISN comply with this directive.

i. **VA Medical Facility Director.** The VA medical facility Director is responsible for

1. Ensuring that the appropriate level of care coordination services is available to all transitioning Service members and Veterans that meet clinical eligibility criteria for that level of coordinated care, according to paragraph 7 of this directive.

2. Authorizing a VA medical facility executive (e.g., Nursing/Social Work Chief, Assistant Chief, or Executive) to serve as the CC&ICM Sponsor, who in turn authorizes the assignment of a social worker and nurse, with expertise in levels of coordinated care, to colead the establishment of an integrated framework and its ongoing operations.

3. Implementing a level of care coordination stratification methodology to ensure effective use of VA medical facility level care coordination resources, according to paragraph 8 of this directive.

4. Maintaining adequate staffing levels to safely and appropriately provide the necessary CM services for Veterans with complex level of care coordination needs.

5. Ensuring health informatics resources are made available to support ongoing data collection and analyses of CM across the Healthcare System (HCS), and CM metrics are monitored.

NOTE*: For implementation guidance related to CC&ICM responsibilities, please see* https://dvagov.sharepoint.com/sites/VHACMSWS/CMI_Taskforce/ICM_Toolkit/GovernanceCouncil/Communications/SitePages/Start-your-CC&ICM-Journey.aspx. *This is an internal VA website that is not available to the public.*

j. **VA Associate Director of Patient Care Services.** The Associate Director for Patient Care Service (ADPCS) or Nurse Executive in every VA medical facility is responsible for overseeing the professional practice of nursing provided by all nursing staff employed by the VA medical facility.

k. **VA Medical Facility Care Coordination and Integrated CM Sponsor.** The VA medical facility Executive Leadership member (e.g., ADPCS, Chief of Social Work, or Executive, Chief of Staff) who will serve as the VA medical facility CC&ICM Sponsor is responsible for

1. Assigning Nurse and Social Worker CC&ICM Co-Champions to implement CC&ICM framework and serve as ongoing subject matter experts on coordinated care.
2. Advocating to their service line or department supervisor that CC&ICM Co-Champions have the necessary resources and time allotted to achieve CC&ICM initiative goals.
3. Ensuring effective communication and collaboration exists among VA medical facility care coordination, care management, and CM service areas and programs (e.g., Patient Aligned Care Team [PACT], Specialty Care), GEC, Mental Health, and Home Telehealth) through
    a. Sharing basic CM clinical eligibility criteria across programs and services to ensure Veterans' equal access to, and safe transitions of, care between and from CM service, as defined by this directive.
    b. Ensuring regularly scheduled CCRT are held monthly, at minimum.
    c. Ensuring LC assignment via the CCRT is acknowledged, accepted, and executed by the program/service supervisor.

***NOTE**: For implementation guidance related to CC&ICM Sponsor, please see* https://dvagov.sharepoint.com/sites/VHACMSWS/CMI_Taskforce/ICM_Toolkit/GovernanceCouncil/Communications/SitePages/Start-your-CC&ICM-Journey.aspx. *This is an internal VA website that is not available to the public.*

l. **VA Medical Facility CC&ICM Co-Champions.** The VA Medical Facility CC&ICM Co-Champions are responsible for

1. Serving as consultants and subject matter experts on CM practice, including keeping abreast of VA policies, laws, and regulations that affect CM delivery to Veterans, their families, and caregivers.
2. Coordinating and collaborating with the VA medical facility level Sponsor(s), care coordination, care management, and CM service area and program leads.
3. Collaborating with internal stakeholders to assess CM composition, structure, and services to identify promising practices and gaps in CM services and identifying opportunities to enhance communication, collaboration, and coordination across the care continuum.
4. Facilitating the completion of a Readiness Assessment located at: https://dvagov.sharepoint.com/:x:/r/sites/VHACMSWS/CMI_Taskforce/ICM_Toolkit/GovernanceCouncil/Communications/_layouts/15/Doc.aspx?sourcedoc=%7BE42CAD9B-14CC-43EA-A3BD-8836312B3E3D%7D&file=CC&ICM%20Readiness%20Assessment.xlsx=&action=default&mobileredirect=true&DefaultItemOpen=1 for the purpose of identifying VA

medical facility strengths and gaps in CM services. The tool is designed to foster communication and information sharing among key stakeholders and reveal opportunities for improvements across the care coordination continuum. ***NOTE:*** *This is an internal VA website that is not available to the public.*

5. Ensuring a CCRT is in place to facilitate safe transitions of care from one level of care coordination or setting to another and with the appropriate assignment of staff as LC.
6. Establishing collaborative relationships with all clinical disciplines and all support staff to foster a culture wherein care coordination is the responsibility of all staff.
7. Developing procedures and processes to support cost-effective, high quality CM across the VA medical facility to eliminate duplication of services where appropriate.
8. Serving as a VA medical facility consultant regarding quality assurance pertinent to monitoring CM performance measure and meeting CM performance metrics.
9. Contributing to the community of practice across VHA through use of a data-driven quality improvement approach to CM practice with established goals and outcomes to evaluate and document CM effectiveness.
10. Identifying and monitoring CM metrics in collaboration with health informatics and preparing program and performance metric reports for VA medical facility leadership on a quarterly basis.
11. Facilitating and coordinating trainings on nationally recognized CM standards of practice to ensure delivery of professional CM services across the healthcare continuum in accordance with paragraph 6 in this directive.
12. Researching community resources (i.e., local, State, and national) available to provide continuity of care and to enhance the quality of life for the Service member or Veteran and disseminating this information annually to Care Coordinators, Care Managers, and Case Managers within the VA medical facility.
13. Establishing and maintaining contact with other CC&ICM Champions to ensure sharing of best practices and promote standards of practice across VHA.

NOTE: *For implementation guidance related to CC&ICM Co-Champions, please see* https://dvagov.sharepoint.com/sites/VHACMSWS/CMI_Taskforce/ICM_Toolkit/GovernanceCouncil/Communications/SitePages/Start-your-CC&ICM-Journey.aspx. *This is an internal VA website that is not available to the public.*

m. **LC.** The LC is a role that can be fulfilled by Care Coordinators, Care Managers, or Case Managers. Case Managers who serve as LCs are responsible for

1. Providing responsive, integrated care coordination to Service members and Veterans in collaboration and coordination with other care team members who also provide services directly to them. The LC responsibilities include but are not limited to: serving as the primary point of contact and facilitating an exchange of information among care team members, implementing care plans in collaboration with care team members; delivering evidence-based practice interventions, and monitoring Veterans health outcomes and effectiveness of interventions delivered by an interprofessional team. Frequency of monitoring is determined by clinical need and the Veteran's preference.
2. Communicating with the Service member or Veteran, their family member, or caregiver on an ongoing basis and providing them with contact information for other members of the care team. Documenting all communication utilizing recommended VHA CM templated notes and codes to ensure capture of health factors and Relative Value Units. Veterans' Comprehensive Care Plan functional status is quantified within LC documentation to indicate progress, no change, or decline.
3. Facilitating the proper phasing of care, benefits, and services to establish, support, and maintain health goals.
4. Referring or procuring indicated services for the Service member or Veteran, family, or caregiver and ensuring that follow-up communication is documented in the EHR. ***NOTE:*** *When assisting VA Community Care with coordinating care for Veterans outside VHA, the Case Manager LC will rely upon the VA Community Care Coordinator to coordinate the technical and business aspects of community care. The LC role is to serve as the upfront point of contact for a Veteran and their family or caregiver who responds to requests for advocacy or information.*
5. Following both VHA CM Practice (paragraph 6) and Process (paragraph 7) standards.

NOTE: *For implementation guidance related to LCs, please see* https://dvagov.sharepoint.com/sites/VHACMSWS/CMI_Taskforce/ICM_Toolkit/GovernanceCouncil/Communications/SitePages/Start-your-CC&ICM-Journey.aspx. *This is an internal VA website that is not available to the public.*

n. **Federal Recovery Consultant (FRC) Office Consultants.** FRCs serve in the role defined for Joint Recovery Consultants in the overarching 2014 VA/DoD Interagency Complex Care Coordination Memorandum of Understanding (MOU). FRCs have agreed to

1. Provide enterprise-level consultation and assistance to VA and DoD LC and Care Management Teams (CMTs).

2. Provide clinical and nonclinical assistance and advice about DoD, VA, other Federal agencies, community, and other resources available to support the Service member or Veteran and the family or caregiver.

6. Veterans Health Administration Standards of Practice for Case Managers

VHA CM standards of practice equip VHA Case Managers with the ability to respond both effectively and consistently to the whole healthcare needs of Veterans, regardless of discipline, program specialty, or care setting. VHA Case Manager standards are organized around key attributes of responsible practice: advocacy, accountability, professionalism, and facilitation, and each attribute is comprised of and further defined by a specific set of standards. VHA Case Managers are responsible for emulating the attributes and meeting the standards outlined herein as well as the associated CM tasks outlined in the paragraph 7, VHA CM Process Standards.

a. **Advocacy.** Case Managers will support and promote the rights, interests, and decisions of Service members and Veterans with individuals, groups, and institutional systems to: protect and advance their dignity, autonomy, wishes, and whole health; remove barriers to care; lend voice to diversity and multicultural concerns and challenges; and seek out new services, resources, and opportunities for growth and well-being.

1. **Self Determination.** Case Managers will, to the maximum extent possible, support Veterans' autonomy and right to be involved in the shared decision-making and determination of their own plan of care to include provision of and education on Living Wills and Advance Directives. ***NOTE:*** *See VHA Handbook 1004.02, Advanced Care Planning and Management of Advance Directives, dated December 24, 2013.* Case Managers recognize and respect Veterans' lifestyle choices and behaviors that conflict with professional recommendations or Veterans' health and wellness goals. There are circumstances, however, when Case Managers must counsel, strongly advise, and even redirect Veterans when Veteran decisions or actions compromise their own safety or the safety of others.

2. **Safety.** Case Managers will, to the extent possible, help ensure a Veterans' well-being, rights, and decisions within all domains of living (physical, emotional, environmental, financial, intellectual, occupational, social, and spiritual) are free of influence, exploitation, or coercion by other individuals that may include: health and non-healthcare professionals, friends, family, or caregivers. Case Managers will obtain all required safety training, including training related to suicide risk reduction and working safely with high-risk Veterans, in all settings (see paragraph 9, Training and Competency Requirements). Case Managers will adhere to

local and national VHA policies and procedures related to management of high-risk safety issues. ***NOTE:*** *See VHA Directive 1071, Mandatory Suicide Risk and Intervention Training for VHA Employees, dated December 22, 2017.* Case Managers will follow their discipline's and VHA reporting requirements on abuse and neglect to include intimate partner violence. ***NOTE:*** *See VHA Directive 1199, Reporting Case of Abuse and Neglect, dated November 28, 2017.*

3. **Multiculturalism and Diversity.** Case Managers will work respectfully and inclusively with all Veterans regardless of their demographics or backgrounds, as well as incorporate such multivarious factors and sensitivities into all assessment and care plan interviews and documentation. Case Managers must display and promote tolerance for cultural differences and diversity within all VHA settings.

b. **Professionalism.** Case Managers will carry out all duties expected, per their assigned service or program role and functional statement, with technical proficiency and integrity to instill Veteran confidence, trust, and credibility in both CM and VA. Professionalism aligns competency and practice with the mission of the organization. In VHA, professionalism specifically encompasses:

1. **Ethical Conduct.** Case Manager practice and behavior will be in accordance with their discipline's specific code of ethics and VHA ideals, codes, and standards. Case Managers should act with beneficence, demonstrate truthfulness and non-malfeasance, and maintain appropriate boundaries with both Veterans and colleagues. ***NOTE:*** *To identify a staff member from the Integrated Ethics program who can address healthcare ethics questions or concerns, please go the National Center for Ethics in Health Care's website at:* h ttps://vaww.ethics.va.gov. *This is an internal VA website that is not available to the public.*

2. **Education.** VHA Case Managers, and clinical staff functioning as Case Managers, are encouraged to participate in ongoing training and professional development to build and maintain CM competencies, including evidence-based practices that promote positive health outcomes and cost-effective care, including, but not limited to motivational interviewing, cognitive behavioral therapy, and health coaching. ***NOTE:*** *See the CC&ICM Portal on VA SharePoint: (*https://dvagov.sharepoint.com/sites/VHACMSWS/CMI_Taskforce/ICM_Toolkit/Govern*anceCouncil/Communications) for specifics on VA Social Work and Registered Nurse Case Manager Competencies and Functions. This is an internal VA website that is not available to the public.*

c. **Accountability.** Case Managers will demonstrate shared accountability that is intrinsic to collaborative practice and follow through on commitments made to Veterans, their families and caregivers, and interprofessional teams. Case Managers must work within their scope of practice and abide by all applicable

Federal, State, and local laws and regulations, which have full force and effect of law. In VHA, accountability specifically encompasses

1. **Privacy and Confidentiality.** Case Managers will safeguard Veteran personal health information by complying with all Federal, State, and local laws and regulations as well as VHA Directive 1067, Confidential Communications, dated November 10, 2015, and VHA Directive 1605.01, Privacy and Release of Information, dated August 31, 2016, and procedures governing patient privacy and confidentiality.

2. **Documentation and Coding.** Case Managers will document all information in a Veteran's EHR or any VHA-approved EHR within 48 hours, in accordance with VHA Handbook 1907.01, Health Information Management and Health Records, dated March 19, 2015. Documentation is the key means of communication among the healthcare team, and hence, Case Managers must write clearly, logically, and with proper use of VHA acronyms. The Veteran Health Information Exchange (VHIE) technology is available to VHA staff through EHR and Joint Legacy Viewer (JLV) for viewing community health data on their Veteran patients to support CM (https://www.va.gov/vler/). ***NOTE:*** *For further elaboration of CM documentation and coding requirements, see Appendix B.*

d. **Facilitation.** Case Managers will establish rapport and build and maintain therapeutic relationships with Veterans to foster trust and engage them in care and empower and equip them in self-care and self-management with the goal of improving positive health and wellness outcomes. Case Managers will utilize facilitation throughout the process of working with the Veteran to organize, streamline, and expedite service delivery. In VHA care, facilitation specifically encompasses

1. **CM Process.** Case Managers will follow the professionally recognized and VHA-adopted framework for evidence-based CM practices, with a sequential set of steps and associated tasks that include: identification, screening, assessment, care planning, implementation, monitoring, care transitions, and program and outcome evaluation. Case Managers will document completion of these steps in the Veteran's EHR.

2. **Communication, Collaboration, Coordination.**

   a. Case Managers will facilitate proactive, patient-centric communication and information sharing between the Veteran or Service member, their family or caregiver, providers, and other care team members, to enhance awareness and clarity, reduce misunderstandings, increase process efficiencies, and improve care plan efficacy.

   b. Case Managers will facilitate collaboration among Veterans, their family or caregiver, providers, and other care team members to engage in shared decision-making, and develop a safe, integrated, and whole healthcare plan that considers the best scientific evidence available as well as the Veteran's values and preferences.

c. Case Managers will facilitate the coordination of care by developing integrated, well-sequenced care plans, assisting Veterans with system navigation, and linking them in a timely manner, to needed health, mental health, health education, self-management and social services, community-based resources, or benefits, as clinically indicated.

3. **Therapeutic Engagement.** VHA Case Managers will engage, develop, and maintain therapeutic relationships with both the Veteran, families, and caregivers, utilizing resiliency-based, recovery-oriented, Veteran-centered communication, and practice techniques (e.g., Health Education, Health Coaching, Shared Decision-Making, Motivational Interviewing, Solution Focused Work, Psychosocial Problem-Solving, Strength-Based work) to facilitate progress, growth, and positive lifestyle changes.

NOTE: *VHA CM Standards of Practice ensure Veterans' experience of CM is reliable and synchronized within and across HCSs. VHA CM standards are based on the Case Management Society of America (CMSA) 2016 Standards of Practice* (http://solutions.cmsa.org/acton/media/10442/standards-of-practice-for-case-management), *American Case Management Association Standards of Practice and Scope of Services (2013)* (https://www.acmaweb.org/forms/Case_Management_SoP_SoS.pdf), *and National Association of Social Work Standards for Social Work Case Management Practice (2013)*

(https://www.socialworkers.org/LinkClick.aspx?fileticket=acrzqmEfhlo%3D&portalid=0). *These linked documents are outside of VA control and may not be conformant with Section 508 of the Rehabilitation Act of 1973. The aforementioned professional organizations' standards align well with VHA mission, values, and evolving priorities.*

VHA standards are an amalgamation of those standards most consistent, agreed upon by the three CM professional organizations, and are organized around key attributes of responsible practice: advocacy, accountability, professionalism, and facilitation.

7. Veterans Health Administration Case Management Process Standards

a. The CM process represents the steps and tasks associated with the functions of a Case Manager. VHA's framework depicts the overall patient/provider process flow to ensure the delivery of comprehensive, timely, high-quality services is aligned with professional expectations and practice standards. To fulfill the VHA Case Manager functions, a Case Manager must be able to demonstrate competency with associated professional responsibilities and tasks in their clinical documentation, per note content and coding (see Appendix B for further details). Each step in the process builds upon the previous step and benefits the Veteran, their family and caregiver, and employee experience when consistently performed within and without VHA. ***NOTE:*** *It is for VA medical facility leadership to determine the manner in which standardization occurs per size, complexity, alignment, and resources of their HCS.*

b. The CM process is dependent on patient progress and thus is cyclical and not linear in nature, and previous steps and actions may need to be revisited. The major goal of the CM process is to increase Veteran autonomy and decrease the long-term dependence on the Case Manager. ***NOTE:*** *VHA's CM process is adapted from the Case Management Society of America's (CMSA, 2016) Standards of Practice guidelines.*

c. The steps and tasks within VHA's CM Framework are

1. **Early Identification.** Veterans are identified for the potential need for CM through self-referral, referral from a family member or caregiver, referral through PACT or other VHA staff such as TCM, referral from VA Liaisons for Healthcare, referral through other government (DoD Military Treatment Case Manager/LC, FRC), and referrals from community agencies. The goal is to identify Veterans in need of CM services as early as possible and develop a mechanism/procedure that facilitates the process (e.g., EHR Clinical Reminder or Templated Note triggered consults, VHA Support Service Center, and other health system portals).

2. **Screening for Clinical Eligibility Criteria.** Veterans are screened for clinical eligibility criteria for CM services. The use of a standardized level of care coordination tool ensures there is consistency among providers, patient stratification, and validity of scoring. Veterans found not to require the frequency and intensity of CM services are recommended for either care management or care coordination services through PACT or another clinical area.

3. **Case Manager Assignment.** Following a thorough screening of needs, qualifying Veterans identified as appropriate for CM will be offered CM services from a Nurse or Social Work Case Manager within a care setting or program (e.g., PACT, Mental Health, Specialty CM Program (e.g., Polytrauma, HUD-VASH, TCM), Geriatrics and Extended Care, Home Telehealth, VHA Community Care [VACC]) per the predominate need of Veteran and their location within the system. For Veterans with a complex level of care coordination need, more than one Case Manager may be involved in care planning and service delivery. In these instances, assignment of a LC is recommended to coordinate CM service delivery, as well as reduce confusion, fragmentation, and unnecessary duplication. ***NOTE:*** *A close, collaborative relationship between multiple Social Work and Nursing Case Managers provides the most comprehensive approach to CM services.* Such a consultative relationship minimizes unnecessary handoffs to ensure that all the Veteran's biopsychosocial needs are met with the least interruption.

4. **Informed Consent.** As a best practice, Case Managers should obtain a Veteran's authorization for CM services as part of the case initiation process. To ensure the Veteran is appropriately informed, the CM must provide a clear definition of CM and its process including: purpose, roles, and responsibilities (of both Veteran and Case Manager), benefits, and risks. If the Veteran, or surrogate, agrees to CM services, it is best practice for the Case Manager to indicate that the CM process is a collaborative one because without collaboration, the ability to provide some services may be challenging.

5. **Comprehensive Assessment.** A Case Manager completes a comprehensive assessment of the Veteran's needs and goals. The assessment and subsequent reassessments are created in collaboration with the Veteran, their family or caregiver, and interprofessional team, as clinically indicated. Assessments are documented in the EHR and include, but are not limited to, the following elements: military history, social supports, housing, transportation, education and employment, income and finances, and care plan. ***NOTE:*** *See national note template titled, "Social Work Comprehensive Assessment" in EHR. Following the initial comprehensive assessment, reassessment is required at each subsequent contact as part of the monitoring and evaluation process.*

6. **Need Identification.** The key concerns, needs, and preferences of the Veteran and their family or caregiver are identified. This information is used to determine the most appropriate CM intervention(s).

7. **Problem-Solving and Goal(s) Identification.** Problem-solving is initiated, and the Veteran and Veteran's family or caregiver's desired or expected goal(s) and outcome(s) are recognized, organized, and prioritized through a brokered process between the Veteran, family or caregiver, and Case Manager. This negotiation ensures goals and objectives are not only agreed upon, but also specific, measurable, action- oriented, realistic, and timebound.

8. **Resource Assessment.** A resource assessment is completed to identify available assistive options and appropriate services and benefits. ***NOTE:*** *From the strength-based perspective, consideration of previous successes, existing natural supports, and internal skills and coping mechanisms is primary.*

9. **Planning and Implementation.** Planning and implementation are accomplished through coordination, collaboration, and communication with the interprofessional team including: The Veteran, the family or caregivers, and VHA and community providers. The intensity and duration of CM services are dependent on the Veteran's care needs. Available natural and community resources (e.g., decision aids, self-care and self-management support programming) are obtained to ensure the best Veteran, family, caregiver, and organizational outcomes. All elements combine to comprise the Veteran's Care Plan.

10. **Referrals and Transition.** Access to the appropriate level of care is ensured by coordinating effective and timely referrals, transitioning the Veteran to VHA, DoD, other Federal, State, and local home and community-based services. Timeliness varies and is dependent on what is considered clinically indicated. Case Managers provide referrals to various service resources along a continuum of care to restore or maintain Veterans independent functioning fully possible. Case Managers manage the delivery of an array of labor-intensive services to meet the needs of target populations.

11. **Monitoring and Evaluation.** Monitoring and evaluation of the care plan is critical to ensure the right care, at the right time, in the right place, at the right cost, is continuous and coordinated each time. Reassessment is necessary to ensure that intervention and CM services are appropriate, effective, timely, efficient, evidence-based and equitable, promote safety, and are agreed upon by the Veteran or healthcare decision maker.

12. **Program and Outcome Evaluation.** Case Managers will use CM best-practice processes, procedures, tools, and templates in their work to allow for better tracking, monitoring, and reporting of quality and performance metrics. Program evaluation and reporting allows for continuous performance improvement to ensure a high quality and sustainable CM program. ***NOTE:*** *See Appendix B for more information on performance metrics.*

8. Veterans Health Administration Levels of Care Coordination Stratification

a. **Stratification Methodology.** To ensure patients are consistently receiving the right care, at the right time, and in the right place, a validated stratification methodology—wherein a Veteran's capacity to self-manage (complexity) is evaluated and matched with an associated service—requires the current care facilitation services (i.e., care coordination, care management, and CM) to align along a seamless continuum based on a measurable denominator common to all—the activity of care coordination. ***NOTE:*** *See paragraph 3 for the conceptual definition of stratification.*

b. **Levels of Care Coordination.** VHA's facilitation services of care coordination, care management, and CM will respectively be delineated and defined by the type and intensity of care coordination interventions provided from basic to moderate to complex. ***NOTE:*** *Within complex care coordination, Case Managers will need to further stratify their patients into tiers of CM that clarify the intensity of interventions and the frequency contact.* The three VHA levels of care coordination are

   1. **Basic.** Basic level of care includes system navigation, information, and referral.

2. **Moderate.** Moderate level of care includes basic care coordination, plus disease management and prevention, health promotion and education, and resource management. Moderate Care Management are typically provided by Care Managers or Specialty Care Coordinators (e.g., Cancer Care Coordinators).

3. **Complex.** Complex (also known as Chronic) level of care includes moderate care coordination, plus biopsychosocial rehabilitation, which emphasizes coaching/mentoring and counseling/treatment aspects of the patient/clinician relationship. Complex/Chronic is provided by qualified, clinical staff with competencies in CM and who adhere to the CM practice and process standards.

NOTE*: For implementation guidance related to Levels of Care Coordination, please see* https://dvagov.sharepoint.com/sites/VHACMSWS/CMI_Taskforce/ICM_Toolkit/GovernanceCouncil/Communications/SitePages/Start-your-CC&ICM-Journey.aspx. *This is an internal VA website that is not available to the public.*

c. **Tiers of CM.**

1. VHA CM Programs further stratify Veterans receiving complex care coordination into "tiers" or "levels" per the type of CM interventions (e.g., intensive, stabilization, progressive/maintenance, supportive) and corresponding "frequency of contact" (e.g., weekly, monthly, and quarterly) by the Case Manager. The nomenclature and interventions used to describe a tier or level of CM as well as the number of tiers or levels of CM varies across specialty CM Programs. The qualitative determination of CM level is based on a Case Manager's or LC's clinical judgment and is applied in conjunction with their respective program's administrative requirements.

2. As a Veteran's level of complexity abates (i.e., biopsychosocial needs stabilize and ability to self-manage improves), it is anticipated that less intensive services and thus fewer contacts with the Case Manager/LC will be required with eventual graduation from CM services. It is also expected, however, that Veterans who have progressed in the continuum may experience significant life events, resulting in a return to a complex level of care coordination (i.e., CM tier). The CM tiers or levels include

   a. **Intensive CM.** Intensive CM requires at least weekly Veteran contact and family or caregiver contact, as appropriate, whenever there is transition of care or major change in the Veteran's clinical, psychosocial, functional status, such as: a new diagnosis, newly identified cognitive and/or behavioral health change, notable change in lifestyle, and/or major access to care concerns. It entails maximum assistance with system navigation and biopsychosocial support from a Case Manager to regain stability.

b. **Stabilization CM.** Stabilization CM requires at least two times per month Veteran contact and family or caregiver contact, as appropriate, to support the Veteran's ability to gain stability following their transition of care or major change in their clinical, psychosocial, functional status. It entails moderate assistance with system navigation and biopsychosocial support from a Case Manager to maintain stability and progress.

c. **Progressive or Maintenance CM.** Progressive or maintenance CM requires at least monthly Veteran contact and family or caregiver contact, as appropriate, to ensure a support system and plan of care is in place. The Veteran is clinically stable, but still needs ongoing intervention for psychosocial or other clinical issues to ensure continuous coordination of care and access to services. Moderate changes in functional status or level of natural supports or concerns with access to care could arise. Entails occasional assistance with system navigation and support from a Case Manager to maintain stability and progress.

d. **Supportive CM.** Supportive CM requires, at a minimum, quarterly Veteran contact and family or caregiver contact, as appropriate, to allow for the monitoring of the Veteran's care plan when the Veteran's clinical and psychosocial issues are stable. Quarterly contact also allows the CM to ensure that the Veteran is well-established in the system of care. Minor changes in functional status or level of natural supports and/or minor concerns with access to care may be observed. This entails only minimal assistance with system navigation and support from a Case Manager to maintain stability and progress.

e. **Transitions of Care (Admission/Transfer/Discharge).** During transitions of care, Veterans may be discharged from care or transferred to a lower level of care coordination when specific clinical disposition criteria and CM process steps are satisfied. ***NOTE:*** *There are specific Veteran populations that may progress in treatment, but due to persistent, chronic, or serious mental health or medical issues, require additional clinical consideration prior to any transition to a lower frequency of contact/complexity rating or discharge from long-term CM services.*

3. **Disposition.** Veteran can be transferred, graduated, or discharged when one of the following criteria is met:

   a. If the Veteran is deceased or becomes incarcerated.

   b. If the Veteran has shown ongoing stability over a cycle greater than 90 days and has accomplished care plan goals. ***NOTE:*** *Time frame may vary according to specialty CM Program.*

c. If the Veteran prefers to no longer participate in the collaborative process, as evidenced by

1. The Veteran's verbal or written request to withdraw from services or

2. The Case Manager's inability to contact the Veteran following outreach efforts and completion of the specialty CM Program's outreach protocol. ***NOTE:*** *Ensure that Case Managers follow any VISN or local policy on Veterans outreach for inability to contact.*

4. **Process.** In addition to disposition criteria being met, Case Managers/LC, to fully transfer or discharge Veterans from CM, must complete the following steps and actions:

   a. The Veteran is notified, or attempted to be notified, in advance of plan to discharge or transfer care and again at time of discharge or transfer.

   b. If the Veteran is transferring LC services, the receiving LC is notified and proactively involved in the transition and acknowledges and accepts responsibility for ongoing LC services. ***NOTE:*** *Disputes regarding the transfer of Veterans must be referred to the VA medical facility's CCRT or in their absence, the VA medical facility's CC&ICM Co-Champion(s) and Sponsor for remediation. For implementation guidance related to the LC, CCRT, and CC&ICM Co-Champions and Sponsor, please see* https://dvagov.sharepoint.com/sites/VHACMSWS/CMI_Taskforce/ICM_Toolkit/GovernanceCouncil/Communications/SitePages/Start-your-CC&ICM-Journey.aspx. *This is an internal VA website that is not available to the public.*

   c. The Veteran's healthcare team is notified of the plan to discharge or transfer care.

   d. Plans to modify level of care coordination and efforts to discharge are clearly reflected in the Veteran's EHR. Discharge from CM/LC services, transition to lower level of coordinated care, or receipt of accepted care by the LC are documented within the Discharge/Transfer Summary Note.

5. **Readmission to CM Services**. If further healthcare complexities or acuities or barriers to care arise in the future, Veterans can and should be referred again for CM screening and reinitiation of services.

9. Training and Competency Requirements

Case Managers will obtain all required safety training related to suicide risk reduction and working safely with high-risk Veterans, in all settings. These include, but are not limited to, Suicide Risk Management Training for Clinicians or S.A.V.E. Training and

Refresher Training. Training in evidence-based CM practice is required. Registered Nurse and Social Worker CM functions related to standards of practice, core competencies and competency requirements, and training and educational materials are provided on the Care Coordination and Integrated CM Portal VA SharePoint. ***NOTE:** See paragraph 11, References, and VHA Directive 1071.*

10. Records Management

All records regardless of format (e.g., paper, electronic, electronic systems) created in this directive shall be managed per the National Archives and Records Administration (NARA) approved records schedules found in VA Records Control Schedule 10-1.

Questions regarding any aspect of records management should be addressed to the appropriate Records Manager or Records Liaison.

11. References

a. VHA Directive 1010, Transition and Care Management of Ill or Injured Servicemembers and New Veterans, dated November 21, 2016.

b. VHA Directive 1067, Confidential Communication, dated November 10, 2015.

c. VHA Directive 1110.02, Social Work Professional Practice, dated July 26, 2019.

d. VHA Directive 1120.02, Health Promotion and Disease Prevention Core Program Requirements, dated February 5, 2018.

e. VHA Directive 1140.11, Uniform Geriatrics and Extended Care Services in VA Medical Centers and Clinics, dated October 11, 2016.

f. VHA Directive 1162.05(1), Housing and Urban Development Department of Veterans Affairs Supportive Housing Program, dated June 29, 2017.

g. VHA Directive 1172.01, Polytrauma System of Care, dated January 24, 2019.

h. VHA Directive 1176, Spinal Cord Injury and Disorders System of Care, dated October 1, 2010.

i. VHA Directive 1199, Reporting Case of Abuse and Neglect, dated November 28, 2017.

j. VHA Directive 1411, Home-Based Primary Care (HBPC), Special Population Patient Aligned Care Team (PACT) Program, dated June 5, 2017.

k. VHA Directive 1605.01, Privacy and Release of Information, dated August 31, 2016.

l. VHA Handbook 1101.10(1) Patient Aligned Care Team Handbook (PACT), dated February 5, 2014.

m. VHA Handbook 1120.04, Veterans Health Education and Information Program Requirements, dated September 24, 2015.

n. VHA Handbook 1160.01, Uniform Mental Health Services in VA Medical Centers and Clinics, dated September 11, 2008.

o. VHA Handbook 1162.01(1), Grant and Per Diem Program, dated June 12, 2013.

p. VHA Handbook 1162.09, Health Care for Homeless Veterans (HCHV), dated May 8, 2014.

q. VHA Handbook 1163.06, Intensive Community Mental Health Recovery Services, dated January 7, 2016.

r. VHA Handbook 1174.03, Visual Impairment Services Team (VIST) Program Procedures, dated November 5, 2009.

s. VHA Handbook 1907.01, Health Information Management and Health Records, dated March 19, 2015.

t. American Case Management Association (ACMA) Standards of Practice and Scope of Practice: https://www.acmaweb.org/forms/Case_Management_SoP_SoS.pdf. ***NOTE:*** *This linked document is outside of VA control and may not be conformant with Section 508 of the Rehabilitation Act of 1973.*

u. Care Coordination and Integrated Case Management Portal on VA SharePoint (https://dvagov.sharepoint.com/sites/VHACMSWS/CMI_Taskforce/ICM_Toolkit/GovernanceCouncil/Communications). ***NOTE:*** *This is an internal VA website that is not available to the public.*

v. Case Management Society of America (CMSA) Standards of Practice: http://solutions.cmsa.org/acton/media/10442/standards-of-practice-for-case-management.

w. Congressional Research Service, The Number of Veterans that Use VA Health Care Services Fact Sheet, dated June 3, 2014: https://fas.org/sgp/crs/misc/R43579.pdf. ***NOTE:*** *This linked document is outside of VA control and may not be conformant with Section 508 of the Rehabilitation Act of 1973.*

x. Kathol, Roger G., Andrew, Rachel L., Squire, Michelle, Dehnel, Peter J. (2018). The Integrated Case Management Manual: Assisting Complex Patients Regain Physical and Mental Health. New York: Springer Publishing Company.

y. National Association of Social Work (NASW) Standards for Social Work Case Management Practice: https://www.socialworkers.org/LinkClick.aspx?fileticket=acrzqmEfhlo%3D&portalid=0 ***NOTE:*** *This linked document is outside of VA control and may not be conformant with Section 508 of the Rehabilitation Act of 1973.*

z. National Social Work Program VA Care Management and Social Work CPT Codes for Social Workers, March 2018 and Frequently Asked Questions CPT Codes for Social Workers, March 2017: https://dvagov.sharepoint.com/sites/VHACMSWS/SocialWork/Data%20Management/Forms/AllItems.aspx?viewid=233127ad%2Dff41%2D43c4%2Da98d%2Dd03e6226bd99&id=%2Fsites%2FVHACMSWS%2FSocialWork%2FData%20Management%2FKDM%20Publications. ***NOTE:*** *This is an internal VA website that is not available to the public.*

aa. VHA Homeless Programs Hub: http://vhaindwebsim.v11.med.va.gov/hub2/hp/initiatives.html. ***NOTE:*** *This is an internal VA website that is not available to the public.*

Collaborative Case Management

1. Collaboration With Social Work Service

The National Social Work Program Office serves as the lead authority for the provision of social work practice across VHA. Social workers are assigned to treatment programs across the continuum of care, including medical, mental health, community-based settings, research, and provide social work services to Veterans, their families, and caregivers. A Social Work Chief or Executive at each Department of VA medical facility is responsible for the professional social work practice of all social workers employed within the HCS. The Social Work Chief or Executive will support Collaborative Case Management (CCM) through the following:

a. Veterans and transitioning Service members referred to VA social workers will be proactively screened for CM.

b. Referrals to VHA Specialty CM services and social work are bidirectional.

c. Social work representation and participation in the CCRT. ***NOTE:*** *For implementation guidance related to the CCRT, please see* https://dvagov.sharepoint.com/sites/VHACMSWS/CMI_Taskforce/ICM_Toolkit/GovernanceCouncil/Communications/SitePages/Start-your-CC&ICM-Journey.aspx. *This is an internal VA website that is not available to the public.*

2. Collaboration With Office of Nursing Service

The ONS serves as a leader in clinical practice and education to support patient care and healthcare delivery across VHA. Nurses are assigned to service lines and programs across the continuum of care to provide clinical nursing services to Veterans, their families, and caregivers. Nurses support healthcare delivery in both the inpatient and outpatient settings and in the following areas: ambulatory, acute, specialty, mental health, research, geriatrics, and community-based care. An ADPCS or Nurse Executive is in every VA medical facility and is responsible for the professional practice of nursing provided by all nursing staff employed by HCS. The ADPCS or Nurse Executive will support CCM through the following:

a. VHA Nurse Care Managers and Case Managers work collaboratively to promote Veterans' timely access to care to support their continuing care needs. Timeliness is based on what is clinically indicated in the Veteran's EHR.

b. Veterans and transitioning Service members referred to VA nurses are proactively screened for CM.

c. VHA nurses support seamless transitions in care within VA and between VA and community providers.

d. Referrals between VHA Specialty CM services and Nursing services are bidirectional.

e. Professional nurse representation and participation in the CCRT. ***NOTE:*** *For implementation guidance related to the CCRT, please see* https://dvagov.sharepoint.com/sites/VHACMSWS/CMI_Taskforce/ICM_Toolkit/GovernanceCouncil/Communications/SitePages/Start-your-CC&ICM-Journey.aspx. *This is an internal VA website that is not available to the public.*

3. Collaboration With Patient Aligned Care Team

a. Primary Care oversees the PACT model and promotes team-based, patient-centered care focusing on a personalized, integrated, and coordinated approach to healthcare. Integrated with PACT, the Health Promotion and Disease Prevention (HPDP) Program offers a variety of health education programs and services that support PACT. For more information, see VHA Directive 1120.02, HPDP Core Program Requirements, dated February 5, 2018, and VHA Handbook 1120.04, Veterans Health Education and Information Core Program Requirements, dated September 24, 2015.

b. The PACT RN) Care Manager and PACT Social Work Case Manager are two interprofessional team members who may screen and refer to specialty CM due to their role in the provision of care coordination services. The following is a description of the intersection of CC&ICM and PACT services when Veterans are referred to specialty CM and assigned a Case Manager or LC. ***NOTE:*** *For elaboration of the role and responsibilities of the LC, see paragraph 5, Responsibilities.*

   1. Case Managers and LCs collaborate with the PACT RN to harmonize healthcare services for the Veteran, avoiding duplication of care, preventing miscommunication, providing comprehensive care, and maintaining continuity of care.

   2. Veterans will continue to receive care management services from their PACT RN while receiving specialty CM services. The Case Manager/LC defers to the PACT RN Care Manager's expertise in facilitating care management-related activities (e.g., completion of Primary Care consults). Concurrent, non-primary care-related concerns are addressed directly by the Case Manager/LC (e.g., psychosocial issues). ***NOTE:*** *Following a warm handoff, PACT Social Work Case Manager discontinues the provision of CM services when Veterans are assigned to a specialty Case Manager/LC, to prevent unnecessary duplication of CM services.*

4. Transitions and Transfers

a. When Veterans no longer meet criteria for "specialty" CM, but still require CM services, the specialty Case Manager/LC transfers Veteran to the PACT Social Work Case Manager through a warm handoff for continued CM services. The

PACT Social Work Case Manager becomes the new LC for the Veteran at that time, and their family and/or caregiver.

b. When Veterans no longer meet clinical eligibility for CM services and are ready to be safely maintained with the provision of a lower level of care coordination, the specialty Case Manager/LC transitions the Veteran to the PACT RN for care management services. The PACT RN functions as the LC for Veteran and their family and/or caregiver regarding the Veteran's care.

c. For elaboration of the CC&ICM framework, see the CC&ICM Portal on VA SharePoint. ***NOTE:*** *For implementation guidance related to CC&ICM, please see* https://dvagov.sharepoint.com/sites/VHACMSWS/CMI_Taskforce/ICM_Toolkit/GovernanceCouncil/Communications/SitePages/Start-your-CC&ICM-Journey.aspx. *This is an internal VA website that is not available to the public.*

d. For elaboration of the VHA PACT model, see VHA Handbook 1101.10(1), VHA PACT Handbook, dated February 5, 2014.

5. Collaboration With Specialty Population Programs/Services

a. Referral for specialty CM services should be considered to ensure all resources are appropriately utilized. Case Managers may receive the assigned role of LC and would collaborate on the coordination of care and prevent duplication of services with specialty Case Managers through regular assessment and communication, and if necessary, clear deferment to one source of CM by another.

b. Specialty Case Managers can be found in programs such as: Polytrauma; HUD-VASH; Health Care for Homeless Veterans (HCHV); HUD-VASH; Grant and Per Diem (GPD); SCI; TCM; Mental Health Intensive Case Management (MHICM); Visual Impairment Services Team (VIST); GEC; Home Based Primary Care (HBPC); as well as other VA medical facility and/or community-based programs. ***NOTE:*** *CM policies for the programs can be found in various VHA directives and handbooks at* https://www.va.gov/vhapublications/.

1. **Collaboration with Homeless Program Office.** VHA's Homeless Programs constitute the largest integrated network of homelessness housing, prevention, and rehabilitation services in the country. These programs are designed to help Veterans live as self-sufficiently and independently as possible. The foundation for these programs is based on the principles of Housing First with supportive services to ensure Veterans are able to end the cycle of homelessness. Homeless and at-risk Veterans are assessed by VHA staff and referred to CM, residential, and other services as their needs indicate.

2. **Collaboration with TCM Program.** The TCM program serves as the initial point of contact for newly enrolled Post 9/11-era Veterans. TCM works closely with the National VA Liaison Program and/or DoD Case

Managers to ensure the continuity of care and transition into the VA system of care is timely, high quality, and safe. Transitioning Veterans are screened for CM needs and are referred to the appropriate services. VA medical facilities may choose to assign a member of TCM to serve as LC or Case Manager during their own DoD/VA CM Review Team meetings. The CM model can be found in VHA Directive 1010, TCM of Ill or Injured Servicemembers and New Veterans, dated November 21, 2016.

3. **Collaboration with Suicide Prevention Program.** As established by department Memorandum, "Mental Health Funding for Suicide Prevention Coordinators," every VA medical facility has at least one suicide prevention coordinator, whose responsibilities include the tracking of Veterans identified as high-risk for suicide through a computerized EHR high-risk flagging system, providing crisis interventions, developing Veteran Safety Plans, and conducting outreach efforts. VHA Case Managers can play a vital role in the agency's multipronged approach to reducing Veteran suicide rate and effectively implementing a public health model of suicide prevention. Case Managers provide

   a. Increased monitoring, communication, and collaboration with the Veteran, their family, their caregiver, and the interprofessional team through whole healthcare plan integration.

   b. Augmented one-on-one psychosocial rehabilitative engagement and reinforcement (e.g., coaching, mentoring, and counseling) of the Veteran's clinical treatment plan.

   c. Referrals between VHA CM services and Suicide Prevention Program are bidirectional. Suicide Prevention Coordinators continue to be involved and assist with Veterans' cases; however, it is the Case Manager that will serve as the easily identifiable point of contact responsible for developing, orchestrating, and synchronizing the comprehensive care plan.

4. **Collaboration with Caregiver Support Program.** Caregivers play a vital role in the health and well-being of Veterans of all eras. VHA's Caregiver Support Program offers training, resources, and extensive tools to help support caregivers of Veterans throughout the caregiving journey. VHA Caregiver Support Coordinators (CSCs) are located at every VA medical facility and are the clinical experts on caregiver issues regarding VA and non-VA resources. CSCs help ensure caregivers are collaborative partners in the care of Veterans.

   a. All Veterans enrolled in the Caregiver Support Program and/or receiving caregiver support services should be screened for CM.

   b. Referrals between VHA specialty CM services and the Caregiver Support Program are bidirectional.

c. CSCs may continue to be involved with a Veteran's case as it relates to the needs of their caregiver. The Case Manager serves as the point of contact responsible for developing, orchestrating, and synchronizing the comprehensive care plan for the Veteran. Linkage to resources needed by the Veteran is carried out by the Case Manager.

5. **Collaboration with VACC Program.** The VHA OCC goal is to provide Veterans with the right care, delivered at the right time, at the right place, and by the appropriate provider. In some cases, Veterans may need to receive care from a local community care provider where efficient care coordination is paramount for seamless transitions of care. Care coordination is a Veteran-centered, team-based activity designed to assess and meet the needs of Veterans, while helping them navigate effectively and efficiently through the continuum of care inside and outside VA medical facilities. VA OCC is committed to collaborating with the community stakeholders to ensure that our partners understand current processes, are informed of future enhancements, and receive excellent customer service. These interactions continue throughout the episode of care to identify risk factors and allow VA staff to engage Veterans across different points of care.

6. **Collaboration with Federal Recovery Consultant Office (FRCO).** FRCs serve in the role defined for Joint Recovery Consultants in the overarching 2014 VA/DoD Interagency Complex Care Coordination MOU. FRCs provide enterprise-level consultation and assistance to VA and DoD LCs and CMTs, providing clinical and nonclinical assistance and advice about DoD, VA, other Federal agencies, community, and other resources available to support the Service member or Veteran and the family or caregiver. FRCs do not perform direct CM but may engage as early as the time of CMT establishment, as reflected in the Interagency Comprehensive Plan (ICP), at the discretion of the attending physician and upon request of the LC, assigned military headquarters leadership, or senior VA official. Stationed at key military treatment facilities, headquarters for the military's wounded warrior programs, and select VHA polytrauma centers, FRCs oversee a small subset of the population requiring high-intensity management and provide a channel of communication for field level staff to assist VISN, VA Central Office leadership, and assigned military headquarters leadership in identifying, validating, and implementing improvements for care and benefits coordination and processes.

Case Management Documentation, Workload, and Performance Metrics

1. Case Management Documentation

Documentation is a key means of communication among interdisciplinary team members. Documentation contributes to a better understanding of a Veteran and their family members' or caregiver's unique needs and allows for interdisciplinary service delivery to address those needs while reflecting the accountability and involvement of the Case Manager in Veteran care. The Case Manager is responsible for

a. Completing and documenting a comprehensive CM assessment. The documentation in the EHR must include time spent providing the service, details of the assessment/reassessment with diagnosis, plan of care, and changes in CM intensity when clinically indicated. Documentation must also adhere to The Joint Commission, Commission on Accreditation of Rehabilitation Facilities (CARF), and professional CM organization standards.

b. Ensuring all workload and encounter data utilizes appropriate current procedural terminology (CPT), international classification of diseases, and stop codes.

c. Ensuring all documentation occurs in the Veteran's EHR. ***NOTE:*** *Specialty CM programs, such as TCM and Homeless Programs, utilize additional web-based systems for program-specific tracking and reporting.*

2. Workload, Coding, and Performance Measures

Accurate coding describes the scope of services delivered and demonstrates the quality of care. Specialty Program directives, handbooks, and publications provide guidance on productivity and coding (these documents are listed in the last paragraph of this appendix). Decision Support System (DSS) identifiers are composed of a primary stop code and a secondary (i.e., credit) stop code. Two DSS identifiers that are used to collect and evaluate CM data including the number of Veterans who received CM and CM workload are as follows:

a. **DSS Identifier Number 182. Telephone CM.** DSS Identifier Number 182 includes CM for an interdisciplinary care plan via the telephone. All elements of Veteran assessment, monitoring, and treatment or care planning must be documented in the Veteran's EHR. Staff utilizing this code must have documented competencies in CM.

b. **DSS Identifier Number 184 (this is a secondary stop code and must be used with a primary stop code). Care or CM (Office Visit).** DSS Identifier Number 184 records Veteran care or CM activities in accordance with an interdisciplinary plan of care. The episode of care is a face-to-face clinical office encounter between the Veteran and the Case Manager and must include elements of Veteran assessment, monitoring, and treatment or care planning. Staff utilizing this code must have documented competencies in CM.

c. **CPT.** Use of appropriate CPT coding is also vital to accurate workload capture. CPT Code, T1016, is documented in 15-minute increments and applies to direct patient care (face to face visits only with the patient) that is not psychotherapy. Clinical content should include a minimum of one the following: assessment, care planning, referral and related activities, and monitoring and follow-up.

d. **Performance Measures.** CM program leaders must be data-driven and utilize performance measures and metrics to monitor the quality, effectiveness, and efficiency of their program. The application of national quality improvement principles is needed to ensure program growth aligns with the strategic direction of the organization. CM program-specific metrics may vary, but may be linked by overarching, national CM metrics. The identification of specific quality metrics is beyond the scope of this directive.

NOTE: *See VHA Directive 1010, TCM of Ill or Injured Servicemembers and New Veterans, dated November 21, 2016; VHA Directive 1140.11, Uniform GEC Services in VA Medical Centers and Clinics, dated October 11, 2016; VHA Directive 1162.05(1), HUD-VASH Program, dated June 29, 2017; VHA Directive 1176.01, SCI/D System of Care, dated October 1, 2010; VHA Directive 1411, Home-Based Primary Care (HBPC), Special Population PACT Program, dated June 5, 2017; VHA Handbook 1162.01(1), GPD Program, dated June 12, 2013; VHA Handbook 1162.09, HCHV, dated May 8, 2014; VHA Handbook 1163.06, Intensive Community Mental Health Recovery Services, dated January 7, 2016; and VHA Directive 1172.01, Polytrauma System of Care, dated January 24, 2019.*

Case Manager Caseload

1. Review of literature on CM and guidance from professional organizations, such as the CMSA and the National Association of Social Workers (NASW), shows that there is an inconsistent approach to establishing caseloads.
2. Veterans frequently have complex clinical and psychosocial issues. Determining an appropriate caseload for these patients is dependent on many factors:
   a. Case severity/complexity (case mix index) and intensity of the care plan requirements.
   b. Availability of community-based services and network development.
   c. Communication and coordination between Department of VA, Veterans Benefits Administration (VBA), DoD, and community resources and partners.
   d. Case Manager role (including requirements of other duties as assigned, especially if the Case Manager has major responsibilities to another program area).
   e. Intensity of support needed by the family or caregiver.
   f. Accessibility to necessary and supportive information.
   g. Amount of administrative support.
   h. Benefit provisions.

i. Types of CM interaction with beneficiaries (e.g., face-to-face, telephone, V-tel, VA Video Connect).

j. Professional experience and knowledge of the patient population.

Resources

1. Commission for Case Manager Certification Case Management Body of Knowledge: https://www.cmbodyofknowledge.com/content/case-management-knowledge-2

2. Tahan, H. and Treiger, T. Case Management Society of America Core Curriculum for CM, 3rd edition. 2017. Philadelphia: Wolters Kluwer.

3. Hudson, C. et al. Case Management in Primary Care for Frequent Users of Health Care Services: A Mixed Methods. Study Annals of Family Medicine. May/June 2018; vol. 16. no. 3, 232–239.

4. Kathol, Roger G., Andrew, Rachel L., Squire, Michelle, Dehnel, Peter J. (2018). The Integrated Case Management Manual: Assisting Complex Patients Regain Physical and Mental Health. New York: Springer Publishing Company.

5. Care Coordination Measures Atlas Update. Chapter 2. What is Care Coordination? Content last reviewed 2014. Agency for Healthcare Research and Quality, Rockville, MD. http://www.ahrq.gov/professionals/prevention-chronic- care/improve/coordination/atlas2014/chapter2.html.

6. Mawn, Barbara. Trends in Case Management Acuity Determination. Occupational Medicine and Health Affairs; 2013; Oct; Vol 1, No. 132, 132–144.

7. Tahan, H., Watson, A., Sminkey, P. What Case Managers Should Know About Their Roles and Functions, A National Study from the Commission for Case Manager Certification: Part 1. Professional Case Management, 2015; Vol 20, No. 6, 271–296.

8. Hudon, C. et al. Key factors of case management interventions for frequent users of healthcare services: a thematic analysis review. British Medical Journal. 2017; Vol 7.

9. Watson, A. Evaluating and Measuring Quality and Outcomes: A New "Essential Activity" of Case Management Practice. Professional Case Management. January/February 2016; Vol 21. Issue 1, pp. 51–52.

10. Case Management Model Act. *Revised 2017*. Retrieved from http://solutions.cmsa.org/acton/attachment/10442/f-0464/1/-/-/-/-/2017%20Model%20Care%20Act_Final%209.27.pdf. ***NOTE:*** *This link is outside of VA control and may not be conformant with Section 508 of the Rehabilitation Act of 1973.*

11. Congressional Research Service, "The Number of Veterans That Use VA Health Care Services: A Fact Sheet," dated June 3, 2014, available from https://fas.org/sgp/crs/misc/R43579.pdf. ***NOTE:*** *This linked document is outside of VA control and may not be conformant with Section 508 of the Rehabilitation Act of 1973.*

12. Carr, D. Building collaborative partnerships in critical care: The RN Case Manager/Social Work Dyad in Critical Care, Professional Case Management. May-June 2009; Vol 14, No. 3, 121–132.

APPENDIX N

Emotional Intelligence Questionnaire

Emotional Intelligence Questionnaire (Self)

Complete the questionnaire.

On a scale from 1 to 5, using the following categories:

5. Strongly Agree
4. Agree
3. Neither Agree or Disagree
2. Disagree
1. Strongly Disagree

Please rate the following statements about yourself:

_____ 1. I am emotionally aware and recognize my emotions and their effects.

_____ 2. I am able to accurately assess myself and know my strengths and limitations.

_____ 3. I am self-confident and have a strong sense of self-worth and my capabilities.

_____ 4. I am able to maintain self-control and keep any disruptive emotions and impulses in check.

_____ 5. I am trustworthy and maintain high standards of honesty and integrity.

_____ 6. I am conscientious and take responsibility for my personal performances.

_____ 7. I am able to easily adapt by being flexible and effectively handling change.

_____ 8. I am innovative and comfortable with new and novel ideas, approaches, and new information.

_____ 9. I have a need to achieve and strive to improve or meet standards of excellence.

_____ 10. I make commitments and align myself with the goals of the group, agency, or organization.

_____ 11. I show initiative and readily act on opportunities.

_____ 12. I am optimistic in pursuing goals and persist despite obstacles and setbacks.

_____ 13. I have a good understanding of others and sense their feelings, grasp their perspectives, and take an active interest in their concerns.

_____ 14. I am good at developing others by recognizing their needs and strengthening their abilities.

Source: Created by Jon Simon Sager based on the work of Goleman, D. (1998). *Working with emotional intelligence.* Bantam Books.

_____ 15. I have a strong service orientation and anticipate, recognize, and meet client and consumer needs.

_____ 16. I cultivate and increase my opportunities through diverse and different kinds of people.

_____ 17. I have good political awareness and understand an individual's or group's emotional undercurrents and power relationships.

_____ 18. I am good at influencing others by using effective tactics of persuasion and attitude change.

_____ 19. I am a good communicator by being open, actively listening, and send clear understandable messages.

_____ 20. I have good conflict management skills and can negotiate and resolve disagreements.

_____ 21. I am able to inspire and guide individuals and groups.

_____ 22. I often initiate and can manage change.

_____ 23. I am good at nurturing important and instrumental relationships.

_____ 24. I am cooperative and collaborate, often working with others concerning shared goals.

_____ 25. I am good at teamwork and can create synergy and pursue collective goals.

Source: Created by Jon Simon Sager based on the work of Goleman, D. (1998). *Working with emotional intelligence.* Bantam Books.

Emotional Intelligence Questionnaire (Other)

On a scale from 1 to 5, using the following categories:

5. Strongly Agree
4. Agree
3. Neither Agree or Disagree
2. Disagree
1. Strongly Disagree

Please rate the following statements as they pertain to____________:

_____ 1. is emotionally aware and recognize their emotions and their effects.

_____ 2. is able to accurately assess themselves and know strengths and their limitations.

_____ 3. is self-confident and has a strong sense of self-worth and their capabilities.

_____ 4. is able to maintain self-control and keep any disruptive emotions and impulses in check.

_____ 5. is trustworthy and maintain high standards of honesty and integrity.

_____ 6. is conscientious and takes responsibility for their personal performances.

_____ 7. is able to easily adapt by being flexible and effectively handle change.

_____ 8. is innovative and comfortable with new and novel ideas, approaches, and new information.

_____ 9. has a need to achieve and strive to improve or meet standards of excellence.

_____ 10. makes commitments and aligns themselves with the goals of the group, agency, or organization.

_____ 11. shows initiative and readily acts on opportunities.

_____ 12. is optimistic in pursuing goals and persists despite obstacles and setbacks.

_____ 13. has a good understanding of others and senses others' feelings, grasps their perspectives, and takes an active interest in their concerns.

_____ 14. is good at developing others by recognizing their needs and strengthening their abilities,

_____ 15. has a strong service orientation and anticipates, recognizes and meets client and consumer needs.

Source: Created by Jon Simon Sager based on the work of Goleman, D. (1998). *Working with emotional intelligence.* Bantam Books.

_____ 16. cultivates and increases their opportunities through diverse and different kinds of people.

_____ 17. has good political awareness and understands individual's or group's emotional undercurrents and power relationships.

_____ 18. is good at influencing others by using effective tactics of persuasion and attitude change.

_____ 19. is a good communicator by being open, actively listening, and sends clear understandable messages.

_____ 20. has good conflict management skills and can negotiate and resolve disagreements.

_____ 21. is able to inspire and guide individuals and groups.

_____ 22. often initiates and can manage change.

_____ 23. is good at nurturing important and instrumental relationships.

_____ 24. is cooperative and collaborates, often working with others concerning shared goals.

_____ 25. is good at teamwork and can create synergy and pursue collective goals.

Source: Created by Jon Simon Sager based on the work of Goleman, D. (1998). *Working with emotional intelligence.* Bantam Books.

Scoring Instructions

Scoring the questionnaire is simple. There are five component scores, two basic category scores, and an overall score.

This emotional intelligence questionnaire has the following five components. Score them as follows (this will yield a mean score for each of the five components):

Column 1

1. Self-Awareness: Sum Questions Q1, 2, and 3 and divide by 3 _____
2. Self-Regulation: Sum Questions Q4, 5, 6, 7, and 8 and divide by 5 _____
3. Motivation: Sum Questions Q9, 10, 11, and 12 and divide by 4 _____
4. Empathy: Sum Questions Q13, 14, 15, 16, and 17 and divide by 5 _____
5. Social Skills: Sum Questions Q18, 19, 20, 21, 22, 23, 24, and 25 and divide by 8 _____

Column 1 represents the mean score for each of the five components.

Score the subscales: Personal Competency and Social Skills as follows:
For Personal Competency, using Column 1, add the three means for components 1, 2, and 3 and divide by 3.
Personal Competency Subscale score _____

For Social Skills, using Column 1, add the two means for components 4 and 5 and divide by 2.

Social Skills Subscale score _____

****

To find your Emotional Intelligence Total Score, add the five component means in Column 1 and divide by 5.

Emotional Intelligence Total score _____

Source: Created by Jon Simon Sager based on the work of Goleman, D. (1998). *Working with emotional intelligence.* Bantam Books.

Index

Printed in the United States
by Baker & Taylor Publisher Services

Printed in the United States
by Baker & Taylor Publisher Services